Medical Ethics
and Law

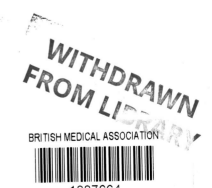

THIRD EDITION

Medical Ethics and Law

A curriculum for the 21st Century

Dominic Wilkinson MBBS, BMedSci, MBioeth, DPhil, FRACP, FRCPCH
Professor of Medical Ethics, Director of Medical Ethics, Oxford Uehiro Centre for
  Practical Ethics, University of Oxford;
Consultant Neonatologist, John Radcliffe Hospital;
Senior Research Fellow, Jesus College, Oxford, UK

Jonathan Herring BCL
Vice-Dean and Professor of Law at Exeter College, University of Oxford, Oxford, UK

Julian Savulescu BMedSci, MBBS, MA, PhD
Uehiro Chair in Practical Ethics, Director, Oxford Uehiro Centre for Practical Ethics
  University of Oxford, Oxford, UK;
Visiting Professorial Fellow in Biomedical Ethics, Murdoch Children's Research
  Institute, Victoria;
Distinguished Visiting International Professorship in Law, University of Melbourne,
  Australia

For additional online content visit ExpertConsult.com

ELSEVIER   Edinburgh   London   New York   Oxford   Philadelphia   St Louis   Sydney   2020

First edition 2003
Second edition 2008
Third edition 2020

The right of Dominic Wilkinson, Jonathan Herring and Julian Savulescu to be identified as authors of this work has been asserted by them in accordance with the Copyright, Designs and Patents Act 1988.

Notices

Practitioners and researchers must always rely on their own experience and knowledge in evaluating and using any information, methods, compounds or experiments described herein. Because of rapid advances in the medical sciences, in particular, independent verification of diagnoses and drug dosages should be made. To the fullest extent of the law, no responsibility is assumed by Elsevier, authors, editors or contributors for any injury and/or damage to persons or property as a matter of products liability, negligence or otherwise, or from any use or operation of any methods, products, instructions or ideas contained in the material herein.

ISBN: 978-0-7020-7596-4

Printed in China

Last digit is the print number: 9 8 7 6 5 4 3 2 1

Content Strategist: Laurence Hunter
Content Development Specialist: Fiona Conn
Project Manager: Julie Taylor
Design: Margaret Reid
Marketing Manager: Deborah Watkins
Cover illustration: "Knot" by John French, johnefrench@hotmail.com, Barcelona

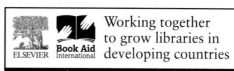

Working together to grow libraries in developing countries

www.elsevier.com • www.bookaid.org

Contents

CONTENTS

Part 3 Extensions — 275

List of Cases

Chapter 1

Chapter 2

Chapter 3

Chapter 4

Chapter 5

Chapter 10

Chapter 11

Chapter 12

Chapter 13

Chapter 14

Chapter 15

Chapter 16

Chapter 17

Chapter 18

Chapter 19

Chapter 20

Preface to the third edition

Does ethics make progress? Does ethics change?

Writing a new edition of a textbook on medical ethics might raise the above challenging questions. In the foreword to the previous edition, we cited Alfred North Whitehead's claim that European philosophy was a series of footnotes to Plato. In many respects, we have sympathy with that claim. The fundamental philosophical and ethical questions at the heart of medicine are ones that have been apparent for two thousand years or longer. What makes life go well? How should we live? What is the goal of medicine? How should health professionals behave? How should doctors relate to patients? In the first chapter of this book we reject the view that ethics is 'relative' – i.e. that it is relative to a particular culture, time or place. However, ethics *is* context-dependent. What is ethical depends on the options available, on our understanding of the effects of our actions and on the values that are held by those affected by decisions. And it is very clear that the context of medicine in the 21st century is changing, and has changed significantly in the last decade. This century is characterized by exponential medical advances outstripping resource availability. At the same time, the community of health professionals and patients is becoming increasingly globalized and diverse in the values they apply to decisions. Value pluralism is different to value relativism: the fact that there are many justifiable values does not imply that any or every value commitment that people hold is justifiable. This century is also characterized by digital revolution. There is an explosion of data, information, misinformation, power and disempowerment. Patients are no longer passive recipients of authoritative decision-making about their interests.

The second edition of this book was published in 2008. There have been important changes in the law and in professional guidance in the last decade. The UK Institute of Medical Ethics (IME) published a revision of its 1998 consensus statement on core topics for medical ethics education in 2010. This edition has been revised and updated to reflect these changes.

In addition, the book includes a new section that provides an extension to the core curriculum focused on four key emerging topics in medical ethics – neuroethics, genethics, information ethics and public health ethics. This new section is aimed at providing material for students who wish to extend their understanding of medical ethics, or undertake a formal extension unit of study. It also aims to keep the textbook fresh and appealing to students by providing material on cutting-edge topics that are frequently in the media, and that we anticipate will be part of a future 'core curriculum'.

The new edition has been extensively rewritten and restructured to help make it engaging for medical students and medical professionals. We have concentrated more in this edition on methods of argumentation and illustration through cases. The reason for this is that more will change between the next edition of the textbook and this current, than changed between this edition and the last. Textbooks will rapidly become obsolete if they do not focus on ways of thinking.

Each chapter is now organized around a set of cases. The majority of these are real cases, drawn from the media or from law reports, or (with some modification to preserve confidentiality) from our own experience. We have identified some key debates across the book and summarized arguments for and against particular positions. We hope that this will encourage readers to think deeper about the arguments on both sides of issues. The chapters include revision questions to help students test their learning, and extension cases designed to encourage further discussion, reading and debate.

The third edition has seen a change of guard – we are extremely grateful to Tony Hope and Judith Hendrick, who contributed enormously to the first two editions but have passed on the baton for this edition. Dominic Wilkinson and Jonathan Herring have joined Julian Savulescu in revising, building on and adding to Tony and Judith's work for this third edition.

One of the challenges of a textbook is that it is difficult to go into depth on any individual issue. There are more than 75 case studies included in the book. The brief descriptions and necessarily concise analyses cannot do justice to the complexity of real ethical dilemmas. For those who share that feeling, this edition is accompanied by a companion book, written by Dominic Wilkinson and Julian Savulescu. 'Ethics, conflict and medical treatment for children: from disagreement to dissensus' provides an in-depth discussion of one of the most controversial cases in UK medical ethics of the last decade. The Charlie Gard case is raised briefly in Chapter 11 (Case 11.4). The companion book delves into the details of the case, and, from opposing sides of the debate about treatment for Charlie Gard, illustrates the challenge of assessing when treatment is in a child's best interests, when experimental treatment may or may not proceed and whether parents' wishes should or should not be respected.

DW, JH, JS

Acknowledgements

The authors are indebted to Tony Hope and Judith Hendrick for their permission to use previous editions of this textbook. Much of the work in this book is drawn from their trail-blazing contributions.

DW and JS would like to particularly acknowledge the generous support of The Uehiro Foundation on Ethics and Education and their President, Mr Tetsuji Uehiro. Without their support, there would be no Chair of Practical Ethics at the University of Oxford, nor Centre for Practical Ethics.

DW and JS would also like to acknowledge the support of the Wellcome Trust and the Wellcome Centre for Ethics and Humanities, who have supported research that has gone into this book.

We would like to thank a number of people who have provided invaluable assistance in putting together this new edition. Alberto Giubilini provided background research and assisted in writing the new chapter (20) on Public Health Ethics. Vic Larcher gave incisive and insightful comments and suggestions on the child safeguarding section in Chapter 11. Libby Rose-Innes, Lydia di Stefano, Lauren Yip, Claudia Brick and Emily Feng-Gu provided very helpful proofreading and comments on chapters of the book.

This edition has been enriched by illustrations from a number of cartoonists who have very kindly given permission for their work to appear here: Marty Bee, Jim Bergman (mooselakecartoons.com), Dave Coverly (speedbump.com), Arend van Dam, Barry Deutsch (leftycartoons.com), Bob Englehart, Professor Craig Froehle, Randy Glasbergen, Sidney Harris (ScienceCartoonsPlus.com), Ryan Lake (chaospet.com), Don Mayne, Don Piraro and Mick Stevens. We are particularly grateful to John French for providing the cover illustration for this book and the companion volume.

We have benefited enormously from the support and encouragement of Laurence Hunter and Fiona Conn at Elsevier. Finally, we would especially like to thank Rocci Wilkinson and Miriam Wood for tireless personal, administrative and research support.

Part 1

Foundations

Chapter 1

Reasoning about ethics

Case 1.1

An 83-year-old woman, Mrs L, is admitted to hospital with pneumonia. She has dementia, and has previously been living at home with family, though they have been struggling with her care. She is malnourished, and after recovery from her chest infection eats little. She repeatedly removes intravenous lines and nasogastric tubes.

Her family wish her to have a gastrostomy inserted, however, the gastroenterology team decline on the grounds that there is no evidence that this would be beneficial, and it is not clinically indicated.

Should Mrs L have a gastrostomy?

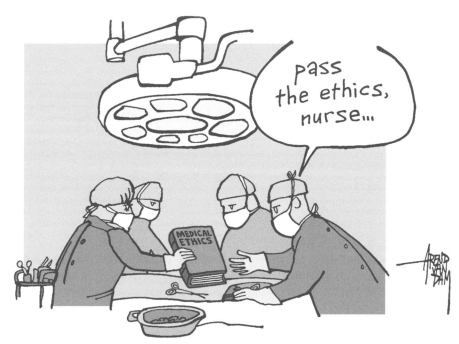

Figure 1.1 Pass the ethics (© Arend van Dam, reproduced with permission)

SCIENTIFIC REASONING IN CLINICAL MEDICINE

Faced with a clinical dilemma, like the case above, health professionals often seek the opinions of medical experts. There is important wisdom to be gained from experience. However, expert opinion is not enough. Doctors are exhorted to provide or cite evidence to support their clinical judgement. That evidence needs to be critically appraised to see how well it supports a particular approach.

Proponents of evidence-based medicine point to examples of useless and even harmful treatments being perpetuated because they were not critically evaluated. In the case of a gastrostomy for Mrs L, the gastroenterology team might cite a Cochrane systematic review from 2009 which concluded that there was no evidence that gastrostomy improves survival, nutritional status or quality of life in patients with severe dementia (Sampson, Candy, and Jones 2009).

In evaluating the evidence about the effects of an intervention, many factors have to be taken into account: the methodological design, the size of the trial, the method of recruitment, the outcomes and the methods used to measure them. For the doctor who is helping the individual patient, it is not enough simply to evaluate the quality and conclusions from the scientific trials; the doctor also has to apply the evidence to the individual case. In doing this, questions arise as to the extent to which this patient does and does not resemble the people who took part in the trial – and judgement is needed in order to decide what features are important in assessing 'resemblance'. For example, how severe was the dementia of those in the trials, and how severe is this patient's dementia? The doctor may also use implicit knowledge gained from experience that suggests that, for this particular patient, there are further factors that may be important in deciding on the best treatment. And, of course, the patient may want to be involved in the decision – so the issue for the doctor may be more about how to help the patient make the decision than about what decision should be (see Chapter 5 for discussion of models of the doctor–patient relationship). Indeed, evidence-based medicine is not value-free. Sometimes the evidence about best treatment will depend on how the patient values different types of outcome and different side-effects.

In Mrs L's case, there is a need to assess whether the evidence applies to her. For example, how severe is her dementia, and does she have other conditions that would make the gastrostomy an advantage or a problem? Further scrutiny of published studies indicates a lack of evidence of benefit, rather than clear evidence of lack of benefit. There have been no randomized controlled trials of feeding tubes in dementia (perhaps because of ethical challenges with such research). Absence of evidence might provide a reason not to proceed with a gastrostomy, but that will potentially depend on the values at stake in the decision. Some have even pointed out that, if gastrostomies do *not* prolong life in patients with dementia, this might be seen as a point in their favour (Regnard et al. 2010) (at least some people would not wish their life to be prolonged in such a state). The point here is not that a gastrostomy should be inserted in Mrs L – rather it is to highlight that scientific evidence alone cannot answer the question.

In thinking of the scientific assessment and justification of medical interventions, a number of key points can be summarized as follows:

1. Most clinical situations and decisions require knowledge gained from scientific evaluation.
2. The fact that doctors 'traditionally' consider that X is the best treatment in these circumstances is not a good reason, and certainly not a sufficient reason, for offering X: the decision should be based on, or at least informed by, best evidence.
3. When a decision is made, it is important to be able to give the reasons and the evidence for that decision.
4. There are structured approaches to assessing evidence and reasons for the scientific aspects of clinical decisions – these 'critical appraisal skills' are vital for health professionals.
5. Evidence may be more or less compelling in a particular set of circumstances (e.g. there are better quality and poorer quality scientific studies). Clinical judgement will normally be needed in interpreting the evidence and relating it to the specific clinical decision and the specific patient.
6. Evidence is not value-free, because it will typically require some relative evaluation of different outcomes. Sometimes the evidence will be such that whatever values people hold within reason, one specific intervention is clearly best in particular circumstances. In many situations, however, the balance of the outcomes from different interventions might be evaluated differently by different patients.

7. What evidence we choose to look for, how we choose to look for it and the success criteria (degree of confidence or statistical significance) we assign are value judgements.

ETHICAL REASONING IN CLINICAL MEDICINE

Ethical reasoning should be just as integral a part of modern medicine as scientific reasoning. The following points concerning the roles of ethics mirror the points made above about science:

1. Many clinical situations and decisions involve reasoning based on ethical values.
2. The fact that doctors traditionally consider that X is the right thing to do is not a good reason, and certainly not *enough* reason to do X: the decision should be based on good ethical reasoning.
3. When a decision is made, it is important to be able to give the reasons for the ethical aspects of that decision, as well as for the scientific aspects.
4. Reasoning about ethics is not simply a matter of personal opinion or a purely introspective and intuitive process. Health professionals need to apply what might be called 'critical appraisal skills in ethical reasoning'. These will be discussed as *tools of ethical reasoning* later in this chapter.
5. Ethical arguments may be more or less compelling. There are good and bad reasons and arguments. Ethical judgement is needed in making final decisions – there is no ethical algorithm that can be applied without judgement.
6. Ethics is not science-free or independent of evidence. Many ethical arguments depend on factual premises. Ethics-based medicine therefore is complementary to evidence-based medicine.

In summary, the ethical aspects of clinical care and decision-making need to be explicit, and reasons have to be given for the decisions taken. This is as true of the ethical aspects as it is of the scientific aspects of clinical care. Society increasingly expects this from doctors as part of the general move towards transparent decision-making and the requirement that professionals should be able to account for and justify their decisions and actions. Health professionals' reasoning about ethical aspects of care will need to be able to stand up to scrutiny – in a court if necessary – just as they need to be able to defend the scientific or technical aspects of decision-making.

THE FACT-VALUE DISTINCTION

The above discussion separates two fundamentally different concepts about the world: the normative and the non-normative (empirical). This is captured by the 'fact-value' distinction, which is central to medicine, and to life. The non-normative or empirical is denoted by the use of words like 'is', 'was', 'will be', 'could be', 'would be', etc. It is about facts. Science is the domain of gaining knowledge about the world and about the living organisms, including humans, within it.

The normative is about value. It is denoted by words like 'should be', 'ought to be', 'right', 'wrong', 'good', 'bad', 'permissible', 'impermissible', 'best', 'worst', etc. It is about ethics. Science can assist ethics: facts are important. But they can never alone decide what is of value.

Every action requires a goal (a value) and facts about how best to achieve that. Ethics is about reasoning about values and goals; science is about discovering facts.

For example, in the case of Mrs L, science can tell us what level of consciousness Mrs L has: persistent vegetative state, minimally conscious, semi-responsive, fully responsive. However, it cannot tell us whether it is good to continue to live, worth living, in that state. That is an ethical or moral issue. Ethics is about how to make a reasoned or rational decision about such value questions.

SCEPTICISM ABOUT ETHICS

There are often areas of uncertainty about the scientific basis of clinical practice, and two doctors may disagree about which course of treatment will be the most effective. In theory, though, it should be possible to answer the question of which treatment is better given agreement over the outcome measures and the relevant patient group. If needed, we can obtain more evidence – and that evidence will settle the disagreement. But the same is not true of ethics. Two people may disagree over the morality of abortion, and no amount of factual evidence will necessarily ever resolve their disagreement, because the dispute is over (moral) values, not over empirical facts.

This lack of a factual basis for ethical values can lead to scepticism about ethics. It seems that there is no ultimate way of deciding whether your values are better than my values. Some people have the impression that all ethical values are mere opinion. There are no right or wrong answers. All views are purely subjective or are relative to a particular culture. This is called relativism about ethics. According to this view, your opinion is as good as my opinion, and if we disagree all we can say is: we beg to differ; end of story. If this were true, there would be no point in our discussing ethical issues at all, except perhaps to identify false beliefs about the facts on which these are based (you might as well close this book now…). It would imply that there was nothing wrong with the values of the Nazis, we just disagree with them, just as we might support a different football team.

This sceptical position is based on two false assumptions. The first is that if, in the end, there is no natural (or divine) truth about ethics, then there is no point to discussion, reasoning and argument about ethics. However, even if ethical values are based finally on our individual personal choices and commitments, or if they are based on social and cultural values, reasoning about ethics is still of crucial importance. The sceptical position also assumes that, if there can be reasonable disagreement about ethical questions, *any* answer is equally valid. However, even if there is not a single right answer to many ethical questions, there can still be *wrong* answers.

Consider first the view that ethical values are personal. Most of us have standards of behaviour and a concern for living in a morally good way. These standards 'can energise us to defend ourselves when those standards are belittled and threatened'

(Blackburn 2001). But where do these come from? How do we know that we have the right ones? The answer is through subjecting them to rational enquiry. Such rational enquiry is helped by engaging with others in argument: trying to defend our own position. But if the counter-arguments are stronger, if there is a contradiction between what we thought our principles were and what we think is right in a specific situation, then we need to resolve that contradiction. Sometimes that will mean changing our mind on a topic – following the arguments wherever they lead us. Other times, this may lead us to go back and review the arguments to identify where they may have gone astray.

Rational analysis is important too if we focus on the social and cultural basis of morality. This is perhaps of particular importance to health professionals, because doctors practise within a highly socialized role. Society allows doctors a degree of personal freedom in making decisions and in their interactions with patients. But in giving doctors that freedom, society expects them to be able to defend their decisions and actions with reasons. Through the legal system, and through guidelines from organizations such as the General Medical Council, society also provides specific ethical principles or concepts within which it expects doctors to work. Doctors must be able to show how their decisions and actions relate to the law and to the norms of their profession.

We live in a complex and diverse society – it is completely unrealistic to imagine that everyone would reach agreement about value-based questions such as the ones discussed in this book. We need to respect that diversity, and respect the range of reasonable points of view about ethics. It is crucial, though, to distinguish between *pluralism* and *relativism*. Pluralism is the idea that there can be more than one value, value system or viewpoint. There can be more than one correct answer. For example, a longer, worse quality of life might be equally valuable, or incommensurate, to a shorter, better quality life. However, there can also be one or more *incorrect* answers. Pluralism does not mean supporting any value or any value system that someone happens to support. It does not mean (as relativism would imply) that all answers are equally acceptable.

Oxford philosopher Isaiah Berlin famously rejected the suggestion that accepting pluralism meant that 'anything goes': 'I am not a relativist; I do not say "I like my coffee with milk and you like it without; I am in favour of kindness and you prefer concentration camps" – each of us with his own values, which cannot be overcome or integrated' (Berlin 1998). We do not think that slavery or the Nazi treatment of the Jews are simply matters of personal opinion, or that they were acceptable just because society at the time thought that they were. A crucial task for ethical analysis is to identify arguments, reasons and answers that should be *rejected* (even if it cannot always tell us which ones must be accepted).

In summary, reasoning is important in coming to a view about what is the right thing to do. The importance of reasoning is not undermined by the point that there might be no natural foundation for ethics. In any case, society increasingly expects doctors to be able to explain, giving the reasons why they acted or decided in the way that they did; and this expectation applies as much to the ethical aspects of clinical practice as it does to the scientific aspects. It is important, therefore, that doctors are able to identify and reason about the ethical aspects of their work and to relate this to guidelines and law. This book aims to help health professionals gain the knowledge and skills to do this.

THE ROLE OF EMOTION IN MORAL ARGUMENT

As will be clear from what we have said, throughout this book we stress the role of reason in ethical argument. Emotion, however, also plays a part, and this can arise in at least three ways:

1. A person's feelings and emotions may be of moral importance in a particular situation. We note in Chapter 14 that withdrawing (stopping) and withholding (not starting) medical treatment are equivalent. However, sometimes families find stopping treatment much harder, or even unacceptable. We have called this phenomenon 'Withdrawal Aversion', and have argued that it does not have direct moral significance (Wilkinson, Butcherine and Savulescu 2019). However, those feelings may be relevant to a decision about starting treatment if they cannot be changed. More generally, patients' wishes are often of crucial significance in medical decisions, and those wishes may be based on the patient's feelings and emotions.

2. Our moral intuition as to particular cases plays an important part in the process of moral reasoning (see below). When there is a mismatch between our theory and our intuition in a particular case, we may adjust either one or the other, or both. The key point in a rational ethics system is that we must bring the two into line. It does not mean that a purely intellectual theory always trumps our gut responses to individual situations. Indeed, ethical reasoning often involves challenging a theoretical position by showing that it leads to conclusions in specific cases that few people would find intuitively acceptable. Emotions are often involved in such intuitive responses.

3. The ability to respond to, and have feelings towards, other people is important. Indeed, it is one of the most important aspects of our lives. We may well feel that a health professional who does not have such emotional responses towards patients is missing something important – and may, indeed, be less likely to be able to help patients. In the medical setting, communicating effectively and making the right decisions often depends on appropriate emotional responses.

Emotional responses and moral intuitions, however, need to be subjected to rational analysis. An initial feeling of disgust (the so-called 'yuck factor') may be irrational. For example, the idea of faecal transplantation (transferring faeces from a healthy donor to a sick patient) might generate a visceral sense of revulsion. However, if the treatment works and is safe, there is no ethical basis for concern. Our 'yuck' response has no foundation. Other times, such responses may be the result of prejudice or social conditioning, and should be actively rejected. For example, arguments from repulsiveness have at times been used to justify sexist, racist or homophobic laws. Still other times, a deep sense of moral disquiet may be helpful in identifying an ethical problem (Savulescu 2010).

REFLECTIVE EQUILIBRIUM WITH DIALOGUE

Two caricatures of moral reasoning: the mathematical and the scientific models

All of us have gut reactions as to what we think is morally right in particular situations. Such reactions are a result of our previous experience, of our upbringing and education, perhaps, on occasion, of our genetic inheritance and, in the case of medical decisions, of our apprenticeship learning. Such gut reactions need to be exposed to the crucible of rationality. But this raises the question of what is the relationship, within the context of rational argument, between our intuitive ethical responses to specific situations and our more general principles and theories.

There are two caricatures of moral reasoning. The first might be called the 'mathematical model', because it works top-down from general theory to particular cases. According to this caricature, moral reasoning begins by examining the major moral theories and principles (see Chapter 2) and selecting that theory which you believe is right. This theory is then applied to individual situations in order to decide what it is right to do. For example, if you decide that utilitarianism is the right moral theory, you can solve a dilemma in resource allocation by applying that theory. The problem with this mathematical model is that moral theories are not taken on board once and for all. They may need to be modified or even rejected. An ethical dilemma is a test of a moral theory, and not simply to be solved from the perspective of that theory.

The 'scientific model' sees moral reasoning as moving bottom-up from observation of particular cases to generating general theories (although this is itself a caricature of the scientific process). According to this view, precedence is given to our moral intuitions in particular circumstances. If there is a clash between our moral theory and what we believe to be right in particular circumstances, then the theory needs to be revised. Thus, moral theories are, in effect, an organization or summary of our moral intuitions. The problem with this model is that it gives precedence to our intuitions, and effectively precludes a reasoned or principled approach to ethics. Furthermore, our intuitions, or gut reactions, will come from our previous experience and upbringing. They are not an infallible guide to right or wrong. Rational morality requires that we test these gut reactions with reasons.

Reflective equilibrium

Ethical reasoning (like scientific reasoning) needs to combine both the mathematical and the scientific models. It requires a continual moving between our moral responses to specific situations and our moral theories. This process of moving back and forth between theory and individual situations is what political philosopher John Rawls called 'reflective equilibrium' (Rawls 1999). The idea is partly that we need to balance theory with our 'considered convictions'.

Rawls described the qualities of people who should be engaged in reflective equilibrium. They should be knowledgeable about the relevant facts. Importantly, they should be 'reasonable', meaning: (i) willing to use inductive logic, (ii) disposed to find reasons for and against a solution, (iii) having an open mind and (iv) making a conscientious effort to overcome intellectual, emotional and moral prejudices. Lastly, they are to have 'sympathetic knowledge … of those human interests which, by conflicting in particular cases, give rise to the need to make a moral decision' (Rawls 1951).

Dialogue

In this process of reflective equilibrium, we are attempting to ensure that our beliefs about what is right in various individual situations, and our theories, are consistent with each other. This involves developing principles (such as the best interests principle and those of distributive justice) and concepts (such as well-being and a life worth living), but crucially revising these in line with intuitions about specific cases (see for example the case of Charlie Gard (Wilkinson and Savulescu 2018)). During the process both the theories and the beliefs can undergo revision. When there is lack of agreement, there is no algorithm, or automatic way, to tell us which or what we must change. That has to be a matter of judgement. This process of reflective equilibrium can be undertaken by an individual person, but dialogue – discussion with others – can help the process. Discussion of ethical issues is important for several reasons:

1. It helps us identify inconsistencies between our moral views; between our views in one situation and another; and between our theories and our intuitions.
2. It helps ensure that we are aware of the perspectives of different moral theories.
3. It helps ensure that we are aware of the perspectives of different people – and in the medical setting this can be particularly important.

In reading this book, we would encourage you to discuss the cases with others. The 'Up for Debate' sections in many chapters could be used as a starting point for a discussion. For an example of ethical dialogue – on a controversial case on which two authors of this book disagree – see Wilkinson and Savulescu (2018).

TOOLS OF ETHICAL REASONING

In the remainder of this chapter, we will outline various 'tools' of ethical reasoning and end with a discussion of the 'slippery slope argument', which is frequently used within ethical discussion. You probably already use many of the tools in discussions about ethical issues, though you may not be able to name or classify the particular method of argument. You may want to skip the rest of this chapter and get straight on with reading about particular clinical settings (see Part 2). However, when faced with an ethically problematic issue, it can be valuable to consciously consider whether one or more of these tools might be particularly helpful. We pick out seven tools of ethical reasoning that we find particularly helpful.

Tool 1: Distinguishing facts from values

In making medical decisions, particularly in difficult situations, it can be important to distinguish clearly between medical facts and moral evaluations.

It will typically be the case that rather different types of argument and evidence bear on the factual components compared to the evaluative components of a medical decision. Consider the following case:

Case 1.2

Mr B is 55 years old and has a persistently raised diastolic blood pressure of 105 mmHg. A blood pressure of this level is associated with a significantly increased risk of an earlier death within the next 20 years. Treatment, leading to a lowering of this blood pressure to less than 90 mmHg, will increase Mr B's likely lifespan. National guidance recommends that doctors should offer anti-hypertensive drug treatment to patients with stage II hypertension.

Should the doctor offer blood-pressure lowering treatment to Mr B and try to persuade him to take the treatment?

The key factual statements are: that Mr B's blood pressure is of a particular level; that such a level is associated with an increased mortality rate; that lowering the pressure with treatment is associated with a reduced population risk of early death; and that national guidelines recommend this. The skills in assessing these statements are largely those of assessing empirical evidence – the skills of evidence-based medicine.

The key evaluative statements are that the increased mortality rate is 'significant', and that the facts justify trying to persuade Mr B to a certain course of action (to take the medication). The term 'significant' has two meanings, which can be confused. The first is a technical one in statistics, referring for example to the probability of obtaining the observed results if the null hypothesis is true. The second meaning is that of normal language, meaning that the results have some importance. The second meaning in particular incorporates values. Whether someone agrees with it will depend on how important they judge the effect of treatment (particularly compared with the cost or side-effects). For example, one estimate is that it would be necessary to treat 120 patients like Mr B to prevent one stroke in the next 5 years (Kaplan 2001). Is that 'significant'? Does that justify the doctor trying to persuade Dr B to take the treatment? You might well think that it does (we do), but assessing these evaluative statements takes us into the realm of moral argument.

Tool 2: Clarifying the logical form of the argument

An argument is a set of reasons supporting a conclusion. A particular form of argument – a 'deductive', or logical, argument – is a series of statements (called premises) that lead logically to a conclusion. A 'valid' argument is one in which the conclusion follows as a matter of logical necessity from the premises. If the premises are correct, and the argument is valid, the conclusion must be correct.

Box 1.1 summarizes some of the types and elements of formal logical arguments.

When testing our own arguments, or those of others, it can be helpful to summarize the argument in logical form. This enables the premises (sometimes

Box 1.1 Valid and invalid forms of argument

The basic form of deductive argument is called a syllogism. It is an argument that can be expressed in the form of two propositions, called premises, and a conclusion that results, as a matter of logic, from those premises. There are two main types of valid syllogism.

1 Modus ponens

A syllogism of the following form:

Premise 1 **(P1)**	If **p** then **q**	(if statement **p** is true, then statement **q** is true)
Premise 2 **(P2)**	**p**	(statement **p** is true)
Conclusion **(C)**	**q**	(therefore statement **q** is true)

An example:

P1	If a fetus is a person it is wrong to kill it.
P2	A fetus is a person.
C	It is wrong to kill a fetus.

2 Modus tollens

A syllogism of the following form:

Premise 1 **(P1)**	If **p** then **q**	(if statement **p** is true, then statement **q** is true)
Premise 2 **(P2)**	**Not q**	(statement **q** is false)
Conclusion **(C)**	**Not p**	(therefore statement **p** is false)

An example:

P1	If a fetus is a person it is wrong to kill it.
P2	It is not wrong to kill a fetus.
C	A fetus is not a person.

3 An example of an invalid argument

Premise 1 **(P1)**	If **p** then **q**	(if statement **p** is true, then statement **q** is true)
Premise 2 **(P2)**	**Not p**	(i.e. statement **p** is false)
Conclusion **(C)**	**Not q**	(therefore statement **q** is false)

This argument is invalid – the conclusion does not follow from the premises.
An example:

P1	If a fetus is a person it is wrong to kill it.
P2	A fetus is not a person.
C	It is not wrong to kill a fetus.

This argument is invalid because there might be other reasons why it is wrong to kill a fetus even if it is not a person. (The argument could be made valid by changing the first premise to the following: – 'If and only if a fetus is a person, it is wrong to kill it'.)

See Chapter 13 for further discussion about the ethics of abortion

including hidden assumptions) to be clearly identified – and examined – and will help expose any fallacy in the argument itself (Box 1.2).

Tool 3: Analyzing concepts

An important component of valid reasoning is conceptual analysis.

Philosophers are sometimes caricatured as replying to every question with the words 'it all depends on what you mean by…'. The fact is that it often *does*. Lack

> **Box 1.2**   Some fallacies in argument (see Warburton (2007) for many further examples)
>
> **Ad hominem move**
>
> Shifting the argument from the point in question to an irrelevant aspect of the person who is making the argument.
>
> **Arguments from authority**
>
> Arguing that a statement or position or argument is true simply on the grounds that someone in authority has said that it is true.
>
> **Begging the question**
>
> An argument in which the conclusion, or the point that is in dispute, has already been assumed in the reasons given in favour of the conclusion. The argument is therefore a circular one. An example might be: the death penalty is wrong because killing is wrong.
>
> **But-there-is-always-someone-who-will-never-agree diversion (Flew 1989, p. 23)**
>
> The fact that there are people who are not convinced by an argument or set of reasons does not in itself show that the argument is not valid.
>
> **Confusing necessary conditions for sufficient conditions**
>
> A necessary condition for some states of affairs is one that is *required* for that state of affairs to obtain. For example, for a doctor to be found liable in negligence it is necessary for that doctor to have a relevant duty of care (see Chapter 4). However, this is not a sufficient condition, because other conditions are also required. Conversely, a patient request not to be resuscitated would be a sufficient condition for completing a DNACPR (Do Not Attempt Cardio-Pulmonary Resuscitation) form – however, it is not necessary, as a DNACPR can still be appropriate without patient agreement, e.g. if the doctor believes it is not in the patient's best interests (see Chapter 14).
>
> **The-intention-wasn't-bad-so-the-action-isn't-wrong fallacy**
>
> Judging people and judging acts or beliefs are two quite different things.
>
> **Motherhood statements**
>
> Bland statements that are used as rhetorical devices to gain agreement from others, often as a cloak to then gain agreement to more contentious statements without proper argument. For example: 'all humans are equal' (so it would be wrong to withdraw treatment from a patient in a persistent unconscious state).
>
> **Overgeneralization**
>
> A fallacious argument which provides some examples that illustrate a point and uses those examples to conclude a much more general statement.
>
> **The ten-leaky-buckets tactic**
>
> This is: '… presenting a series of severally unsound arguments as if their mere conjunction might render them collectively valid: something that needs to be distinguished carefully from the accumulation of evidence, where every item possesses some weight in its own right' (Flew 1989, p. 287).

of clarity about the meanings or definitions of key concepts in an argument can be a rhetorical device used to make an unsound argument persuasive. Consider the following argument:

It is murder to kill another human being. A human fetus is a human being. Doctors who terminate a pregnancy are murderers. They should be given life imprisonment, not an NHS salary.

A first stage in analyzing this argument is to define key terms. The term 'murder' normally means an *unlawful* killing, and a 'murderer' is someone who has committed murder. In English law, it is not unlawful for a medical practitioner to kill a fetus when terminating a pregnancy, so this is not normally murder (see Chapter 13). In the argument above, the words 'murder' and 'murderer' are being used with a different meaning (perhaps to mean 'morally wrong killing') for rhetorical effect. The term 'human being' also needs to be defined.

Definition, however, is often only a first, and a rather small, step. In the example above, a definition of 'human being' may be readily agreed. What is at issue is not whether the fetus is a human being, but whether that fact alone provides a convincing reason as to why killing the fetus is, from a moral point of view, like killing, say, a 10-year-old child. In order to examine this issue, it is necessary to go beyond definition and carry out some elucidation, or further analysis, of key concepts. In debates about termination of pregnancy, or embryo experiments, the concept of a 'person' has played a key role (see Chapter 13).

In addition to definition and elucidation, conceptual analysis may involve 'splitting' or 'lumping'. Splitting is the making of distinctions. In a discussion of the morality of euthanasia, it is important to make distinctions between the different types of euthanasia (see Chapter 14). This is because the relevant ethical issues bear differently on these different types.

Lumping involves clarifying similarities between things that are usually considered to be quite different. For example, the argument might be made that there is no clear conceptual difference between withholding and withdrawing life-extending treatment (see Chapter 14).

Tool 4: Reasoning from principles and theory

There are a number of principles relevant to many situations in medicine and which are endorsed as important by many moral theories (see Chapter 2). Four principles in particular have been identified (Beauchamp and Childress 2012, Gillon 1986); these are summarized in Box 1.3. When faced with an ethical problem in medical practice, it can often be helpful to apply each of the four principles. This can help in clarifying and distinguishing the key moral issues that are relevant.

Tool 5: Using case comparison

Perhaps the most powerful strategy in developing moral argument is the use of consistency. Consistency is a fundamental ethical value – one that is shared by many ethical and religious traditions. The principle of treating 'like cases alike' is, arguably, part of the very concept of justice. If you believe that in two similar

Box 1.3 Four principles in medical ethics

1 Respect for patient autonomy (see also Chapter 3)

Autonomy (literally: self-rule) is the capacity to think, to decide and to act on the basis of such thought and decision, freely and independently (Gillon 1986). Respect for patient autonomy requires health professionals (and others, including the patient's family) to help patients come to their own decisions (for example, by providing important information) and to respect and follow those decisions (even when the health professional believes that the decision is wrong).

2 Beneficence: the promotion of what is best for the patient (see also Chapter 3)

This principle emphasizes the moral importance of doing good to others, and, in the medical context, doing good to patients. Following this principle would entail doing what was best for the patient. This raises the question of who should be the judge of what is best for the patient. This principle is often interpreted as focusing on what an objective assessment by a relevant health professional would determine as being in the patient's best interests. The patient's own views are captured by the principle of respect for patient autonomy.

In most situations, respecting the principle of beneficence and the principle of respect for patient autonomy will lead to the same conclusion, as most of the time patients want what is (objectively) in their best interests. The two principles conflict when a competent patient chooses a course of action that is not in his or her best interests.

3 Non-maleficence: avoiding harm

This principle is the other side of the coin of the principle of beneficence. It states that health professionals should not harm patients. In most situations this principle adds little to the principle of beneficence. Most medical treatments have some chance of doing harm. It does not follow from this that such treatments should always be avoided. Rather, the potential benefits and harms and their probabilities need to be weighed up at the same time to decide what is overall in the patient's best interests. The main reason for retaining the principle of non-maleficence is that it is generally thought that health professionals have a *prima facie* duty not to harm anyone, whereas they owe a duty of beneficence to a limited number of people (their patients).

4 Justice (see also Chapter 10)

Time and resources do not allow every patient to get the best possible treatment. Health professionals have to decide how much time to spend with different patients, and at various levels within a healthcare system, because of limited resources, decisions must be made about limitations on treatments that can be offered in various situations. The principle of justice emphasizes two points: first, that patients in similar situations should normally have access to the same health care; and second, that in determining what level of health care should be available for one set of patients we must take into account the effect of such a use of resources on other patients. In other words, we must try to distribute our limited resources (time, money, intensive care beds) fairly.

situations you should do different things, then you must be able to point to a morally relevant difference between the two situations. Otherwise you are being inconsistent.

The method of case comparison is one use of the idea of consistency. It can be used as a method for deciding what it is right to do in a problematic situation. This method involves comparing the problematic case with cases that are more straightforward – or already decided. This contrasts with other methods of ethical analysis, such as applying an ethical principle or a particular moral theory. Case comparison is used extensively in legal decisions, where the legal position may be judged by comparing the case under examination with one that has already been decided (see Chapter 4). The key question is whether the two cases are sufficiently similar in relevant ways for the earlier case to act as precedent for the later case.

Tool 6: Thought experiments

Sometimes, if we are engaging in case comparison, there may be value in considering hypothetical, or even unrealistic, examples. Philosophers frequently use imaginary cases in testing arguments and in examining concepts. These are called 'thought experiments'. Like many scientific experiments, they are designed to test a theory in controlled settings. For example, to work out how important a particular factor is, you might consider a variant of the current case without that factor. Or a hypothetical case might be designed to isolate a particular element. There are several examples of thought experiment in this book (e.g. the case of the connected violinist (see Case 13.3)).

Some practically minded people, including doctors, are sceptical of thought experiments because the cases do not describe real situations. Such scepticism can miss the point. Suppose that person A justifies her view that euthanasia is wrong by appealing to the general principle that intentional killing is always wrong. Person B might use a thought experiment to challenge this general principle. He might, for example, describe the situation of the trapped lorry driver (see Chapter 14). In this situation, the driver will either burn to death with much suffering, or might be killed painlessly. The power of this thought experiment is that it provides a convincing example of when it would seem right, at least to many people, to kill. If you believe that it would be right to kill the trapped lorry driver, then you need to modify your general principle that it is always wrong to kill. Your objection to euthanasia will need to rest on a less general principle, and you will need either to give reasons that justify distinguishing, morally, between the two cases or to change your position with regard to one of the situations. The fact that the case of the lorry driver is imaginary does not render it irrelevant as a test of the general principle.

Tool 7: Rational decision theory

In life, we are often faced with making decisions in complex situations. There are different ways of making these decisions. In some situations, we may use a simple rule that is fairly easy to apply: 'buy the best', for example, for items we value and are comfortably within our budget. In other situations, we may search for the item we want until we find one with the features that are satisfactory to us – not worrying about whether we might find a better alternative if we went on looking. In still other situations our concern may be to avoid a particular bad outcome. We avoid this one risk, other considerations being of little importance to us. It is useful to understand these different approaches to decisions, because they sometimes help explain why (for example) patients might make a different decision from the one that doctors feel would be right for them.

Where the outcome of a decision is uncertain, one approach is to use something called rational decision theory. This is a method derived from the systematic application of a *consequentialist* approach to decisions (see Chapter 2). It seeks to identify which option will maximize the expected value (or utility), as we see it, of the decision (for a more detailed discussion see Savulescu 1994).

Consider a simple example. I am offered the opportunity to take part in the following bet on the outcome of the throw of an unbiased die: if I throw a 1 or a 2, then I will win £15; if I throw any other number (a 3, 4, 5 or 6), then I must pay £10. Is it financially sensible to throw the die?

I have two options: either to refuse the offer and not to enter the gamble or to enter the gamble and throw the die. If I take the first option and do not gamble, then the expected 'value' of the outcome will be neither to win nor to lose any money: £0.

If I take the second option and gamble, then there are two possible outcomes: to throw a 1 or 2 and win £15; or to throw a 3, 4, 5 or 6 and lose £10. Thus, I have a one in three chance of winning £15 and a two in three chance of losing £10. Overall, the expected value of taking part in the bet will be:

$$(1/3 \times £15) + (2/3 \times -£10) = 5 - 6.67 = -£1.67$$

The expected value if I join the gamble is -£1.67; the expected value of not joining the gamble is £0. As it is better not to lose anything than to lose £1.67, it is better (according to rational decision theory) not to bet.

What has this to do with ethics? In the above example the value of each outcome was calculated in terms of money. But the same general method can be applied to whatever kind of evaluation we want: people's happiness for example, or some moral evaluation. If we can ascribe both values and probabilities to the various possible outcomes of the various different choices that we might make in a given situation, then rational decision theory can help us in coming to a decision.

Consider the following medical example:

Case 1.3

Mr S is an elderly patient admitted to a general ward with pneumonia on a background of generally declining health and past cardiac problems. The medical team are concerned that he is at risk of suffering a cardiac arrest. They discuss with Mr S what he would want done in that eventuality – would he wish to be resuscitated? Mr S is unsure and asks for advice from the doctors.

What should they recommend?

The question is whether resuscitation should be attempted for Mr S – what would be best? Suppose that the likely effects of resuscitation are as follows: there is a 10% (i.e. probability (p) = 0.1) chance of successful resuscitation with a reasonable life afterwards; a 40% (p = 0.4) chance of successful resuscitation with a very poor life afterwards (return of circulation, admission to intensive care, but either death before hospital discharge or survival with severe neurological impairment); and a 50% (p = 0.5) chance of immediate death. If no resuscitation were attempted, he would certainly die immediately.

In order to use rational decision theory, values must be given to these various possible outcomes. Let us give the value 0 for immediate death. For the sake of illustration, we could imagine that Mr S gives a value +5 for the 'reasonable life'. However, he is very concerned to avoid the 'very poor life' and assigns it a value of -10 (that is a value worse than death). Given these values we can calculate the 'expected utilities' of both attempting and not attempting resuscitation:

- The expected value (probability multiplied by value) of not attempting resuscitation is 0 (1 × 0).
- The expected value of attempting resuscitation is the sum of the various possible outcomes:

$$(0.1 \times 5) + (0.4 \times -10) + (0.5 \times 0) = -3.5.$$

On the given assumptions, not attempting resuscitation has greater expected utility than attempting resuscitation. How is this helpful? It might assist Mr S's doctors in advising him what decision he should make. If the above values accurately reflect Mr S's own evaluation, non-resuscitation would be the most rational choice for him to make. Alternatively, in other situations, this sort of analysis might be helpful in understanding a decision a patient has already made. If another patient with similar prospects to Mr S chooses resuscitation, that could suggest that she places a different value on survival with or without disability. (For example, she may not view it as a negative to survive with disability.) Or, it may suggest that she intuitively believes her chances of recovery are higher than the doctor's estimate.

THE SLIPPERY SLOPE ARGUMENT

The slippery slope argument is frequently used in moral discussion. It is important to judge when its use is valid. The core of the argument is that, once you accept one particular position, then it will be extremely difficult, or indeed impossible, not to accept more and more extreme positions. Thus, if you do not want to accept the more extreme positions you must not accept the original, less extreme position.

One example of the use of such an argument is against the practice of voluntary active euthanasia. Suppose, for example, that a proponent of such euthanasia gave an example of a situation when it seemed plausible that euthanasia is acceptable. The case of mercy killing carried out by Dr Cox (see Chapter 14) could be such an example. The slippery slope argument might be used as providing grounds against such mercy killing, not on the grounds that it would be wrong in this

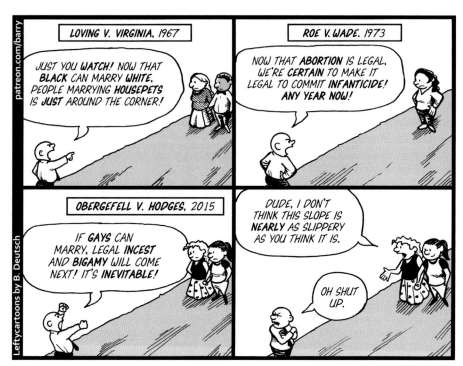

Figure 1.2 The slippery slope (© Barry Deutsch, reproduced with permission)

case, but instead on the basis that allowing killing in Dr Cox's situation would inevitably lead to killing in other situations where it would be wrong.

The main response to the slippery slope argument is to claim that there is no inevitable slide from acceptable to unacceptable cases. To extend the metaphor, the slope is not necessarily slippery (Fig. 1.2): a barrier could be placed partway down the slope, or instead there are a series of steps and it may be possible to stop at any point.

There are two types of slippery slope argument: a logical type and an empirical type. We will consider each separately.

The logical type of slippery slope argument

The logical type of slippery slope argument can be seen as consisting of three steps:

- **Step 1** Proposition p is closely related to proposition q. If you accept that p is ethical, then you must also accept q. Similarly, if you accept q then you must accept proposition r, and so on through propositions s, t, etc.
- **Step 2** This involves showing, or gaining agreement from the other side in the argument, that at some stage in this series the propositions become clearly unacceptable, or false.
- **Step 3** This involves applying formal logic (*modus tollens*; see Box 1.1) to conclude that, because one of the later propositions (proposition t, for example) is ethically unacceptable, it follows that the first proposition (p) must be unacceptable.

The first step in the argument is what is special about slippery slopes. The crucial component is to establish a series of closely related propositions such that there can be no reasonable grounds for holding one proposition true (or false) and its adjacent proposition(s) false (or true).

Slippery slope arguments have apparent force because many (perhaps most) of the concepts we use have a certain vagueness: if a concept applies to one object, then the concept will still apply if there is a very small change in that object. Here is an example:

An adult is someone who has reached full physical (and perhaps emotional and cognitive) maturity. No-one reaches adulthood overnight. If someone is an adult on a particular day, they must have been an adult a day earlier. If they were an adult a day earlier, then (since they did not become an adult overnight) they must have been an adult a day prior. However, if this series is continued, it seems to imply that a newborn infant is an adult…!

There are two different ways of dealing with vague concepts. The first is to deny that the concept has to be either completely true or completely false when applied to a particular object. For example, we may say, perhaps of someone aged 15 years, that she is partly a child and partly an adult – and that the same is true at 16 years, although she is then more of an adult and less of a child. The second way is to choose a point at which one concept ceases to apply. We stipulate, for example, that for many purposes a human is a child until the age of 18 years and then becomes an adult. The precise point, of course, is arbitrary. However, if it is important to make the distinction (for example in deciding when to provide a driver's license), arbitrariness may not matter.

Similarly, there are two ways of dealing with the logical form of slippery slope argument. Consider the following example of such an argument:

P1 It is ethical to terminate a pregnancy at 10 weeks' gestation, even if there are no foetal abnormalities.
P2 A single week of gestation cannot make a crucial difference to moral status because there are no dramatic changes in a fetus' development from one week to the next.
C1 It is ethical to terminate a pregnancy at 11 weeks' gestation, even if there are no foetal abnormalities.

This argument could be repeated (12, 13, 14 weeks, etc.) all the way up to 40 weeks' gestation. Since most people think that it would certainly be wrong to terminate a pregnancy of a normal fetus at 40 weeks' gestation (perhaps with the exception of a life-threatening condition in the mother), that could be interpreted to mean that the first step should be rejected. According to this slippery slope objection, there is no point after conception at which termination would be permissible, without allowing termination even at full term.

One response that could be made to this slippery slope argument is that terminating a pregnancy becomes increasingly problematic with increasing age of gestation. At 10 weeks the wrong in terminating the pregnancy is so slight that the reasons that outweigh such wrong can also be quite slight – maternal wishes, for example. In contrast, at 36 weeks' gestation the wrong of terminating a pregnancy is considerable. There would have to be very good reasons to justify so doing – significant risk to the mother's life, for example. Between these two ages of gestation the weight of justification gradually changes. Perhaps there is even an intermediate phase when termination is neither clearly ethical, nor clearly unethical.

The alternative approach is to draw a line at some age of gestation, such that prior to that age it is generally acceptable for termination to be carried out and after that age it is generally unacceptable. The precise drawing of the line is arbitrary; but it is not arbitrary that a line is drawn. In order to ensure clear policy (and clear laws) it is often sensible to draw precise lines, even though the underlying concepts and moral values change more gradually.

The empirical form of slippery slope argument

The second form of slippery slope argument is empirical, not logical. An opponent of voluntary active euthanasia might argue that if we allow doctors to carry out such euthanasia, then, as a matter of fact, in the real world, this will lead to non-voluntary euthanasia (see Chapter 14). Such an opponent might accept that there is no logical reason to slip from the one to the other, but in practice such slippage will occur. Therefore, as a matter of policy, we should not legitimize voluntary active euthanasia even if such euthanasia is not, in itself, wrong.

This empirical form of argument depends on making assumptions about the world, and therefore raises the question of how compelling the evidence is for such assumptions. There may be disagreement about whether available evidence supports such a slippery slope or not. What will happen if a particular practice is permitted is often likely to depend on how precisely the policy is worded. It may be possible to prevent slipping down the slope by putting up a barrier (as is done in abortion law with regard to 24 weeks' gestation; see Chapter 13) or by carefully articulating the circumstances under which an action is or is not legitimate (as might perhaps be done with euthanasia).

REVISION QUESTIONS

1. All ethics is relative. Do you agree? Why? Why not?
2. A large systematic review of well-conducted trials shows that treatment A is associated with better outcomes than treatment B. Therefore, doctors should offer treatment A rather than treatment B. Is this conclusion warranted? What are the facts and the values in such a decision?
3. Plagiarism is a form of academic misconduct. Therefore, you should not plagiarize. Is this argument valid? Is it missing something?
4. Up for Debate Box 1.1 includes a debate between Dr Smith and Dr Jones around inserting feeding tubes in patients with dementia. Analyze the arguments on each side. Can you spot any problems?

Up for Debate Box 1.1 Should patients with dementia receive a gastrostomy? (Are there any problems with these arguments?)

Dr Jones

Doctors should not insert gastrostomies in patients with dementia for multiple reasons. First, there is no evidence that gastrostomies benefit patients – that was the conclusion of a Cochrane systematic review. Inserting gastrostomies would be flying in the face of evidence-based medicine. Second, doctors have an ethical obligation not to harm patients. The principle of 'do no harm' has been a core value of medicine for hundreds, if not thousands, of years. Third, it isn't medically indicated to perform a gastrostomy on a patient with dementia. Fourth, what about informed consent? It is unethical for doctors to perform surgery without consent, but patients with dementia cannot consent to having a feeding tube inserted.

Dr Smith recommends feeding tubes, but he is a member of a right-to-life group. What do you expect? It is all very well for doctors to respect patient wishes, but most patients don't even want gastrostomies. The push to insert feeding tubes in patients with profound dementia is medicine gone mad. What is next? Inserting feeding tubes in patients who are brain dead? Forcing doctors and nurses to put feeding tubes in patients with dementia would go against their conscience and lead to good people abandoning the profession.

Dr Smith

We should reject Dr Jones' arguments. Patients with dementia have human rights – they are still people. Doctors who want to deny them feeding tubes are treating them as second class citizens. The first principle of the NHS constitution states that patients should receive care irrespective of gender, race, disability, age, sexual orientation, religion, belief, gender reassignment, pregnancy and maternity or marital or civil partnership status. It would therefore be illegal and unconstitutional for doctors to decide not to provide treatment to a group of disabled patients.

Dr Jones is just trying to save money for the NHS. In his other writing, he has even supported active euthanasia, which is illegal and contrary to the core values of medicine. If doctors decide not to put feeding tubes in patients with dementia, who else will be denied treatment: adults with progressive neurological problems? Children with disabilities? This is a symptom of a world view that devalues people with disability.

Extension case 1.4   Organ sales

Jane is a healthy student from a low-income family who is keen to travel overseas to attend a prestigious university to obtain higher education. She has been unsuccessful in obtaining a scholarship to travel for her degree, but has found a wealthy donor who has offered to pay a substantial amount in exchange for her donating a kidney. Jane has sought independent medical advice about the risks of kidney donation, and judges them to be small compared with the benefit of travelling and getting her degree.

What are the ethical arguments in favour of and against allowing Jane to sell her kidney?

Critics of organ sales sometimes claim that this would be a form of commodification or a threat to human dignity.

Continued

For example, read Andorno (2017) and Wilkinson (2000). How do Andorno and Wilkinson define commodification? Can you set out the logical form of Andorno's commodification argument against organ sales? Why does Wilkinson argue that the commodification argument fails?

For the best treatment of organ sales, and a reasons-based approach, see Richards (2012).

REFERENCES

Andorno, R. 2017. "Buying and Selling Organs: Issues of Commodification, Exploitation and Human Dignity." *Journal of Trafficking and Human Exploitation* 1 (2): 119-27. doi: 10.7590/245227717X15090911046502.

Beauchamp, T. L. and Childress, J. F. 2012. *Principles of biomedical ethics*, 7th ed. New York; Oxford: Oxford University Press.

Berlin, I. 1998. "On pluralism." *New York review of books*. https://www.cs.utexas.edu/users/vl/notes/berlin.html.

Blackburn, S. 2001. *Ethics: a very short introduction*. Oxford; New York: Oxford University Press: 2003.

Flew, A. 1989. *An introduction to western philosophy: ideas and argument from Plato to Popper*. Revised ed. Thames and Hudson.

Gillon, R. 1986. *Philosophical medical ethics*. Chichester: Wiley.

Kaplan, R. C. 2001. "Treatment of hypertension to prevent stroke: translating evidence into clinical practice." *Journal of Clinical Hypertension* 3 (3): 153-6.

Rawls, J. 1951. "Outline of a decision procedure for ethics." *Philosophical Review* 60 (2): 177-97.

Rawls, J. 1999. *A theory of justice*. Rev. ed. Oxford: Oxford University Press.

Regnard, C., Leslie, P., Crawford, H., Matthews, D. and Gibson, L. 2010. "Gastrostomies in dementia: bad practice or bad evidence?" *Age and Ageing* 39 (3): 282-4. doi: 10.1093/ageing/afq012.

Richards, J. R. 2012. *The ethics of transplants: why careless thought costs lives*. Oxford: Oxford University Press.

Sampson, E. L., Candy, B. and Jones, L. 2009. "Enteral tube feeding for older people with advanced dementia." *The Cochrane Database of Systematic Reviews* (2): CD007209. doi: 10.1002/14651858.CD007209.pub2.

Savulescu, J. 1994. "Treatment limitation decisions under uncertainty: the value of subsequent euthanasia." *Bioethics* 8 (1): 49-73.

Savulescu, J. 2010. "Julian Savulescu on 'Yuk'." In *Philosophy bites*, edited by D. Edmonds and N. Warburton. Oxford: Oxford University Press.

Warburton, N. 2007. *Thinking from A to Z*, 3rd ed. London: Routledge.

Wilkinson, D., Butcherine, E. and Savulescu, J. 2019. "Withdrawal aversion and the equivalence test." *American Journal of Bioethics* 19 (3): 21-8. doi: 10.1080/15265161.2019.1574465.

Wilkinson, D. and Savulescu, J. 2018. *Ethics, conflict and medical treatment for children: from disagreement to dissensus*. Elsevier.

Wilkinson, S. 2000. "Commodification arguments for the legal prohibition of organ sale." *Health Care Analysis* 8 (2): 189-201. doi: 10.1023/A:1009454612900.

Chapter **2**

Ethical theories and perspectives

Case 2.1

Joe is a senior paediatrician at a specialist hospital. He sees a family for follow-up whose child, Thomas, died last year following a sudden catastrophic illness. The parents remain intensely distressed and are struggling to cope with the loss of their child. During the consultation, the parents express that one of their few sources of consolation is that Thomas was able to donate his kidneys. They mention that they often think about the other child who has Thomas' kidneys and wonder how that child is doing. They ask Joe if he can find out. Out of a desire to help the grieving parents, Joe promises to see if he can and says that he will call them with any news.

The next week, Joe asks one of his renal colleagues at the hospital how he could find out about the result of the transplantation. He mentions the timing and circumstances of Thomas' death, and the renal colleague hesitates before informing Joe that he remembers the case well. In fact, the transplant did not go ahead. Due to a surgical mistake at the time of harvesting Thomas' kidneys, the blood vessels were damaged. When the transplant team reviewed the kidneys, they found that they could not be salvaged.

Joe now finds himself in a difficult position. He wishes to console Thomas' parents, and believes that the news of the unsuccessful transplant will cause them distress and compound their grief. He wonders whether he should lie to them, for example by telling them that the transplant went well and that the other child is thriving, or that he was unable to find details about the result of the transplant. Alternatively, he could simply fail to call them as promised.

Should doctors ever lie to prevent harm to their patients?

THE ROLE OF ETHICAL THEORY

In the last chapter, we described a number of 'tools of reasoning'. One of the tools (tool 4) involved reasoning from principles and theory. We also discussed the interaction between ethical theories and our intuitive responses to specific situations, introducing the idea of 'reflective equilibrium'. We did not, though, say much about ethical theory itself. In this chapter, we will outline some of the different theoretical approaches that moral philosophers take to ethical questions.

What role should ethical theory play in practice? As mentioned in the last chapter, one approach to medical ethics (the 'mathematical approach') starts from a particular ethical theory and then attempts to derive answers to ethical dilemmas. For example, you could outline a Kantian approach to informed consent. Or you might identify a utilitarian perspective on euthanasia. However, this sort of analysis is not always helpful. It will not help people who do not already subscribe to that ethical theory or who do not know which theory is the right one. Another approach to ethics applies a range of different ethical theories to a problem, for example by contrasting utilitarian, deontological and virtue ethics approaches to research ethics (Box 2.1 compares duty-based ethics, consequentialism and virtue ethics). That can be valuable, and indeed we will do this in some places in this book. However, this strategy risks being formulaic or overly simplistic. There are often multiple different versions of these theories, or different views about what they imply for specific practical issues. It can also sometimes lead to cherry-picking of

---

Box 2.1 A comparison of deontological ethics, consequentialism and virtue ethics (adapted from Hursthouse 1997)

Deontological ethics

1. An action is right if, and only if, it is in accord with a moral rule or principle.
2. A moral rule is one that (for example):
    - is laid on us by God
    - is required by reason
    - would be chosen by all rational beings.

    The theory thus depends critically on the concept of rationality (or, alternatively, on understanding God's will).

Consequentialism

1. An action is right if, and only if, it promotes the best consequences.
2. An account must be given of how different states of affairs (consequences) can be morally evaluated and ranked.

    The theory thus depends critically on the concepts used to evaluate states of affairs (such as happiness, in the case of hedonic utilitarianism).

Virtue ethics

1a. An action is right if, and only if, it is what a virtuous agent would do in the circumstances.
1b. A virtuous person is one who exercises virtues.
2. A virtue is a character trait a human being needs in order to flourish.

    The theory thus depends critically on the concept of human flourishing.

ethical conclusions – it suggests that, for difficult problems, you can just select whichever theory gives the ethical answer that fits with your prior view about a particular problem.

In most of the clinical situations that raise problematic ethical issues, the key arguments do not require discussion of general ethical theory. While these theories are useful for moral philosophers, for the most part they can be seen as underlying theory, providing a foundational basis for ethics rather than an ingredient of rational debate over day-to-day issues in practical medical ethics. General ethical theories can perhaps be seen as analogous to general statistical theory, as opposed to the particular statistical tests that are used in assessing specific sets of data. In most circumstances, you can apply statistical tests without needing to refer to the theory. Sometimes, though, if there is a new problem (where the tests do not apply), or if the tests appear to be giving answers that do not seem to be right, it might be important to go back to the underlying theory.

We will start this chapter by looking at three different approaches or types of ethical theory: consequentialism, duty-based (deontological) theories and virtue theory. We will then outline two perspectives on ethics (communitarian and feminist ethics) that have been influential in debates in medical ethics. We will not defend any individual theory in this book, partly for reasons of space, but also because it may not be necessary to all agree on which is the right moral theory. It is perhaps useful to mention the view of one of the great moral philosophers of the 20th century, the brilliant Oxford philosopher Derek Parfit, who argued that, despite appearances, there were not deep irresolvable differences between these theories; ultimately, they were working towards the same destination. Parfit suggested that '[t]hese people are climbing the same mountain on different sides' (Parfit 2011).

CONSEQUENTIALISM

Consequentialist theories of ethics hold that that an action is right if, and only if, it will lead to the best outcome. This can be put in a more practical form: out of all the possible actions in a given situation, you should choose the one with the best overall consequences.

According to consequentialist theories, the only morally relevant features of an act are its consequences. Features such as what someone *intended* by acting, or the nature of an action (e.g. the fact that an act involves lying), are not in themselves morally relevant. This does not mean that consequentialists are indifferent about lying, but for the consequentialist it is only the consequences of lying that are morally important.

There is an ambiguity in the formulation presented above. Is the right action the one that will, as a matter of fact, lead to the best outcome, or is it the one that the agent, at the time of acting, has good reason to believe will lead to the best outcome? Most theorists would argue that, in applying consequentialist theories and in judging whether someone has acted rightly or wrongly, it is the *foreseeable* consequences that are important.

We can see some of these differences when thinking about Case 2.1. One of the outcomes that Joe might consider is the possibility that if he lies to Thomas' parents, they will find out the truth anyway. They may discover that the transplant did not go ahead, be devastated as a result, and be even more upset because a paediatrician who they trusted lied to them. Perhaps Joe foresees this could happen and decides (in order to avoid that possibility) to reveal the difficult news about the unsuccessful organ harvesting. However, let us imagine that, in actual fact, the parents would not have found out on their own. Joe could not have known, but Thomas' parents are tragically killed in an unrelated car accident a month after his meeting with them. We might conclude that, in retrospect, it would have been better for Joe not to tell the truth because the parents would have been less miserable in the last month of their lives. However, since there was no way for Joe to predict this eventuality, it could not be relevant to Joe's decision.

There are two different broad types of consequentialism. In specific cases, we can look at the outcome of particular actions; or, we could look at the outcomes of certain ways of acting in general. *Act-consequentialism* looks to assess and promote the consequences of specific acts. *Rule-consequentialism*, in contrast, is concerned about which rules should be followed, and which would be best to follow overall.

We might also reflect differently on the case above if we are an act- or rule-consequentialist. In this particular situation, Joe might be very concerned about the psychological well-being of Thomas' parents. He might judge their mental health to be very fragile and be concerned that they may even harm themselves if he tells them the news that he has uncovered. Or perhaps he has good reason to think that they will never know the actual truth. Perhaps the family are from out of town and have no other contacts in the hospital. According to act-consequentialism, it might be that lying to the parents would lead to the best foreseeable outcome. However, we could also be concerned about what doctors should do in general in cases like this. There might be good reason, for example, to have a strong rule against doctors lying. The GMC indicates in its Good Medical Practice guidance: 'You must be honest and trustworthy in all your communication with patients and colleagues' (General Medical Council 2013). Even if it would sometimes be better in individual cases, doctors lying to patients might lead to erosion of patient trust and lead to worse outcomes for patients overall. Exactly what rule-consequentialism would recommend to Joe will depend on what we have reason to believe the consequences would be of doctors lying in some situations. It will also depend on how broad or narrow a rule we are considering. We might be thinking about cases of doctors faced with bereaved parents and unpalatable truths that would cause predictable distress. Or we might be concerned about general rules relating to disclosure of medical error.

Utilitarianism: an example of a consequentialist theory of ethics

The best known specific consequentialist theory is utilitarianism. See Up for Debate Box 2.1 for some of the arguments for and against utilitarianism as applied to medical ethics. There at least three different versions of utilitarianism: hedonistic, preference and ideal. Each of these theories differ in what they judge the good (or utility) is to be maximized. In effect, they hold three different theories of well-being. What they recommend in a specific case might vary.

> ✕ **Up for Debate Box 2.1** Should doctors be utilitarians?
>
> **Yes**
>
> Until fairly recently, medical ethics was based either on religious teaching or on professional rules that had been handed down (e.g. the Hippocratic oath). However, those rules cannot be the basis of modern medical ethics. Our societies now include people from a range of different faiths. We cannot base ethics on tradition either – though traditional rules can be useful, some will need changing.
>
> The only rational basis for ethics is concern for what happens as a consequence of what we do. Doctors are concerned, fundamentally, about the outcome for their patients. Evidence-based medicine teaches doctors to critically evaluate medical treatments – to seek those treatments that will do the most good and least harm. We should apply a similar evidence-based strategy to ethics. Doctors should act to do the most good for their patients, and the least harm. If following rules would lead to less benefit, or more harm, the rules need to change.
>
> **No**
>
> Utilitarians teach that the right action is the one that will cause the most 'utility', and understand that to mean the most happiness and the least pain. However, in many circumstances, it simply isn't clear what action will lead to the greatest happiness. It is all very well to look for evidence about medical treatments, but there are no randomized controlled trials of different ethical rules or policies. What is more, the utilitarian concern to maximize happiness seems to be missing something of fundamental importance. Doctors shouldn't be spending their whole time thinking about whether treating patients nicely, not lying to them or spending time with them is going to generate the most utility. Medicine is about caring, not calculating.
>
> Finally, a utilitarian approach to medicine would appear to generate some simply unacceptable answers. For example, on utilitarian grounds, it would be wrong to provide expensive medical treatments to patients with severe disabilities, as this would not generate enough QALYs (quality-adjusted life years). It would be acceptable to conduct harmful experiments on some people (even against their wishes) if that would generate a life-saving treatment for many others.
>
> (See Smart and Williams 1973.)

Case 2.2

Margo is an older woman with advanced dementia living in a nursing home. She gains pleasure from a range of activities (reading, listening to music), though has little memory of events from one day to the next (she listens to the same piece of music over and over). She does not seem to be in pain. Some years ago, when she had full capacity, Margo completed a formal advance directive indicating that if she ever developed Alzheimer's disease she would not wish medical treatment for any life-threatening illness. Subsequently, Margo develops pneumonia, from which she is likely to recover if treated. Should she receive antibiotics or other treatments for her pneumonia?

(The case of Margo was originally described by medical student Andrew Firlik and discussed by philosopher Ronald Dworkin in his book *Life's Dominion*. Dresser (1995), Dworkin (1993), Firlik (1991), Hope (1996))

Hedonistic utilitarianism

According to classical hedonistic utilitarianism, the best consequences are those in which (human) happiness is maximized. In 1863, John Stuart Mill argued that 'actions are right in proportion as they tend to promote happiness, wrong as they tend to produce the reverse of happiness' (Mill, Bentham, and Ryan 1987).

Overall, 'utility' on this theory is seen to be the balance of pleasure over pain. According to this theory, assuming that the positive experiences in Margo's current and future life outweigh the negative ones, it would appear to be good to give Margo treatment for her pneumonia. (We have not considered here any impact of treating Margo on other people, e.g. family members, staff or the wider community.)

Preference utilitarianism

Some utilitarians (e.g. R M Hare and Peter Singer (in his early works)) think that what matters is not purely a question of happiness/unhappiness, but also a question of people's desires or preferences. On this view, human well-being is: 'the obtaining to a high or at least reasonable degree of a quality of life which on the whole a person wants, or prefers to have' (Hare 1998).

For these utilitarians, it might be bad to keep Margo alive because it conflicts with a previous strongly-held preference. Whether or not they think Margo should be treated will depend on how they weigh up her past strong desire not to be kept alive with dementia compared with her current desires to continue to read, listen to music and live.

Ideal/objective utilitarianism

One problem for preference utilitarianism is that sometimes people might have mistaken desires, or might have desires for things that seem to be bad for them. According to other utilitarians, what matters is not mere happiness or getting what we want, but doing things that are worthwhile.

> [C]ertain things are good or bad for people, whether or not these people want to have the good things or avoid the bad things. The good things might include moral goodness, rational activity, the development of one's abilities, having children and being a good parent, knowledge and the awareness of true beauty. The bad things might include being betrayed, manipulated, slandered, deceived, being deprived of liberty and dignity, and enjoying either sadistic pleasure, or aesthetic pleasure in what is in fact ugly (Parfit 1984, p. 499).

Whether it would be good to treat Margo on this sort of utilitarian view might depend on which features of life are seen to be morally valuable, and how they are weighed up.

Each of these theories has its strengths and weaknesses as an account of what is good for people. Some philosophers have argued that what is good is a combination of all three of these elements (Parfit 1984). We will return to some of these theories about well-being and best interests in the next chapter.

DEONTOLOGICAL MORAL THEORIES

There are ethical theories that consider aspects other than consequences as relevant to ethics. Many of these focus on duties, rules or rights (these theories are often called 'deontological' (from the Greek *deon,* duty)).

The key element of deontological ethical theories is that certain acts are wrong in themselves, independent of what is predicted to happen as a result. Such acts may be morally unacceptable even if they are carried out in the pursuit of morally admirable goals. According to deontological theories, the question of which action is right is not answered by looking at the consequences of the possible actions, but by looking at the nature of the actions themselves.

For example, one potential duty is that doctors should not lie to patients. In Case 2.1, Joe might reflect on whether lying to Thomas' parents would cause them less distress, and might even prevent serious harm. According to a deontological theory, it may be wrong for Joe to lie even if this would be better overall for the parents. Indeed, even if Joe knew with certainty that telling the truth would be harmful, he might have an obligation (on some theories) not to lie.

Deontological theory (like *consequentialism*) is a type of ethical theory – it is not in itself a specific theory. In order to guide action, the duties that are morally relevant must be specified.

Some deontological theories are framed around what people *must do,* or *must not do.* In practice, these duties are often phrased as a set of prohibitions, like the Ten Commandments. Religions involve deontological codes. Other deontological theories are based on what must be done, or must not be done, *to people.* These are often phrased in terms of individuals' *rights.* Such rights are sometimes positive, and generate obligations in other people (for example, a right to education or healthcare). More often, the rights are negative and serve to prevent other people acting in certain ways (e.g. a right to privacy, a right to freedom of speech).

Challenges for deontological theories include explaining their source (where do a set of duties or rights come from?), understanding what exactly is required to uphold a duty or right and what to do when duties, rights or rules conflict.

Some deontological rules arise from traditions, historical teaching (e.g. the Hippocratic oath) or divine command (most religious approaches to medical ethics are deontological). Others find their justification in an understanding of the nature of rational beings (e.g. natural law theory) or rationality itself (Kantian ethics). Another prominent contemporary school of deontological theory seeks to identify principles that everyone would agree to if they had to hypothetically decide what the rules should be. For example, philosopher John Rawls sought to provide an account of distributive justice (the question of how money and other goods should be distributed between people in a society) (Rawls 1999). Rawls approached this question by considering which society we would choose if we did not know what place we would have within society (i.e. without knowing whether you would be rich or poor, healthy or ill, etc.). This is called the 'veil of ignorance'. It is a form of contractualism (which kind of social contract would we choose from behind a veil of ignorance). Rawls sought to develop a theory about what is right from those principles that would be chosen by rational people. For example, what rule would we wish to be followed if we were competing for limited life-saving resources and we did not know if we would have a longer life, a worse quality life or were unlikely to benefit? In some cases, contractualism and utilitarianism converge (Savulescu 2013).

According to consequentialist theories, there will usually be one right act in any given situation. In contrast, for duty-based theories there will usually be many right acts. The list of duties – mainly prohibitions – will define some acts as wrong; but any act that is not wrong is one possible right act. However, if rules or duties conflict, it may not be clear what the individual should do. According to some theories, there is one single rule from which all others are derived. The famous German philosopher Immanuel Kant adopted such an approach (see below). Others try to rank the principles or duties into a hierarchy such that, if there is conflict, then that which is highest in the hierarchy should be followed. Still other theories accept that we have a range of duties, and when they conflict in a particular situation one has to make a judgement in order to decide the most important duty in that specific situation. The theory of *prima facie* duties is of this type.

W D Ross developed a duty-based approach to ethics that has influenced the 'four-principle' approach to medical ethics (see Chapter 1) (Ross and Stratton-Lake 2002). Ross calls the various duties *'prima facie* duties'. By this he means that, in any specific situation where there is a clash between different duties, we have to decide whether it is morally more important to follow one duty or another. Deciding where the balance lies is, inescapably, a matter of judgement. There is no general ranking of the duties.

Kantian ethics: an example of a deontological theory

Immanuel Kant (1724–1804) aimed to develop fundamental moral rules that would tell us what we ought to do (Kant, Hill, and Zweig 2002, O'Neill 1993). His minimal assumption was that a moral principle has to be a principle for all people.

Kant distinguished two kinds of rule (or imperative): hypothetical and categorical. A hypothetical imperative is of the form: 'Do this in order to achieve that'. A categorical imperative is one that expresses a command that is unconditional, and is of the form: 'Do this!'. Kant sought to identify a categorical imperative that would be accepted by any normal, sane person on rational reflection. If he could identify such an imperative, then that would provide the basis for a morality derived from pure reason.

Kant described the fundamental moral rule (categorical imperative) in a number of ways, and it is not clear that they are all equivalent. The best known of these is: 'Act only on that maxim which you can at the same time will that it should become a universal law'. (This is often said to be equivalent to the Christian 'golden rule': do unto others as you would have others do unto you). A second version is: 'So act as to treat humanity, whether in your own person or in that of any other, never solely as a means but always as an end'. This second formulation, with the idea that people should be treated as 'ends in themselves', has been influential in political philosophy. It stresses the liberal principle that people should not have their individual freedom compromised for the sake of some other end, in particular for the good of society more generally. In the context of medicine, it implies that there is a strong obligation to obtain consent for anything which is done to a person.

Kant believed that his categorical imperative could be used to derive the specific moral duties that make up a complete ethical framework. For example, he derived a duty to keep promises. Suppose Joe is considering whether to break his promise to Thomas' parents to call them back. According to Kant, no-one could prescribe promise-breaking (whenever convenient) as a universal law; that would result in a breakdown of the trust that is needed for promises to mean anything at all.

VIRTUE ETHICS

While consequentialism focuses ethical attention on the outcomes of an action (whether they are good), and deontological theories focus on the action itself (whether it is permitted), virtue ethics focuses on the person who is taking the action and what sort of person they are. The ethics of action is only one element of the moral life. Readers of this book may be at least as interested in the question of how they might be a good person, or a good doctor, as they are in what they should or should not do. For them, the ethics of virtue will be of particular interest.

Virtue ethics is often traced back to the ancient Greek philosopher Aristotle (Aristotle 2000), though in the East it is linked to the writings of Mencius and Confucius. In Aristotle's view, the right act is one that a virtuous person would do in the circumstances, and a virtuous person is someone who exhibits the virtues. The 'virtues' are characteristics that ensure that those endowed with them will have the best life overall. The best life, for Aristotle, is that associated with *eudaimonia*, often translated as *flourishing*. Flourishing can perhaps be seen as a kind of deep happiness, less connected with the concept of pleasure that is often thought to underpin utilitarianism. In one sense, Aristotle's theory could be seen as a selfish theory, as it depends ultimately on self-interest – maximizing one's personal *eudaimonia*. However, many of the virtues are not selfish at all in the ordinary sense, for example kindness or generosity. For Aristotle, being kind and generous to others contributes to one's own flourishing – virtue is its own reward. There is some psychological evidence to support this idea (Haidt 2006). Other virtue ethicists understand virtue not in terms of flourishing, but in terms of particular types of motivation or disposition.

In order for virtue ethics to be of practical value, the virtues (and vices) must be specified. There are multiple different virtue theories, just as there are multiple examples of deontological or consequentialist theories. Because of this, it is not straightforward to know what virtue ethics would recommend in Case 2.1. Telling the truth is obviously a virtue, but a virtuous person might accept some rare exceptions when it would not be good to tell the truth (for example, when doing so would cause serious harm). Another element of Aristotle's ethics is the idea of the golden mean – the desirable midpoint between excess and deficiency. Someone who always lied would clearly not be a virtuous person. However, someone who always told the truth, no matter how much harm that might cause, might be thought to place too much emphasis on truth-telling.

How should Joe decide? Aristotle emphasized the idea of *phronesis*, or practical wisdom. This is the idea that wisdom is needed in order to apply the virtues. For example, we might imagine that Joe thinks very carefully before deciding what to tell Thomas' parents. He might even seek advice from colleagues with experience and practical wisdom. If he then concluded, on reflection, that in this case honesty was not the best policy, that *would* arguably be compatible with practical wisdom and being a virtuous doctor. In contrast, if Joe were to reach the same decision rapidly and conclude immediately that he should certainly lie to prevent harm, this might appear to be too quick and hasty a conclusion, and reflect badly on his character as a good doctor.

PERSPECTIVES

We have outlined three major types of ethical theory that are dominant in Anglo-American philosophy. There are two broad perspectives on ethics that are also relevant to current medical ethics: *communitarianism* and *feminism*. These are not theories so much as perspectives that emphasize particular issues and aspects of ethics. They have developed, in part, as a critical response to much of modern medical ethics (and, indeed, other forms of practical ethics), taking issue with what is seen to be an undue emphasis on some issues or approaches and a neglect of others.

Communitarianism

Much of modern medical ethics has focused on individual rights and autonomy. One of the central tenets of a liberal approach to ethics is that each person should be allowed to pursue his or her own life's goals without interference. The only significant limit to this is that such freedom should not interfere with the freedom of others.

Communitarianism, in contrast, emphasizes our individual *responsibilities* as part of a community, together with the responsibilities of communities themselves to care for their vulnerable members. At the theoretical level, communitarianism is at odds with liberalism in that its conception of the common good is held at the public level. According to this view, the public pursuit of shared ends can take precedence over the claims of individuals to pursue their own conceptions of the good. Thus, according to communitarianism, there is a primary idea of an agreed way of life for the community. This provides a standard by which different values can be ranked and a reason for the state to use measures (for example, providing subsidy for some activities) to promote those activities that promote the community's values.

This has practical implications for medical ethics. In Chapter 15 we will discuss the issue of opt-out consent for organ donation. Individualistic approaches to the ethics of organ donation emphasize the idea that patients have a right to decide this matter for themselves. Such approaches tend to address the issue not of what the person ought to do, but of what other people can or cannot legitimately force him to do. From the point of view of communitarianism, however, the most salient feature might be that as a community we stand to gain a great deal from facilitating organ donation, and that because of this each of us might have a *prima facie* moral duty to donate our organs if we can do so at little or no personal cost. (After all, if you are going to die anyway, your organs will otherwise go to waste.) The communitarian approach to the allocation of medical resources would emphasize the importance of reaching consensus at the public level on what the goals of health care are. Thus, we have to work not at the level of individuals but at the level of consensus within communities (Zwart 1999).

A communitarian perspective may lead to specifying particular moral duties or valuing certain types of consequences. It is not an alternative to the general types of ethical theory described above, but a perspective that can inform the values of specific ethical theories. It is not clear, for example, that there is a distinctly communitarian answer to how Joe should act in Case 2.1. However, a communitarian might shift the focus of discussion. They might identify the ongoing distress of Thomas' parents and point out that grieving parents often struggle to find support within contemporary societies. Perhaps the key question is not what Joe ought to do, but why Thomas' parents are suffering so greatly. They might point to the community's responsibility to care for people who are distressed and bereaved, and the support that they can draw from a network of family, friends and neighbours.

A feminist approach to ethics

One of the motivations for developing a communitarian approach to ethics was a concern that major theories and approaches were too narrowly focused and neglected important perspectives. This concern has been shared by philosophers developing feminist approaches to bioethics.

The feminist approach to ethics has often drawn attention to specific ethical questions that are highly important for women's health care: access to birth control and abortion, pregnancy, representations of gender. It has also been concerned about those who are marginalized in society, for example because of disability, sexuality or race. Feminist insights have often drawn attention to the way in which social structures or representations create or perpetuate disadvantage.

Just as there is not a single consequentialist or deontological theory, there are multiple different feminist perspectives reflecting a wide range of different insights and approaches to ethics. Nevertheless, there are some shared features of a feminist approach. First, it is often suspicious of simplifying the specific situation so as to focus on what are traditionally seen as the essential moral features. This simplification will often remove factors that are important in thinking about the ethical issues. This is because, from the feminist perspective, many of the important factors involve details of the people involved and their relationships, and the details of exactly what interactions people have had. Second, feminism is sceptical of applying principles in the abstract. Again, the details are important. Third, there is concern that it may not be possible to decide what is the right thing to do (e.g. switch off the ventilator) if only the bare essential outline is given. The feminist perspective may emphasize that the right thing to do will often be to discuss the issues with the key people involved, rather than rush into a decision. The right action may emerge from discussion: the key people may come to some kind of consensus. In its application to medical ethics, feminism has tended to criticize an approach that relies on brief summaries of the situation and the application of a theoretical standpoint and argument.

With that in mind, a feminist philosopher might reject any attempt to derive a simple answer to Case 2.1. The description of the case is too thin: we do not have any details of the relationship between Thomas' parents, any clear picture of how much support they are receiving or even where the loss of their child fits into the rest of their lives. Perhaps the question of whether Joe should tell the truth or lie is the wrong question – rather, the real issue might be how best to support this grieving couple. The feminist might draw attention to the marginalization that bereaved parents often experience in societies where child death has become rare. They might also point out that the parents' distress should be seen within broader narratives in society. Such narratives place enormous value on 'successful' parenting and child-rearing, and may even problematically imply that parents should be blamed or criticized if bad things happen to children.

These characteristics of feminist medical ethics overlap with other perspectives. In particular, there are three other perspectives that share many of these features of feminism. These are: narrative ethics, which emphasizes the details of cases; communitarian ethics (see above), which emphasizes the importance of discussion and coming to a negotiated agreement; and the 'ethics of care'.

The 'ethics of care' is a strand of feminist ethics that has developed a life of its own. This approach has been developed particularly by Joan Tronto. It shares some features with virtue ethics in that it approaches many issues in medical (and nursing) ethics from the point of view of what a caring person would do. Tronto identifies four virtues of caring: attentiveness, for example to people's needs; responsibility; competence; and responsiveness (Tronto 1993). In a practical situation, this approach suggests that one asks what each of these virtues requires one to do, rather than asking what is the right final act.

1. Compare two ethical theories that are relevant to medical ethics. How do these theories differ? Which do you find more attractive, and why?
2. Ethical argument is all very well, but at the end of the day human rights are the basis of ethical practice. Do you agree? Why? Why not?
3. What is the distinctive feature of virtue ethics? Give an example of how virtue ethics is relevant to medicine.
4. There are different forms of consequentialism, and these have very different implications for a consequentialist understanding of ethics. Explain.

Extension case 2.3

Dr A is working in the emergency department during an influenza pandemic. Intensive care units are at capacity throughout the city. Two patients are critically ill and in need of invasive respiratory support. There is a single available bed. One of the patients, James, has pre-existing lung disease, such that, if he is given the intensive care bed, it is likely that he will need a prolonged period of respiratory support (estimates suggest that he would need five times longer than the average intensive care stay). The other patient, Jane, does not have pre-existing lung disease, and is likely to require only an average intensive care stay. Dr A elects to intubate and treat Jane rather than James. He reasons that this will allow the intensive care unit to save five lives rather than only one.

Dr B is working as a surgeon in a busy trauma unit attached to a transplant program. There is a shortage of available organs, and Dr B is aware that patients are regularly dying for want of available organs. A young homeless patient, Jonny, is admitted to the emergency room with a traumatic head injury. He has a card in his wallet indicating a desire to be an organ donor. While the injury is treatable, Dr B elects not to treat it, allowing Jonny to progress to brain death. He reasons that this will allow Jonny to donate his organs and to save five lives rather than only one.

What would the different ethical theories say about the actions of Dr A and Dr B? Are utilitarians committed to thinking that the actions of Dr B are morally equivalent to the actions of Dr A?

The Trolley problem: a runaway train is approaching the points on the railway line. If the points are not switched, the train will kill five people who are on that line. If the points are switched, the train will go along a different line where there is one person (different from the five) who will be killed. There is no way of stopping the train, but the one thing you can do is to switch the points.

Read about the Trolley problem and its variations (e.g. Fig. 2.1) (Edmonds 2015a,b). Which trolley problem cases are analogous to the cases faced by Dr A and Dr B? How do hypothetical cases like the trolley problems help us consider ethical theory?

ETHICAL THEORIES AND PERSPECTIVES

ETHICAL THEORIES AND PERSPECTIVES

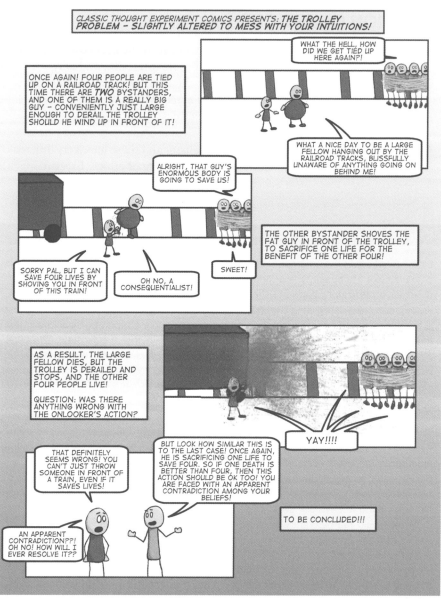

Figure 2.1 Trolley problem cartoon (© Ryan Lake (chaospet.com) with permission)

REFERENCES

Aristotle, R. (Ed.). 2000. *Nicomachean ethics*. Cambridge: Cambridge University Press. Edited by Roger Crisp.

Dresser, R. 1995. "Dworkin on dementia. Elegant theory, questionable policy." *The Hastings Center Report* 25 (6): 32-8.

Dworkin, R. 1993. *Life's dominion: an argument about abortion and euthanasia*. London: HarperCollins.

Edmonds, D. 2015a. "Matters of Life and death." *Prospect Magazine*. https://www.prospectmagazine.co.uk/magazine/ethics-trolley-problem.

Edmonds, D. 2015b. *Would you kill the fat man?: the trolley problem and what your answer tells us about right and wrong*. Princeton: Princeton University Press.

Firlik, A. D. 1991. "A piece of my mind. Margo's logo." *JAMA: The Journal of the American Medical Association* 265 (2): 201.

General Medical Council. 2013. "Good Medical Practice." https://www.gmc-uk.org/ethical-guidance/ethical-guidance-for-doctors/good-medical-practice.

Haidt, J. 2006. *The happiness hypothesis: putting ancient wisdom to the test of modern science*. London: William Heinemann.

Hare, R. M. 1998. *Essays on religion and education*. Oxford: Clarendon.

Hope, T. 1996. "Advance directives." *Journal of Medical Ethics* 22 (2): 67-8.

Hursthouse, R. 1997. "Virtue theory and abortion." In *Virtue ethics*, edited by R. Crisp and M. Slote. Oxford: Oxford University Press.

Kant, I., Hill, T. E. and Zweig, A. 2002. *Groundwork for the metaphysics of morals*. Oxford: Oxford University Press.

Mill, J. S., Bentham, J. and Ryan, A. 1987. *Utilitarianism and other essays*, Harmondsworth, Middlesex, England. New York, NY: Penguin Books.

O'Neill, O. 1993. "Kantian ethics." In *A companion to ethics*, edited by P. Singer. Oxford: Blackwell.

Parfit, D. 1984. *Reasons and persons*. Oxford: Oxford University Press.

Parfit, D. 2011. *On what matters*, vol. 2 vols. Oxford: Oxford University Press.

Rawls, J. 1999. *A theory of justice*, Rev. ed. Oxford: Oxford University Press.

Ross, W. D. and Stratton-Lake, P. 2002. *The right and the good*, New ed. Oxford: Clarendon Press.

Savulescu, J. 2013. "Winchester lectures: Kamm's Trolleyology and is there a morally relevant difference between killing and letting die?". Practical Ethics blog, accessed 26/11/18. http://blog.practicalethics.ox.ac.uk/2013/10/winchester-lectures-kamms-trolleyology-and-is-there-a-morally-relevant-difference-between-killing-and-letting-die/.

Smart, J. J. C. and Williams, B. 1973. *Utilitarianism: for and against*. Cambridge: Cambridge University Press.

Tronto, J. C. 1993. *Moral boundaries: a political argument for an ethic of care*. New York; London: Routledge.

Zwart, H. 1999. "All you need is health: liberal and communitarian views on the allocation of health care resources." In *Ethics and community in the health care profession*, edited by M. Parker. London: Routledge.

FURTHER READING: ETHICAL THEORY

Arras, J. D., Fenton, E. and Kukla, R. 2018. Routledge companion to bioethics.

Ashcroft, R., Draper, H., Dawson, A. and McMillan, J. (Eds.). 2007. *Principles of health care ethics*, 2nd ed. Chichester: John Wiley. *An enormous single-volume collection of specially written chapters covering a wide range of medical ethics explored from many perspectives.*

Ashcroft, R., Lucassen, A., Parker, M., Verkerk, M. and Widdershoven, G. 2010. *Case analysis in clinical ethics*. Cambridge: Cambridge University Press. *A single case from the area of clinical genetics is analysed in detail by 11 authors, each from a different ethical perspective. This book demonstrates how different approaches to medical ethics lead to different analyses.*

Beauchamp, T. L. and Childress, J. F. 2013. *Principles of biomedical ethics*. 7th ed. New York: Oxford University Press. *A well-established, detailed and well-written textbook of medical ethics organized around the four-principle approach.*

British Medical Association Ethics Department, 2012. *Medical ethics today: the BMA's handbook of ethics and law*. 3rd ed. John Wiley and Sons. *More medical in its orientation than most textbooks of medical ethics.*

Dickenson, D., Huxtable, R. and Parker, M. 2010. *The Cambridge medical ethics workbook*. Cambridge: Cambridge University Press. *This provides many cases taken from health care across several European countries, together with in-depth analysis of the cases. A combination of textbook and case book.*

Glover, J. 1977. *Causing death and saving lives*. London: Penguin. *Although this is about end-of-life issues, it is a good introduction to philosophical thinking applied to the medical setting.*

Hope, T. 2004. *Medical ethics: a very short introduction*. Oxford: Oxford University Press. *Intended as an introduction, each chapter makes an argument for a particular ethical position concerning an issue in medical ethics.*

Kerridge, I., Lowe, M. and Stewart, C. 2013. *Ethics and law for the health professions*. 4th ed. Australia: Federation Press. *A good overview of medical ethics and law from an Australian perspective*.

Singer, P. 2011. *Practical ethics*. 3rd ed. New York: Cambridge University Press. *A pithy and readable examination of some of the philosophical issues underpinning medical ethics*.

Steinbock, B. 2009. *The Oxford handbook of bioethics*. Oxford: Oxford University Press.

Chapter **3**

Three core concepts in medical ethics
Best interests, autonomy and rights

Case 3.1

Mohammed has a long-standing psychiatric disorder that has been very difficult to control despite medical treatment. He has spent large parts of his adult life as an involuntary patient in various institutions. When he is psychiatrically unwell, he has elevated mood and is prone to very disinhibited behaviour – frequently exposing himself to passers-by, gambling and consuming alcohol heavily.

In recent years, Mohammed has finally been able to be stabilized on a combination of medications. He has been able to live for some time in supported accommodation without relapse. He attends the local mosque regularly and is deeply devout.

However, during a checkup, Mohammed is discovered to have developed a serious medical complication of his anti-psychotic treatment. This complication is associated with medical risk, which might even be life-threatening. However, there is a high risk that, if Mohammed's medication is reduced or stopped, he may have a relapse of his psychiatric illness that could be very difficult to control.

When asked about the situation, and what his wishes are, Mohammed replies only 'Inshallah' (if Allah wills).

What would be in Mohammed's best interests?

BEST INTERESTS

One of the central ideas of medicine is that doctors or health professionals should help patients – they should benefit them if they can. This is captured in the ethical principle of *beneficence*, and in the notion that doctors should act in patients' *best interests*. The most basic principle of medical ethics is that doctors should offer treatments which are in the best interests of their patients.

For much of medical history, the concept of best interests was equated with medical interests: the treatment and prevention of disease. Effective medical interventions were few. For example, penicillin would be prescribed for a life-threatening streptococcal infection. Patients and doctors broadly agreed about the goals of medical treatment.

But medicine has changed much in the last 50 years. There is an ever-growing panoply of medical interventions with different probabilities of effects on the length and quality of life. New cancer drugs are perhaps the best example, but the age of precision medicine heralds treatment with specific risks and benefits to individual patients. Moreover, the concept of best interests has broadened to reflect the WHO definition of health: 'a state of complete physical, mental and social well-being and not merely the absence of disease or infirmity'.

The concept of best interests forms the core of the doctor–patient relationship (see Chapter 5) and is the legal standard for the treatment of patients who lack the capacity to take part in their own medical decisions (see Chapter 7). However, if you ask people to define what it means to act in a patient's best interests, many will struggle. That is partly because, to work out what course of action would be best for the patient, we need to answer a question that has taxed thinkers for hundreds, if not thousands, of years: what is a good life, and what makes life go well (or badly)? Thinking about Mohammed's situation, it is not clear what would be best for him.

We will start by contrasting some of the different ways that philosophers have tried to answer that question. We will then describe the approach of psychologists and health economists. Finally, we will mention the approach of the law to that question.

The philosophical approach to best interests

In the last chapter, we described three different forms of utilitarianism – hedonic, preference and objective. These are based on three different theories about well-being (what makes life go well). If you are a utilitarian, it is clearly crucial to decide which of these theories is right. However, even for non-utilitarians, it is important to think about well-being. For example, it could determine what we believe would be in Mohammed's best interests.

Mental state theory

According to mental state theories, well-being is solely determined by mental states. At its simplest (hedonism), it is simply a question of the balance between happiness or pleasure and unhappiness or pain. The theory can be enriched and made more complicated by incorporating other states of mind (though this raises the problem of determining which these should be).

For Mohammed, according to the mental state theory, it could be better for him to stop or change his medication, even if that would make him psychiatrically very unstable. Some patients with elevated mood are much happier when they are off treatment. Mohammed might have many more (and more intense) positive mental states if his drugs were stopped. Even if he ended up institutionalized for a long period, that might be better for him from a mental state point of view, particularly if he would live longer.

Objections to mental state theories

1. There are some things that seem to make our lives go well or badly that are not mental states or experiences. For example, imagine if your life-long partner were secretly unfaithful to you, and you never knew. Many might think that this would be bad for you, because it would make your life go worse, even if it did not affect your mental state at all.

2. In 1974 (two decades before this idea was memorably depicted in the film 'The Matrix'), the philosopher Robert Nozick asked us to imagine a virtual reality machine (the 'experience machine') that could provide any set of subjective experiences, including the experience (but not the actuality) of 'writing a great novel, or making a friend, or reading an interesting book. All the time you would be floating in a tank, with electrodes attached to your brain' (Fig. 3.1). Even if you could pick those mental states that we most want, few of us, Nozick believed, would choose to live our life connected to such a machine. This is because we also want to *do* certain things, and we want to *be* a certain way, to be a certain sort of person. (Nozick 1974)

Desire fulfilment theories

According to the next theory, what makes someone's life go well is to have their desires fulfilled. (This is clearly related to the importance of patient *autonomy* – but not exactly the same. See below.) We do often think that it is good for a person if they are able to have the things they want. However, that isn't always the case ('...when the gods wish to punish us they answer our prayers') (Wilde and Bollinger 2012); some modification to the theory may be needed to either limit it to 'rational desires' or to those desires that relate to life as a whole.

In Mohammed's case, it is possible that he would be happier if he went off his anti-psychotic medication. However, it also seems that his behaviour when unwell would be contrary to deeply held views that he holds when more stable. For example, he has strong religious beliefs and a desire to act in accordance with those, e.g. not to drink alcohol or expose his genitals to strangers. It seems that his life would be going very badly when he is mentally ill, not because he is unhappy, but rather because some long-held desires that are important to him are being frustrated.

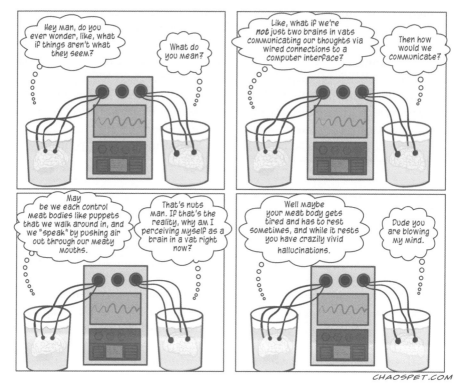

Figure 3.1 Brains in a vat (© Ryan Lake (chaospet.com) with permission)

Objections to desire fulfilment theories

Suppose that I desire something – a particular thing, or an entire 'life plan'. It seems quite reasonable to ask the question, 'Is that something good for me?'. There could be a conflict between what a person most desires and what is good for that person. Imagine, for example, that Mohammed, even when he is well, has a desire to gamble. He might feel, and others might feel, that it would not be good for him to satisfy this desire. If we have such a response, that suggests that there is more to well-being than fulfilling desires.

This is the central question of Plato's dialogue with Euthyphro. Socrates asks Euthyphro, 'Is the pious loved by the gods because it is pious, or is it pious because it is loved by the gods?'. In ordinary life, it is important to not only ask: what do I desire? But also, what *should* I desire?

Objective list theories

According to objective list theories of well-being, certain things can be good or bad for a person and can contribute to her well-being, whether or not they are desired and whether or not they lead to a 'pleasurable' mental state. Examples of the kinds of things that are considered intrinsically good in this way are friendship, significant achievement, important knowledge and autonomy (Hooker 2015). Examples of things that are bad might include being betrayed or deceived, or gaining pleasure from cruelty. Philosophers who have drawn on such theories have sometimes referred to the idea of 'flourishing' (rather than purely 'happiness').

As an example, in Mohammed's case, one way that his life could be going very badly if he became psychiatrically unwell is through the loss of his freedom. It seems that it would be bad for him to become an involuntary patient confined to a psychiatric institution (this might be the case even if he did not have a desire to be more free).

Objections to objective list theories

1. A major problem with objective list theories is that it is difficult to give an account of why one thing is good, and thus contributes to well-being, whereas another thing is bad. How do we work out what should be on the list?
2. If there are multiple different elements that contribute to well-being, it becomes more difficult to know how to combine them. Are they equally important? How should we weigh up different elements on the list?

Composite theories

Each of the three theories of well-being seems to identify something of importance, but none seems to present the full picture. Because of this, we might opt for a composite theory: what is good for a person is objectively valuable activity which the person desires and which makes her happy. This has some practical implications for medical practice. The main implication is that, when considering what is in a patient's best interests, and particularly when these are not clear, we should consider the different aspects of well-being that are highlighted by each of the three theories.

We have mentioned some of the different aspects of well-being that are relevant to Mohammed's case. It is difficult to know what would be best. That is partly related to the medical uncertainty. However, even if we knew for certain what would happen, it might still be very difficult to know what would be in his best interests. Imagine, for example, that the choice is between 2 years of life with mental health (life much as Mohammed has lived in recent times), or 10 years of life with major psychiatric instability – much of it as an involuntary patient. Which of those would be best? That is very difficult to answer. This difficulty in working out what would be in someone's best interests is one reason why the patient's wishes are so important. We will return to those shortly.

Psychologists' approach to measuring well-being

Can science help answer questions about best interests? Would it be possible to scientifically determine whether one medical treatment or another led to greater happiness or flourishing?

The psychological study of human happiness and flourishing has burgeoned in recent years under the broad term of 'positive psychology' (Tiberius 2006). This scientific study has required psychologists (and economists) to develop methods for the measurement of well-being. There are three fundamentally different concepts that psychologists measure. These have some overlap with (but are also somewhat different from) the philosophical theories that we outlined above.

Quantitative hedonism – the 'smiley' approach

Some psychologists (see Kahneman and Riis 2005) identify the basic unit of happiness as *moment utility* (happiness at each particular moment in time). People are asked to give a measure of how happy they feel at a particular moment (for example on a rating scale using smiley faces). Over any particular period of time, total happiness is simply the sum of these *moment utilities*. Kahneman calls this *experienced well-being*.

It is difficult to measure happiness in this way because it requires rather frequent measurements. To overcome this technical problem, you could ask people to give a single average measure over a period of time (e.g. over the previous 24 hours). In practice, however, when people are asked to do this they do not remember (and add up) the *moment utilities*; rather they evaluate, or make a judgement about, their overall well-being – what Kahneman calls *evaluated well-being*. These evaluations can be strange, even illogical. In a famous experiment, Kahneman asked participants to dip their hands in painfully cold water. Participants reported that 60 seconds in very cold water was worse than 60 seconds in identically cold water followed by 30 seconds in still painful (but slightly warmer) water. However, that seems truly illogical! This is an example of what has been called the 'peak-end rule': when evaluating a painful past experience, people are influenced by how bad it was at its worst, and by the level of pain at the end of the experience. Because of this paradox, some have thought that measures of *evaluated well-being* are simply flawed measures of *experienced well-being*.

Life satisfaction and evaluated well-being

However, we might be more interested in how happy people are with their lives overall than simply the sum of pleasurable or painful moments.

Psychologists have measured how satisfied people are with their lives. In answering that question, people express an emotional response to thinking about their life. The literature on life satisfaction has yielded results that might seem surprising to some. Individuals with significant disabilities often express levels of life satisfaction that are similar to non-disabled people. This finding has been referred to as the 'disability paradox' (Albrecht and Devlieger 1999). For example, in a study of patients who had experienced spinal cord injury, motor function did not predict life satisfaction (Hartoonian et al. 2014). A survey of patients with locked-in syndrome found that three quarters reported being happy overall (Bruno et al. 2011).

One potential explanation for some of these findings is *hedonic adaptation*. This is the idea that people's happiness levels tend to be stable over time. After major life events, their level of happiness or life satisfaction will change acutely – but then often return to the baseline level that is normal for them.

A different form of life evaluation asks people to compare their life with others. Psychologists ask people to rank their lives on a scale from the best to the worst possible lives. This tends to yield seemingly objective evaluations of people's material circumstances.

Flourishing

Psychologists who (influenced by Aristotle) are drawn to an 'objective list' approach to the measurement of well-being have sometimes tried to measure elements of flourishing. One example of a scale for measuring well-being based on this approach is that of Ryff (Ryff and Keyes 1995). People may be asked whether they consider their lives to be worthwhile, or to have meaning.

How do these different psychological instruments for measuring well-being interact? They can give contradictory answers (in much the same way that the philosophical theories gave contrasting answers for Mohammed). For example, studies suggest that people who are unemployed have lower levels of evaluated well-being (they report lower life satisfaction), but their actual experienced (hedonic) happiness seems similar to people who are employed (Dolan, Kudrna, and Stone 2017). A very large survey from the US indicated that those who found their life meaningful reported higher levels of happiness (but not necessarily lower levels of stress, tiredness, sadness or pain) (Dolan, Kudrna, and Stone 2017). It isn't clear how to interpret this complicated psychological picture of the different measurable elements of well-being. Like the philosophical version, we might think that some combination of different elements is necessary to get a full picture of well-being.

Paternalism

With the above complex picture of assessing best interests, it might be obvious why there would be something wrong with paternalism. 'Paternalism' refers to a decision that is made for the sake of someone's best interests, against their will. As we will discuss in more detail in Chapter 5, the doctor–patient relationship used to be strongly paternalistic. However, the challenge of determining what would be best for someone provides a good reason for doctors to be cautious before assuming that they know best.

There are some useful distinctions that are often made between different types of paternalism. 'Soft' or 'weak' paternalism refers to situations where a patient's capacity and understanding of a situation are not known. An emergency physician would potentially be justified in intervening urgently on behalf of patient who appears to be behaving erratically and posing a risk to himself. It may not be possible to assess acutely if the patient has capacity. The physician might call security to restrain the patient, or even sedate them until further assessment is possible. Such an intervention would be paternalism, but only soft paternalism. In contrast, 'hard' or 'strong' paternalism refers to situations where a patient's wishes are ignored even though they are known to have the relevant facts and to have capacity. If the erratic patient had just been assessed by a psychiatrist to have capacity, and the emergency physician nevertheless decided to sedate the patient in his best interests, that would be hard paternalism.

The legal approach to best interests

Doctors have a general duty to treat patients in their best interests, although a patient who has capacity (to give or withhold consent) can refuse the treatment offered (see Chapter 6).

The concept of best interests becomes a crucial consideration when patients lack capacity. For patients who are aged 16 years and over, this is governed by the Mental Capacity Act 2005 (MCA) which provides detailed guidance (Box 3.1). For children, this is set out in the Children Act (1989).

How does the law view the above philosophical/psychological debates? The legal concept of best interests is centred primarily around respecting and promoting patient autonomy (see below) – the best interests of a patient who lacks capacity is to do what that patient would choose if he or she were to (magically) gain capacity. In terms of the theories of well-being described above, the legal concept of best interests is closely allied to the 'desire fulfilment theory'. When it comes

---

Box 3.1 Patient's best interests

The Mental Capacity Act 2005 (MCA)

Section four (s.4) of the MCA states how a person's best interests are to be determined, and there is further detailed guidance in the Code of Practice that supplements the Act. The intention behind s.4 is to set out the common factors that must always be taken into account by anyone (e.g. a doctor) who needs to decide what is in the best interests of another person (e.g. a patient) who lacks capacity. Some of the most important points are:

s.4(1): the principle of equal consideration, i.e. no-one should assume a person cannot make a decision just because of their age, disability or how they look. (Note, however, that the Act applies only to patients aged 16 years and over.)

s.4(3): the duty to consider whether the person is likely to regain capacity to make the decision in question; and if so, to put off the decision until then.

s.4(4): permitting and encouraging participation, i.e. ensure that the person is involved in the decision-making process to the fullest possible extent.

One of the section's key provisions is s.4(6), which requires decisions-makers (e.g. doctors) to take into account the following specific factors when deciding what is in a person's best interests. These are:

1. his past and present wishes and feelings (including any written statements)
2. his beliefs and values that would be likely to influence his decisions
3. other factors that the patient would be likely to consider, were he able to do so (e.g. altruistic motives).

Also worth noting is s.4(7), which establishes the right for family members, partners, carers and other relevant people to be consulted on decisions affecting a person who lacks capacity. The primary purpose in consulting relatives is to obtain evidence about the patient's wishes concerning the above three issues (see also Chapter 6).

The Children Act (1989) includes a **Welfare checklist** (see Chapter 11, Box 11.2). This was designed with custody decisions in mind, but has been applied to medical decisions. It includes the child's wishes, but also includes physical, emotional and educational needs; harm or suffering they have experienced; and the effect of any change in circumstances.

to individuals who have never been able to indicate their wishes or express desires (for example, very young children), courts have sometimes struggled to articulate what concept of well-being they are drawing on. Is it just a question of pleasure versus pain, or are there objective interests to be considered? For further discussion of some of the challenges of determining the best interests of children, see Wilkinson and Savulescu (2018). Some have also criticized the overly individualistic legal interpretation of best interests and welfare, arguing that these should be taken as concepts which recognize the importance of relational interests, the performance of obligations and the virtue of altruism (Herring and Foster 2012).

AUTONOMY

The above discussion makes clear that it is sometimes very difficult to know what would be in someone's best interests. Most of the time in medicine, however, doctors do not need to answer that question because there is another ethical principle which takes precedence. The principle of respect for patient autonomy (see Chapter 1) has had an enormous effect in changing attitudes to the doctor–patient relationship over the past 30 years. It has been used to criticize medical paternalism, and has informed the development of 'patient-centred' medicine. It has led to ever-increasing standards in providing patients with information, and to the development of the concept of *informed consent* (see Chapter 6). Some definitions of autonomy are given in Box 3.2.

There are two different reasons for respecting patient autonomy. One reason is that knowing the patient's wishes can be helpful in working out what would be best for them. In Mohammed's case, he isn't able to articulate a clear preference for either continuing or stopping his current anti-psychotic medication. That makes it more challenging. However, it might be possible, from discussion with Mohammed or with those close to him, to work out, for example, how much he values his physical health compared with his mental health, how important his religious beliefs are and how much he values physical liberty. Respecting Mohammed's preferences will help his medical team to act in his best interests.

Box 3.2 Some philosophical explanations, or definitions, of autonomy

1. 'I am autonomous if I rule me, and no one else rules I' (Joel Feinberg, quoted in Dworkin 1988, p. 5).
2. 'To regard himself as autonomous … a person must see himself as sovereign in deciding what to believe and in weighing competing reasons for action' (Scanlon T, in Dworkin 1988, p. 5).
3. 'It is apparent that …"autonomy" is used in an exceedingly broad fashion. It is sometimes used as an equivalent of liberty …, sometimes as equivalent to self-rule or sovereignty, sometimes as identical with freedom of the will … It is identified with qualities of self-assertion, with critical reflection, with freedom from obligation, with absence of external causation, with knowledge of one's own interests … It is related to actions, to beliefs, to reasons for acting, to rules, to the will of other persons, to thoughts and to principles' (Dworkin 1988, p. 6).

The second reason to respect patient autonomy is because of the value placed on individual freedom. This might be expressed in terms of a right to make medical decisions. If we value autonomy in this way, that will sometimes *conflict* with a patient's best interests. We know that people do not always make wise or prudent decisions. Sometimes people are not the best judge of what would be good for them. Nevertheless, it may still be important to respect their choices.

Liberty and freedom

The liberal tradition has placed great emphasis on the moral and political importance of freedom for the individual and, in particular, freedom from the interference of others. This has been expressed by Isaiah Berlin as follows:

> … those who have ever valued liberty for its own sake believed that to be free to choose, and not to be chosen for, is an inalienable ingredient in what makes human beings human. (Berlin 2002)

This freedom includes freedom from unwanted interference, even if the interference is for the good of the person who suffers it. Mill, writing in 1859, argued against paternalism, and in favour of liberty. He wrote:

> … the only purpose for which power can be rightfully exercised over any member of a civilised community, against his will, is to prevent harm to others. His own good, either physical or moral, is not a sufficient warrant. (Mill 2011)

In modern medicine this freedom from unwanted interference is protected by the law relating to consent (see Chapter 6). A competent adult patient has the legal right to refuse any – even life-saving – treatment. On those occasions when a competent adult patient is refusing treatment that is, objectively, good for her, a conflict arises between respecting the patient's wishes and doing what is best for the patient. This is widely seen as a conflict between the principle of respect for patient autonomy and the principle of beneficence (see Chapter 1).

However, 'respecting autonomy' does not necessarily just mean doing what the patient wants. Occasionally respecting what a patient says (e.g. her refusal of treatment) and respecting her autonomy will be in conflict.

Some aspects of autonomy

What conditions need to be met for a person's decisions and actions to be autonomous, i.e. truly their own? It is important to separate out autonomy as an *ideal* from the minimum level required for decisions to count as autonomous. (The minimum level of autonomy – especially the need for rational evaluation – forms the philosophical foundation for 'capacity', as discussed in Chapter 7.) Three aspects of autonomy have been the focus of recent analysis:

1. *To be autonomous one must make evaluations.* The ideal of the autonomous person is the person who forms overarching desires for how her life is to go (life plans) and can act on those desires (Young 1985). To create such a life

plan, we need to make evaluations about the kind of life we should live, or that might be best for us. Someone who makes spur-of-the-moment, impulsive decisions without a clear idea about what is important to them, or what sort of life they wish to lead, would not be autonomous according to this view.

2. *Evaluations should be rational.* If a desire or choice is not based on a rational evaluation, then it is not autonomous. There are three key components of an autonomous evaluation:
   - It is based on a correct understanding of the relevant facts.
   - The facts are evaluated without making a relevant error of logic.
   - The person has been able to imagine what the relevant states of affairs will be like, i.e. the likely states of affairs for the various choice options.

3. *Higher order desires should be respected.* A person may have conflicting desires. For example, Mohammed may simultaneously desire to gamble and at the same time wish that he did not have the desire to gamble. The desire to gamble is a 'first-order' desire, and the wish not to desire gambling is a 'second-order' desire. Some (e.g. Dworkin 1988) have argued that respecting autonomy implies respecting the higher (second-order) desire, on the grounds that this higher desire is the one that is part of the life plan.

What should we do if someone asks for something that doesn't seem fully autonomous in the above senses? Many political liberals, such as Berlin (2002), generally favour respecting what a person says. It is too easy and dangerous, they believe, for a repressive political regime, or for powerful people, to impose their will on the grounds that their will coincides with what the other person really wants, despite his saying to the contrary.

In medicine, if a patient has capacity, their wishes should be respected, even if their desires are not fully autonomous. However, that does not mean that the doctor must simply accept what the patient says. Physicians should engage with the patient, attempt to understand his or her values and higher order desires, and, where a choice appears to conflict with these, attempt to persuade the patient to revise their decision (Savulescu 1995). Doctors should engage patients in a dialogue mirroring reflective equilibrium, in which they together try to decide what is best for this patient in this circumstance at this time. Crucially this will sometimes require that the doctor revise their own conception of what is best for the patient (Savulescu 1997).

Changing decisions and autonomy

In some situations, patients' views may fluctuate.

Case 3.2

Julia is pregnant with her first child. She has been reading extensively about child-birth and wishes to have a natural labour and delivery. She writes a birth plan indicating that she does not wish to have an epidural or nitrous oxide, and wishes to do everything possible to facilitate a vaginal delivery rather than a caesarean section.

However, Julia has prolonged second stage of labour, and, after many hours of labour, exhausted, she asks for an epidural.

There are two different interpretations of autonomy in the face of shifting preferences like Julia's. On the one hand, the desire for analgesia while experiencing the pain of labour might not be viewed as Julia's autonomous desire – it conflicts with her higher order desire not to seek pain relief. On the other hand, Julia's desire to avoid analgesia, when not in labour, might not properly take into account just how bad the pain will be. According to this second interpretation, her prior evaluation was not fully rational because it was based on insufficient imagination of her future state of affairs.

When faced with situations where patients' desires fluctuate, doctors need to decide what, given the patient's general values, is most important overall. In the case of pain during labour, where the analgesia poses little risk to the mother or fetus, ethical reflection is likely to be in favour of analgesia at the time when the mother asks for it. In general, patients' current desires should be respected, unless the patient lacks capacity.

Can one autonomously choose to delegate choice?

Case 3.3

Arnold is 84 and is living independently, though increasingly frail. During a routine checkup he is found to have a large (asymptomatic) abdominal aortic aneurysm. Arnold is referred to a surgeon, Ms S, who advises him that surgery would be possible, but associated with a high risk of complications. Ms S asks Arnold for his views about surgery. Arnold tells the surgeon to 'do what she thinks best'.

In his essay *On Liberty*, Mill (2011) considered whether a liberal society should allow people to sell themselves into slavery. He concluded that this would be contrary to the idea of liberty – a decision to relinquish future freedom could not be autonomous. What would this mean for situations like Arnold's, where a patient appears to be autonomously relinquishing their decisions?

The answer depends on why the patient has chosen to delegate choices. Imagine if Arnold has always been happy passively doing as others do, letting his friends and family decide for him. If Arnold has never deliberately chosen to lead such a life (perhaps in his family and his work he was never given the option to choose for himself), then such a life would not be autonomous. On the other hand, a patient who asks the doctor to choose for him may be acting autonomously if he has good reasons: he trusts the doctor's judgement; finds making choices about his own health difficult; and believes that the doctor's experience about how patients react to different situations is likely to predict his own responses correctly. In general, people should actively make decisions for themselves about their care, though they should take advice and support from doctors, family and others as appropriate.

Relational autonomy

While the notion of individual autonomy has taken a central place in western medical ethics, there are some, less individualistic, concepts of autonomy that

Case 3.4

In a busy outpatient clinic, Dr N is about to meet an elderly patient, Mr Z, who was diagnosed recently with a gastrointestinal malignancy. As Dr N is about to meet the patient, his family gives Dr N a piece of paper that reads 'Please do not tell our father the diagnosis'. When Dr N asks the family about the reason for this request, they explain that they fear that he will take the news badly, and that he will 'give up'.

What should Dr N do?

are favoured by other approaches to ethics. For example, 'relational autonomy' often features in feminist ethics, and emphasizes the social context of individuals and the relationships that are crucial to the person's sense of self and the decisions that they make. Some non-Western approaches to ethics similarly place much greater role on the family in decision-making (e.g. Confucian ethics).

Relational autonomy might be one justification for the family's request in Case 3.4 (though the family would be unlikely to use the term!). Some cultures place much weight on the importance of the patient's individual autonomy, and much more on the family. However, that can create conflicts for the doctor in situations like Case 3.4, where the doctor feels torn between their obligations to the patient and their duty to respect cultural values and the family's (potentially accurate) assessment of what would be best for the patient (McCabe, Wood, and Goldberg 2010). (In other cases, families' concerns relate to particular stigma associated with cancer, or a false belief that communicating the news of a terminal diagnosis will accelerate the death of the patient.)

One approach to the situation in Case 3.4 would be for Dr N to try to assess Mr Z's desire for information about his health. For example, Dr N could say something like this:

'I'm interested in knowing about your views on sharing health information. Some of my patients would like to be given health information on their own. Then they can decide how much they would like to share with their family. Other patients would like their family to be present when they get health information from their doctor. Then the family will know the same things as the patient. Still other patients would like the doctor to give their family all of the health information, and then the family decides how much to pass on to the patient. What do you think about this? Does one of these match your view about how you would like health information to be shared?'

RIGHTS

A competent adult patient has a *right* to refuse any treatment. We could say that a patient has a *right* to the best available treatment. Doctors, too, have rights. It is often claimed that a doctor – an obstetrician, for example – has a right to refuse to carry out a termination of pregnancy on grounds of conscientious objection, although there are varying views about the nature and extent of this right. (We will return to questions about conscientious objection in Chapter 5.) In wider society, claims about rights are frequently made. We hear of animal rights and the rights of the disabled.

We talk of both legal rights and moral rights. The two are often linked, in that a moral right forms the basis for a legal right. The Universal Declaration of Human Rights, for example, seeks to establish moral rights that can then be enforced through legal process involving the Court of Human Rights. These moral rights also form the basis for the Human Rights Act (see Chapter 4).

What are rights?

Rights impose moral (and legal) constraints on collective social goals. If a person has a right, it provides a safeguard so that his or her right is respected even if the overall social good is thereby diminished. Sumner (2000) explains that there is a part of our moral thinking concerned with the promotion of collective social goals. Such thinking is particularly evident in consequentialist moral theories such as utilitarianism, but is also found in duty-based approaches to morality. For example, we may have a duty to bring about some social good. In health care, we may consider that bringing about the best health, either for an individual patient or in the setting of public health (see Chapter 20), is a major ethical duty. However, that ethical duty may be trumped by the moral requirement to respect an individual's rights. For example, an individual's right to refuse treatment might trump the doctor's duty to treat in the best interests of the patient. Similarly, we might believe that there are circumstances when a person has a right to treatment. Someone injured in a road accident, for example, might be considered to have a right to treatment even if the resources needed could be better spent in terms of social goals.

Rights have been politically important in protecting minority groups and those who might be the victims of more powerful groups. In employment law, for example, they help to ensure that certain groups cannot be unfairly discriminated against.

Types of rights

There are several types of right that are sometimes distinguished (Box 3.3).

Are rights absolute?

Rights need not be absolute. One could say that any particular right has a certain strength. This is the degree to which it stands up to other ethical claims. Thus, if a right had no strength in the light of consequentialist moral claims, it would become redundant, and the ethical theory would be purely consequentialist. If, on the other hand, a right had infinite strength, it would mean that the right was absolute. In Sumner's words (2000): 'rights raise thresholds against considerations of social utility but these thresholds are seldom insurmountable', i.e. the rights are seldom absolute. Rights might clash not only with some ethical theory, but also with other rights. Even the most ardent supporter of rights would not be able to claim that two rights were absolute if there were possible situations in which they could come into conflict.

Box 3.3 Types of right

Claim rights

The subject of the right has a claim against another person or people (who are the object of the right). A patient may have a claim right arising from the doctor's duty of care; for example, the patient may be able to claim a certain level of medical care. Contracts normally establish certain claim rights. If I have entered into a contract to sell my house to another for a certain price, then I may have a right to claim the money agreed. Outside the legal sphere, claim rights may arise from a promise. If I have promised to lend you a book, then you have a moral claim against me for the loan of that book.

Liberty rights

Liberty rights give rights of action to the subject rather than the object of the right. The law may give to someone a liberty, or privilege, for example, to seek private medical insurance. Liberties are generally protected by what has been called a 'protective perimeter' of duties imposed on others not to frustrate those liberties. These others are the objects of the right. Property rights usually confer liberty rights (for example the liberty right to use the things you own).

Powers

Many rights provide people with powers to do things. A claim right usually gives the person who holds the right the power to waive the claim, and a property right would include the power to give the property to another.

Immunities

Liberty rights normally give people immunities; that is, they give to the right holder a protection from certain actions of others. My liberty to belong to a political party provides me with immunity from my employer seeking to forbid this.

REVISION QUESTIONS

1. What is paternalism? Is it ever justified for doctors to be paternalistic?
2. What is the disability paradox? How is it relevant to thinking about a patient's best interests?
3. Jeremy Bentham, one of the founders of utilitarianism, rejected the idea of natural rights. He claimed that rights were 'the fruits of the law, and of the law alone. There are no rights without law—no rights contrary to the law—no rights anterior to the law'. Do you agree?
4. A Jehovah's Witness patient, Joshua, has signed an advance directive indicating that he does not want to receive blood products in any circumstances, even if that would lead to him dying. However, two years later Joshua suffers major trauma with life-threatening haemorrhage. In the emergency room, one of the nurses explains to Joshua that he has suffered major bleeding and that he might need a blood transfusion. Joshua indicates that he wishes to receive blood if he needs it; however, shortly after, he loses consciousness. What should the medical team do in this case? Explain the relevance of different theories of best interests and autonomy.

THREE CORE CONCEPTS IN MEDICAL ETHICS

A. Pathologists in a major research institute have retained a heart specimen from a child who died some years ago. The specimen has been kept in formalin and used for teaching doctors.

It transpires that the heart was obtained at post-mortem, but permission from the child's parents was never sought to keep the heart.

B. Medical students in an anatomy class dissect the cadavers of patients who have donated their bodies to science.

Students are told by their tutors to treat the bodies with 'dignity'; however, one student takes a photo of another student posing 'thumbs up' next to one of the cadavers.

What do you understand by human dignity? How is it relevant to these cases?

Some bioethicists claim that dignity is too vague to be useful, and is reducible to respect for patient autonomy or to rights. What do you think?

For further analysis of dignity, read Foster (2011, 2014), Macklin (2003), and Killmister (2010).

REFERENCES

Albrecht, G. L. and Devlieger, P. J. 1999. "The disability paradox: high quality of life against all odds." *Social Science and Medicine* 48 (8): 977-88.

Berlin, I., Four essays on liberty Berlin. 2002. *Liberty: incorporating Four essays on liberty*. Oxford: Oxford University Press.

Bruno, M. A., Bernheim, J. L., Ledoux, D., Pellas, F., Demertzi, A. and Laureys, S. 2011. "A survey on self-assessed well-being in a cohort of chronic locked-in syndrome patients: happy majority, miserable minority." *BMJ Open* 1 (1): e000039. doi: 10.1136/bmjopen-2010 -000039.

Dolan, P., Kudrna, L. and Stone, A. 2017. "The measure matters: an investigation of evaluative and experience-based measures of well-being in time use data." *Social Indicators Research* 134 (1): 57-73. doi: 10.1007/s11205-016-1429-8.

Dworkin, G. 1988. *The theory and practice of autonomy*. Cambridge: Cambridge University Press.

Foster, C. 2011. *Human dignity in bioethics and law*. Oxford: Hart.

Foster, C. 2014. "Dignity and the use of body parts." *Journal of Medical Ethics* 40 (1): 44-7. doi: 10.1136/medethics-2012-100763.

Hartoonian, N., Hoffman, J. M., Kalpakjian, C. Z., Taylor, H. B., Krause, J. K. and Bombardier, C. H. 2014. "Evaluating a spinal cord injury-specific model of depression and quality of life." *Archives of Physical Medicine and Rehabilitation* 95 (3): 455-65. doi: 10.1016/j.apmr.2013.10.029.

Herring, J. and Foster, C. 2012. "Welfare means relationality, virtue and altruism." *Legal Studies* 32 (3): 480-98. doi: 10.1111/j.1748 -121X.2012.00232.x.

Hooker, B. 2015. "The elements of wellbeing." *Journal of Practical Ethics* 3 (1): 15-35.

Kahneman, D. and Riis, J. 2005. "Living and thinking about it: two perspectives on life." In *The science of well-being*, edited by F. A. Huppert, N. Baylis and B. Keverne. Oxford: Oxford University Press.

Killmister, S. 2010. "Dignity: not such a useless concept." *Journal of Medical Ethics* 36 (3): 160-4. doi: 10.1136/jme.2009.031393.

Macklin, R. 2003. "Dignity is a useless concept." *BMJ* 327 (7429): 1419-20. doi: 10.1136/bmj.327.7429.1419.

McCabe, M. S., Wood, W. A. and Goldberg, R. M. 2010. "When the family requests withholding the diagnosis: who owns the truth?" *Journal of Oncology Practice* 6 (2): 94-6. doi: 10.1200/JOP.091086.

Mill, J. S. 2011. *On liberty*. Luton: Andrews UK Limited.

Nozick, R. 1974. *Anarchy, state, and utopia*. Oxford: Blackwell.

Ryff, C. D. and Keyes, C. L. 1995. "The structure of psychological well-being revisited." *Journal of Personality and Social Psychology* 69 (4): 719-27.

Savulescu, J. 1995. "Rational non-interventional paternalism: why doctors ought to make judgments of what is best for their patients." *Journal of Medical Ethics* 21 (6): 327-31.

Savulescu, J. 1997. "Liberal rationalism and medical decision-making." *Bioethics* 11 (2): 115-29. doi: 10.1111/1467-8519.00049.

Sumner, L. W. 2000. "Rights." In *The Blackwell guide to ethical theory*, edited by H. LaFollette. Oxford: Blackwell.

Tiberius, V. 2006. "Wellbeing: psychological research for philosophers." *Philosophy Compass* 1 (5): 493-505, doi: https://doi.org/10.1111/j.1747-9991.2006.00038.x.

Wilde, O. and Bollinger, M. 2012. *An ideal husband*. London: Sovereign.

Wilkinson, D. and Savulescu, J. 2018. *Ethics, conflict and medical treatment for children: from disagreement to dissensus*. Elsevier.

Young, R. 1985. *Personal autonomy: beyond negative and positive liberty*. London: Croom Helm.

Chapter **4**

An introduction to law

Case 4.1

Six men were having cancer treatment which was liable to render them infertile. They had their sperm frozen and stored by the hospital. However, the hospital freezer malfunctioned (the liquid nitrogen supply had not been topped up), and the men's sperm was destroyed.

They brought a legal action against the hospital. But what law could apply to the case?

Was there a relevant statute? While the Human Fertilisation and Embryology Act 1990 did regulate the storage of sperm, it did not give a right to damages for someone whose sperm was destroyed inappropriately. So that argument was not pursued in court.

Could the hospital be sued for negligence? For a medical negligence claim, the patient must have suffered an injury because of the negligence. The court considered whether the men could claim to have suffered a personal injury. They could not find any previous cases which said that harm to bodily material separated from the body could count. The court considered extending the common law to say so, but thought that would create too much uncertainty.

Continued

59

Did the men have a property right in their stored sperm? The court considered whether a claim under bailment was possible (in short, that a person looking after someone else's property had damaged it). The court looked at the traditional common law rule that a body could not be owned, but also the fact that, in several cases, the courts had acknowledged that there could be exceptions to this rule, particularly in relation to separated body parts. Although none of those cases had specifically covered the kind of case the court was looking at, the court found that the men's sperm could be considered to be their property, and consequently that they could claim for damage to it. (This is the case of *Yearworth v North Bristol NHS Trust [2009]*.)

England and Wales share a legal system; Scotland's system is different both in having a different structure of courts (see below) and in having its own parliament. Some statutes (see below) apply only to England and Wales, and others only to Scotland. The Welsh Assembly now has authority to pass legislation in some areas that will impact only Wales. They have done this in relation to organ donation (see Chapter 15). However, unless there is specific Welsh legislation, the law is the same in England and Wales. The same is not true for Scotland. Scottish courts are not generally bound by English court decisions. For these reasons, there are differences between Scottish law and the law in England and Wales, and some of these differences have an impact on medical law. Northern Ireland has a separate system again, with its own appeal court. For the most part, this book describes law that applies to England and Wales. We have, however, attempted to outline the approach taken by Scottish law when this differs significantly from English law in its application to medical practice.

There are two principal sources of law. The most obvious is when a law is passed by Parliament. Such laws are called *Acts of Parliament* or *statutes.* Parliament typically passes about 50 statutes each year. The courts are commonly called upon to interpret the legislation. This means it is often necessary to read not only the Act itself, but also the interpretation of that Act by the courts, in order to fully understand the law. Much English law, however, has not originated from Acts of Parliament, but has been built up on the basis of court decisions over the past nine centuries developing general legal principles (common law).

THE MAIN TYPES OF LAW

One way of dividing the law is into *common (or case) law* on the one hand and *statute law* on the other. The crime of theft is defined by the Theft Act 1968, and is therefore part of statute law. Murder, on the other hand, is a common law crime, as there is no statutory definition.

Another, and quite different, division is between *public law* and *private law* (also called *civil law*) (Box 4.1). Both public law and private law are made up of both statute law and case law. Public law involves the state or government; private law is concerned with disputes between private individuals and businesses. A significant part of public law (see Box 4.1) is criminal law. Thus, the division

Box 4.1 Public law and private law

Types of public law

1. *Criminal law.* This determines the kinds of behaviour that are forbidden (by the State), at risk of punishment. It is normally the State that prosecutes the person who is thought to have committed the crime, and not the victim(s) of the crime. The victim(s) can bring a private prosecution, but the State can intervene and take over.
2. *Constitutional law.* This controls the method of government. If a dispute arises, for example over who can vote or who can become a Member of Parliament, then it is constitutional law that is involved.
3. *Administrative law.* This controls how public bodies such as local councils, government departments or ministers should operate.

Some types of private law (civil law)

1. *Law of contract.* An agreement between two or more persons that is legally binding.
2. *Law of tort.* The word *tort* comes from the French, meaning a wrong. A tort is a civil (not criminal) wrong other than a breach of contract or trust. A tort is a duty fixed by law that affects all persons – it does not arise from a prior agreement. Torts cover negligence, nuisance, trespass and defamation. The most important of these in medical practice are negligence and battery (a part of the tort of trespass).
3. *Law of property.* This covers legal rights to property of all types.
4. *Family law.* This covers the law relating to marriage, divorce and the responsibilities of parents to children.
5. *Welfare law.* This is concerned with the rights of individuals to obtain State benefits, and the rights and duties that arise with regard to housing and employment.

between public and private law is largely that between *criminal law* and *civil law*. The differences between these two key aspects of law are summarized in Table 4.1.

The place of precedent in English law

The idea of judicial precedent is central to case law. This means that court decisions must, where relevant, follow previous decisions of a higher or equivalent level of court. Once a case has been heard, there is a judgement. That judgement not only gives the court's decisions, but also the reasons for those decisions and the principles on which they are based. It is these legal principles that create a 'binding precedent', and which future judges must follow (subject to certain caveats) if that previous decision was made in a court higher in the hierarchy than the court in which the current case is being heard (Box 4.2). A binding precedent must normally be followed even if the judge does not agree with it. A precedent may be 'persuasive' but not binding. Such precedents may originate, for example, from courts lower in the hierarchy, or from decisions of the courts in other countries that use a common law system, notably Canada, Australia and New Zealand. Sometimes when a court is issuing a ruling it makes general statements about the law which are not strictly necessary to resolve the case before it (e.g. a judge might say 'if the facts had been different I would have reached this conclusion...'). Such statements are known as *obiter dicta* ('by the way') and are not binding on subsequent courts, but can be taken into account.

Table 4.1 Distinctions between criminal and civil cases (Martin 2016)

	Criminal	Civil
Purpose	To maintain law and order and protect society	To uphold the rights of individuals
Person originating the case	The State (through the police and Crown Prosecution Service)	The individual whose rights have been affected
Legal name of person bringing the case	Prosecutor	Claimant (formerly plaintiff)
Legal name of person against whom the case is brought	Defendant	Defendant
Courts involved	See Box 4.2	See Box 4.2
Standard of proof	Beyond reasonable doubt	Balance of probabilities
Person(s) making the decision	Magistrates or jury	Judge or panel of judges (very occasionally a jury)
Decision	Guilty *or* not guilty	Liable *or* not liable
Sanction if guilty/ liable	Punishment	Usually compensation (damages)
Powers of court	Prison, fine, probation, discharge, community service order, etc.	Usually an award of damages, but also injunction, etc.

The doctrine of precedent only came to be applied in Scotland in the 19th century. The doctrine recognizes the hierarchy of the Scottish courts (see Box 4.2). Decisions in English courts may form persuasive precedents in Scottish courts. The Supreme Court is the highest UK court for civil cases in the Scottish (as well as in the English and Welsh) court system.

Statute Law (Acts of Parliament)

Statute law is made by Parliament. In the case of major pieces of legislation, there is frequently a consultation period prior to consideration by Parliament. Typically, the relevant government minister produces a consultative document known as a *Green Paper*. Comments on this paper are sought from relevant people and institutions, and changes are made to the original proposals in the light of these comments. This results in the publication of a *White Paper*, which contains firm proposals for the new law to be considered by Parliament.

Not every statute passed in the UK Parliament applies to Scotland. Acts passed since 1707 (the Union of the Parliaments) apply to Scotland unless there is a specific statement to the contrary. Conversely, some Acts apply only to Scotland. These have the word 'Scotland' in brackets in the title. Examples of such Acts are: National Health Service (Scotland) Act 1978, Mental Health (Care and Treatment) (Scotland) Act 2003 and The Adults with Incapacity (Scotland) Act 2000.

Box 4.2 The hierarchy of courts (from highest to lowest)

England and Wales

Criminal cases

European Court of Human Rights
Supreme Court
Court of Appeal (Criminal Division)
Crown Court
Magistrates' Court

Civil cases

European Court of Justice (with regard to EC law only); European Court of Human
   Rights
Supreme Court
Court of Appeal (Civil Division)
The Divisional Courts (two or three judges hear each case)
High Court (which has three divisions: Queen's Bench; Chancery; Family)
County Court
Magistrates' Court

Scotland

The judicial system in Scotland is also based on a division between civil and criminal
   law.

Criminal cases

High Court of Judiciary
The Sheriff Court deals with the more serious summary cases
District courts

Civil cases

Supreme Court (as in the rest of the UK). Two of the Supreme Court Justices are
   Scottish in origin and experience, although there is no binding rule that a Scottish
   Justice must sit on a Scottish case
Court of Session (which consists of an Inner House and an Outer House)
Sheriff Courts. These courts correspond most closely to the English county courts
There are, in addition, specialist courts. For example, cases involving children under
   16 years of age who are alleged to have committed a crime, or who for other
   reasons might be 'in need of compulsory measures of care', are dealt with at
   special Children's Hearings.

THE TORT OF NEGLIGENCE

The single most common reason for doctors to be taken to court is because they
are being sued for negligence. In order for a doctor to be found liable in negligence,
the claimant (see Table 4.1) would need to prove three things:
1. That the doctor owed a *duty of care* to the relevant patient.
2. That the doctor was *in breach of the appropriate standard of care* imposed by
   the law.
3. That the *breach in the duty of care caused the patient harm* meriting
   compensation.

Is there a duty of care?

A duty of care is an obligation on one party to take care to prevent harm being suffered by another. Generally, doctors owe a duty of care to their patients. A hospital Trust would normally owe a duty of care to a patient of a doctor employed by that Trust. If a person comes into the casualty department of a hospital, and the casualty doctor is informed of this, then normally both the hospital Trust and the doctor would owe a duty of care to that person.

Outside a hospital or a doctor's surgery, for example at the scene of an accident, doctors would not normally owe a duty of care if they did not attempt to help. In other words, doctors are not legally obliged to act as 'good Samaritans'. However, once a doctor stops and either says that she is a doctor or starts to act as though she is a doctor, she has taken on a duty of care to that patient. This means that she is now potentially liable in negligence. However, a general practitioner (GP) who is within his geographical practice area does normally owe a duty of care to a person in need of medical help (for example, if the GP is at the scene of an accident). This is a result of the GP's contract with the health authority.

What is the standard of care? – the Bolam test and its aftermath

Case 4.2

Mr Bolam was receiving electro-convulsive therapy (ECT) for a serious illness. This treatment (now used largely for severe depression) is usually carried out under general anaesthetic with the use of a muscle relaxant. The muscle relaxant is important, because ECT causes powerful contractions of skeletal muscle and, without relaxant, this can result in torn muscles and fractured bones. At the time of Mr Bolam's treatment, muscle relaxants were less well established than they are now. The majority of doctors used such relaxants during the administration of ECT, but the relaxants were not without potential risks, and some doctors at the time were of the opinion that they shouldn't be used. Mr Bolam was given ECT without the use of muscle relaxants and without restraining his limbs. He suffered a fractured hip from the contraction induced by the ECT.

Was Mr Bolam's doctor negligent for failing to prescribe a muscle relaxant?

(This is the Bolam case (Bolam v Friern Hospital Management Committee [1957]).)

In most cases of negligence, the key issue is whether the doctor was in breach of the standard of care. The test in English law is whether the doctor fell below 'the standard of the ordinary skilled man exercising and professing to have that special skill. A man need not possess the highest expert skill at the risk of being found negligent. It is a well established law that it is sufficient if he exercises the ordinary skill of an ordinary man exercising that particular art' (Bolam v Friern Hospital Management Committee [1957]). In the Bolam case, the evidence before the court was that, although most doctors with expertise in this area would use either relaxants or limb restraint, there was a body of medical opinion that supported the method used for Bolam.

Where the profession is divided as to what is the appropriate management (as was the case in Bolam), the doctor will not be found negligent simply because the procedure adopted was not approved by the majority of the profession. In the Bolam case the judge said: 'A doctor is not guilty [*sic*] of negligence if he has acted in accordance with a practice accepted as proper by a responsible body of medical men skilled in that particular art'. This is known as the Bolam test. Thus, a doctor will not be found negligent if the court is satisfied that there is a responsible body of medical opinion that would consider that the doctor had acted properly. That responsible body need not be the majority of the profession. The courts, however, do not simply accept what a group of doctors says is acceptable practice. In the case of Hills v Potter [1984], the judge said: 'In every case the court must be satisfied that the standard contended for on their behalf accords with that upheld by a substantial body of medical opinion ...'. Other terms have been employed in other judgements. The judge in Bolam talked not only about a responsible body, but also, elsewhere in his judgement, of a *reasonable* body of opinion. In other judgements, the term *respectable* body has been used. Essentially, therefore, the effect of the Bolam test is that it is difficult to establish that a doctor has breached the duty of care.

However, following the important case of Bolitho v City & Hackney Health Authority [1997], the law's approach is less clear cut.

Case 4.3

P was a two-year-old child admitted to hospital with severe croup. Dr H was notified, but did not attend, and P subsequently had a cardiac arrest and suffered brain damage. If P had been intubated, he would not have arrested, and his mother sued Dr H for negligence. Dr H testified that, even if she had attended, she would not have intubated him (given his clinical features), and it was argued that a reasonable body of professionals would have supported this decision (not to intubate).

(This is based on the Bolitho case.)

In that case, the Law Lords argued that, it was not enough that experts support the doctor's action, that action would have be *reasonable*. One of the Law Lords said:

> ... *the court has to be satisfied that the exponents of the body of opinion relied upon can demonstrate that such opinion has a logical basis... In the vast majority of cases the fact that distinguished experts in the field are of a particular opinion will demonstrate the reasonableness of that opinion ... But if, in a rare case, it can be demonstrated that the professional opinion is not capable of withstanding logical analysis, the judge is entitled to hold that the body of opinion is not reasonable or responsible.*

(In the Bolitho case, the judges did accept the expert opinion to be reasonable, and so the negligence claim was dismissed).

Many legal commentators interpreted the Bolitho decision as representing a radical departure from the courts' traditional deferential approach to doctors. But others were more sceptical and doubted that the courts would play a more active role in reviewing medical decisions and setting the legal standard of care. An analysis of post-Bolitho case law (e.g. Hanson v Airedale Hospital NHS Trust [2003] and French v Thames Valley Strategic Health Authority [2005]) does, however, reveal that judges are much more willing than in the past to scrutinize medical experts, even though it will 'very seldom be right' for a judge to regard competent medical experts' views as unreasonable (per Siber J in M (A Child by his Mother) v Blackpool Victoria Hospital NHS Trust [2003]). In others words, although the Bolam test will usually prevail, it is no longer impregnable. Although clinical judgement will in all probability continue to be endorsed by the courts, the case of Bolitho is important because it shows that, in principle, English courts have determined that they should play a role in reviewing medical decisions and setting the legal standard of care.

It is important to note that the Bolam test is limited to matters of professional judgements (e.g. to diagnosis; decisions concerning treatment; and performance of surgery). It does not apply to the provision of information (see Chapter 6), which the courts (following a case called 'Montgomery') have held *not* to be a question of professional judgement (Montgomery [2015]); for informed consent, the law (rather than professional medical opinion) will determine how much information should be given to a patient. Also, it should be noted there are a few treatments where there is specific legal regulation (such as abortion and organ donation), and where a doctor will be acting negligently if they breach the legal requirement (even if they were somehow to satisfy the Bolam test).

Did the breach of the duty of care cause the patient harm?

In order to show negligence, the patient must prove that, on the balance of probabilities, the harm resulted from the breach in the duty of care. (That was one reason why it was difficult to prove negligence in the Yearworth case, Case 4.1.) In one case (Barnett v Chelsea and Kensington Hospital Management [1968]), for example, three night watchmen came to the casualty department of a hospital with abdominal pains after drinking tea. The doctor told them to go and see their own doctors, without examining them. One man died after leaving the hospital from what was later discovered to be arsenic poisoning. The court found that the casualty doctor owed a duty of care to the patient, and that he had been in breach of the appropriate standard of care. However, the expert evidence was that, even had the casualty doctor acted properly, he would not have been able to save the man's life. The harm (of death) was therefore found not to have been caused by the breach in the duty of care, and so neither the hospital nor the doctor was negligent.

Case law on causation has consistently revealed how difficult a hurdle this element is for any potential claimant to overcome. Thus, it is rare for cases to be as simple as the Barnett case above, where failure to treat a patient made no difference because he would have died anyway (i.e. his death was not caused by the negligence). In practice, most causation cases are far more complex. The aetiology of medical conditions is often unclear, so that it is uncertain whether the injury was 'caused' by the defendant's action (or inaction) or by some other cause (or even multiple causes). Often, too, the situation will be further complicated by the presence of an underlying illness or other pre-existing vulnerability. In such a case, it can be crucial that the claimant show that, on the balance of probabilities, the negligence caused the harm. If the court decides the aetiology is unclear, then that may well mean the claim will fail.

One typical situation is where what the patient has been deprived of (for example, through a missed or delayed diagnosis) the chance of treatment, and what is uncertain is whether the prognosis would have been substantially different had the diagnosis not been missed (see on this Gregg v Scott [2005]). Yet, despite the difficulties of proving causation, several legal commentators (e.g. Laurie, Harmon, and Porter 2016) have suggested that the courts seem increasingly willing to bend causation rules to achieve what they see as a just outcome. This is perhaps why in some cases (albeit rarely), even if it cannot be shown that the harm was caused by a breach in the defendant's standard of care, damages may be awarded. In Chester v Afshar [2004] the House of Lords held that a patient was entitled to damages because she had not been warned about a risk of injury that in fact occurred (although not due to any negligence in how the operation was performed). As a result of that failure she underwent surgery (which she would not have had at that particular time had she been properly informed). The Supreme Court, controversially, found that the negligence in nondisclosure caused the risk. The reasoning being that, if the patient had had the surgery on another occasion, then she would not have suffered the injury that she did.

In Scottish law, liability in negligence rests on the principle of 'delict' or 'reparation' rather than tort. A key Scottish case was that of Hunter v Hanley [1955], which predates the Bolam case in England (see above) and which established that a doctor's conduct, in the setting of negligence, should be judged against the normal and usual practice of his profession. In practice, the law regarding negligence in Scotland is similar, although not identical, to that in England and Wales.

Reform of the law of negligence

The law of negligence has long been criticized as a system of compensation. The most common criticisms are that the law is too complex, unfair, slow and costly. It also fosters a climate of blame and confrontation that undermines the doctor–patient relationship and discourages the reporting of errors (see also Department of Health 2003).

One response to these criticisms was the NHS Redress Act 2006. Under the Act, patients would no longer have to go to court to get compensation, care or an investigation when something goes wrong. They would instead be entitled to receive a more consistent, speedy and appropriate response to their claims of negligence. There was a proposed upper limit to claims of £20000 (although this could increase). The new redress scheme was designed to give claimants an alternative to litigation rather than to replace court proceedings. Over a decade after being passed, the Act has not been put into effect, although many

NHS Trusts do run procedures to deal with complaints that are designed to avoid litigation.

TRESPASS TO THE PERSON

There are three forms of trespass: trespass to the person, trespass to goods and trespass to land. The most important of these for health professionals is trespass to the person. Trespass to the person can consist of assault, battery or false imprisonment. It is the first two that concern us here. Assault is when a person causes someone else to fear that force will be used imminently against their body. Most cases will involve a situation where one person has threatened violence against another. Battery occurs when the act goes beyond a threat, and the person is touched without consent. Battery can also occur if the touching is indirect, as, for example, if a person throws an object at another person and hits her.

Assault and battery are both potentially criminal offences, but they can also give rise to civil actions (in the tort of trespass to the person). In the setting of medical practice, it is the tort (i.e. civil action; see Box 4.1) of battery that is of most significance. If a surgeon, for example, removes a patient's uterus, for justifiable medical reasons but without the consent of the patient, the surgeon may be successfully sued for battery, and the patient may be awarded damages. It is very unlikely that criminal proceedings would be taken against the doctor, unless he or she was trying to harm the patient or was grossly negligent. In one bizarre case, a surgeon was convicted of battery after using an argon beam to put his initials on a patient's liver. More commonly, doctors are convicted of sexual assault when they touch a patient sexually for non-medical reasons.

The tort of battery is of considerable importance in medical practice. It establishes that a doctor can touch a patient only with that patient's consent, unless the patient lacks capacity to give or withhold consent. Because examination, investigations and many treatments involve the doctor touching a patient, this requirement means that a patient can in general refuse medical help and treatment, even if this results in considerable harm or death. This issue is discussed in detail in Chapter 6.

EUROPEAN COURTS AND THE HUMAN RIGHTS ACT 1998

At the time of writing, Brexit is looming. However, it is far from clear what the relationship between European Law and the law in the UK will be after the UK leaves the European Union.

The European Court of Justice (also called the Court of Justice of the European Communities)

This is the judicial branch of the European Union. It reviews the legality of the acts of the Commission and the Council of Members of the European Union, for example concerning issues involving disputes over trade or environment. Rulings made by the Court are binding on the member states, including both England and Wales, and Scotland (see Box 4.2). The Court is located in Luxembourg.

The European Court of Human Rights

The purpose of this court, which is located in Strasbourg, is to protect rights set out in the European Convention on Human Rights. It does not deal with any other set of issues. The Convention and the Court are established under the Council of Europe (not to be confused with the European Union). Individuals can take cases to the Court, usually against the state (country) of that individual. The court has no legal power to enforce its decisions (in contrast to the European Court of Justice). However, most states that belong to the Council of Europe (which currently has 46 members) would follow its rulings. The ultimate sanction available to the Council of Europe would be to expel the offending member state. However, an important development in English law is the Human Rights Act 1998.

The Human Rights Act 1998 (HRA)

The Human Rights Act 1998 (HRA) came into force in October 2000. The Act makes the rights and freedoms that are set out in the European Convention of Human Rights (ECHR) enforceable in English (and Scottish) courts. It means that it is unlawful for a public authority to act in a way that is incompatible with a Convention right. It also means that, in interpreting domestic law, the UK courts should, so far as is possible, interpret any ambiguities in the law in a way which is compatible with the ECHR. Some predicted that the HRA would have an enormous impact on medical law. In fact, its effect has been modest. The Act has been used successfully to ensure that procedural safeguards are in place to protect patients' rights. In Glass v UK [2004], for example, the ECHR held that treating a child against its parents' wishes was a breach of the child's right to respect for its private and family life under Article 8(1).

Three of the Rights in particular may be relevant to clinical practice.

The right to life (Article 2 of the Convention)

According to this Article, everyone's right to life shall be protected by law, and no-one shall be deprived of their life intentionally. The European Court has interpreted this as placing a positive obligation to protect life, and not simply as guaranteeing the negative obligation not to take life. This might have implications for the allocation of resources, because it might allow a patient to take legal action if denied expensive treatment that could save life (for example, expensive chemotherapy). Individual patients or their relatives might be able to challenge the withdrawal or withholding of life-prolonging treatment. The courts, however, ruled that there was no breach of Article 2 either in a case involving the withdrawing of artificial nutrition and hydration in two patients in persistent vegetative state (NHS Trust A v M and NHS Trust B v H [2001]) or in another case involving excluding the resuscitation of a 19-month-old child who was dying (A National Health Trust v D [2000]) or withdrawal of life-sustaining treatment from a seriously ill baby (Gard v UK [2017]).

The prohibition of torture (Article 3 of the Convention)

This Article states that '[n]o one shall be subjected to torture or to inhuman or degrading treatment or punishment'. It is well established through decisions of the European Court that there is an obligation to provide adequate medical treatment for patients who are detained (for example, in prison or in a psychiatric hospital). This Article may also be interpreted as implying that experimental medical treatment could amount to inhuman treatment, in which case it could have implications for clinical research. Furthermore, it could be relevant to the provision of information in the context of consent to treatment and research. In a key case, Diane Pretty, who suffered from motor neuron disease, argued that, when the time came, her husband should be able to assist her suicide. The European Court, however, confirmed the House of Lords' ruling, that Section 2 of the Suicide Act 1961, which makes assisting suicide a crime, is not incompatible with Article 3 (Pretty v United Kingdom [2002]).

Right to respect for private and family life (Article 8 of the Convention)

This Article states that '[e]veryone has the right to respect for his private and family life, his home and his correspondence'. Whether this will set a standard for confidentiality that is different from that already set by the law and the General Medical Council is unclear. The leading case on breach of confidence is now Campbell v MGN [2004]. Here the House of Lords emphasized that the protection of confidential information is about respecting the autonomy and dignity of individuals. The court also emphasized that the right to respect for private and family life under Article 8 should be regarded as underpinning the law's protection of confidentiality.

It is possible to justify interfering in an Article 8 right where it 'is in accordance with the law and is necessary in a democratic society in the interests of national security, public safety or the economic well-being of the country, for the prevention of disorder or crime, for the protection of health or morals, or for the protection of the rights and freedoms of others'. Hence, breach of confidentiality could be justified if necessary to protect a child from abuse. Similarly, in Pretty v United Kingdom [2002] it was held that, while making decisions about the end of your life did fall within the right to respect for private life, the law could restrict that right by prohibiting assisted dying, as a necessary means of protecting vulnerable people.

UNDERSTANDING LEGAL REFERENCES AND REPORTS

Cases

Doctors are used to the system of citing references in terms of author, date, title of article, journal (or book), volume number and page numbers. References to legal cases can appear puzzling, and even daunting. The most authoritative legal reports are those produced by the Incorporated Council of Law Reporting and published as a general series known as the *Law Reports*. There are four series of reports, depending on the type of case and the court: Appeal Cases (AC), Chancery Division (Ch), Queen's Bench (QB) and Family Division (Fam). These Law Reports are referenced by name of case, year, the law report series abbreviation and the starting page. For example, the reference to the House of Lords hearing of the 'Gillick' case (see Chapter 11) is: **Gillick v West Norfolk and Wisbech AHA [1986] AC 112**. The two parties concerned in the action were Mrs Gillick and the West Norfolk and Wisbech Area Health Authority, and this provides the name of the case. The 'v' stands for the Latin *'versus'*, i.e. against. AC refers to the fact it is found in the Appeal Cases, and 1986 is the year of the reporting. The 112 refers to the page number in the volume. Sometimes a case arises not because one party is suing the other, but because one party wants a court ruling on some issue, or an injunction to prevent something from happening. A hospital may, for example, in unusual circumstances, want a court to determine whether a treatment can be imposed on a patient. Typically, in such instances, the person who is the subject of the case is referred to by an upper-case single letter of the alphabet, and the name of the case will include a brief description. For example, the case name might be **Re B (A minor) (Wardship: Medical Treatment)**.

Although bound paper copies of law reports can be found in law libraries, they are generally now found online. The Government has a website which has many recent judgements (https://www.judiciary.gov.uk/judgments/). The BAILII (British and Irish Legal Information Institute) provides a free resource which is widely used (http://www.bailii.org/). There are also popular subscription legal databases, the two best known being LexisNexis and Westlaw. All of these websites allow you to search for cases using the name of the parties or by keywords. The subscription databases can provide sophisticated search tools including, for example, references to every case which has mentioned a particular decision or Act of Parliament.

Statutes

Statutes are Acts of Parliaments. The most authoritative publication of statutes is the *Public General Acts*, duplicated in the *Law Reports Statutes*, which are published by the Incorporated Council of Law Reporting. These are both arranged chronologically. Nowadays research is primarily done online using the Government's database (http://www.legislation.gov.uk/), although statutes can also be found in the subscription databases.

REVISION QUESTIONS

1. Briefly describe the doctrine of precedent.
2. Assess the impact of the Human Rights Act 1998 on medical law.
3. Summarize what needs to be proved to establish a claim in the tort of negligence.
4. What role is there for ethics when judges write legal judgements?
5. Would it be more accurate to say that the law sets the minimum standards doctors must reach (while hoping that doctors will exceed these expectations), or that the law aims to direct how doctors should act?

Many years ago, Mrs L had a biopsy for cancer of the cervix. The specimen was given to a cancer researcher who noted that the cells reproduced very rapidly and could be kept alive in culture for a long time, allowing further study. After Mrs L died, the researcher obtained more cells from her body, and was able to establish a cell culture line.

The cell culture derived from Mrs L became widely used in medical research and contributed to many breakthroughs. There are many patents based on the cultured cells.

Does Mrs L's family have any claim to the medical breakthroughs that arose from her cells? Could they claim a property right in her cells? What about Mrs L's genome? Do patients have property rights in their genetic sequences?

(This Case is based on the case of Henrietta Lacks. See Skloot 2010.)

REFERENCES

A National Health Trust v D [2000] 2 FLR 677.

Barnett v Chelsea and Kensington Hospital Management Committee [1968] 1 All ER 1068.

Bolam v Friern Hospital Management Committee [1957] 1 WLR 582.

Bolitho v City and Hackney HA [1997] 4 All ER 771 HL.

Campbell v MGN [2004] UKHL 22.

Chester v Afshar [2004] UKHL 41.

Department of Health. 2003. *Making amends: a consultation paper setting out proposals for reforming the approach to clinical negligence in the NHS* Online. Available: http://www.dh.gov.uk.

French v Thames Valley Strategic Health Authority [2005] EWHC 459.

Gard and Others v United Kingdom (application no. 39793/17) [2017] European Court of Human Rights.

Glass v UK [2004] ECHR 102.

Gregg v Scott [2005] UKHL 2.

Hanson v Airedale Hospital NHS Trust [2003] CLY 2989 (QBD).

Hills v Potter [1984] 1 WLR 641.

Hunter v Hanley [1955] SC 200.

Laurie, G. T., Harmon, S. H. E. and Porter, G. 2016. *Mason & McCall Smith's law and medical ethics*. 10th ed. Oxford: Oxford University Press.

Martin, J. 2016. *The English legal system*. London: Hodder & Stoughton.

M, Re (A Child by his Mother) v Blackpool Victoria Hospital NHS Trust [2003] EWHC 1744.

Montgomery v Lanarkshire Health Board [2015] UKSC 11.

NHS Trust A v M and NHS Trust B v H [2001] 2 WLR.

Pretty v United Kingdom (Application No. 2346/002) [2002] 2 FLR 45.

Skloot, R. 2010. *The immortal life of Henrietta Lacks*. London: Pan.

Yearworth and others v North Bristol NHS Trust [2009] EWCA Civ 37.

Chapter **5**

Doctors and patients
Relationships and responsibilities

We have discussed some of the ethical theories and principles that provide a background for understanding medical ethics. In the next part of the book we will move on to examine some practical ethical questions. But before doing that we should look at one of the fundamental interactions in medicine: the relationship between doctors and patients, and the roles and responsibilities of each participant.

Case 5.1

Laura is 33, and is pregnant with her second child. She is still in the early stage of pregnancy when she is diagnosed with breast cancer. In women who are not pregnant, surgical treatment options would include mastectomy or breast-conserving surgery (lumpectomy) followed by moderate-dose radiotherapy. However, in Laura's case, radiotherapy would pose significant risks for her fetus.

Laura's surgeon, Ms S, believes that mastectomy is clinically indicated, as that would give her the best chance of long-term survival. She regards Laura's situation as an absolute contraindication to breast-conserving surgery. However, Laura is not happy to have a mastectomy because of the effect that she fears it would have on her appearance and her image of herself. Another option would be for Laura to terminate her pregnancy, but Ms S (who is a devout Muslim) is strongly opposed to that option.

How should Laura's surgeon counsel her about treatment?

THE DOCTOR–PATIENT RELATIONSHIP

Medical students, who have sat in on many different consultations, might reflect back on the different ways in which the doctors and surgeons they have observed would approach the above consultation. Some might be more directive, others more hands-off in their counselling. These different styles can represent different views of the medical consultation, the values of well-being and autonomy, and the nature of ethical dialogue. Table 5.1 summarizes four different points on the spectrum of shared decision-making.

The paternalistic (traditional) model

The idea of a 'paternalistic relationship' is derived from the traditional relationship between a father and his child. The father believes that he knows what is best for his child and may override the child's own wishes or choices for the child's own good.

As discussed in Chapter 3, in the past, doctors' relationships with patients were largely paternalistic. A doctor would make the main decisions about health care, often with little or no discussion with the patient. According to this model, the doctor can decide what is in the patient's best interests from knowledge of the medical facts alone. The doctor's role in the consultation is to reach a diagnosis

Table 5.1 Four models of the doctor–patient relationship (based on Emanuel and Emanuel 1992)

	Informative	Interpretative	Deliberative	Paternalistic
Conception of doctor's role	Competent technical expert	Counsellor or adviser	Friend or teacher	Guardian
Patient values	Defined, fixed and known to the patient	Inchoate and conflicting, requiring elucidation	Open to development and revision through moral discussion	Objective and shared by the physician and patient
Conception of patient's autonomy	Choice of, and control over, medical care	Self-understanding relevant to medical care	Moral self-development relevant to medical care	Assenting to objective values
Doctor's obligation	Providing relevant factual information and implementing the patient's selected intervention	Elucidating and interpreting relevant patient values, as well as informing the patient and implementing the patient's selected intervention	Articulating to the patient and persuading the patient of the most admirable values, as well as informing the patient and implementing the patient's selected intervention	Promoting the patient's well-being, independent of their current preferences

and to plan management. In Laura's case, Ms S would decide how Laura's breast cancer should be managed.

One advantage of the paternalistic model is that it emphasizes the importance of the best interests and well-being of the patient. It draws attention to a doctor's duty to do what is best for the patient, and not what is best for the doctor, or for society more broadly. The paternalistic model works best in clinical situations where it is unlikely that any set of patient values would make a difference to the treatment, and where the illness interferes with the patient's ability to take part in the decision-making process. When doctors provide urgent life-saving treatment (like resuscitation) for acutely ill patients, they are doing so based on their paternalistic judgement about what would be best.

Some patients prefer this model of medical decision-making. Patients who have trust in their doctor, who do not particularly want to have to think about the details of their condition and its management and who see making decisions as a burden may be particularly satisfied with this model of the doctor–patient relationship.

However, criticisms of the paternalistic model include:

1. It adopts too narrow a meaning of 'well-being' or of the best interests of a patient. Such best interests are not determined by the medical facts alone, but may differ depending on the patient's own values – her views of what are the most important things to her. For example, in many medical decisions towards the end of life there may be a trade-off between quality of life and quantity of life. Does the patient want to live longer, but potentially with reduced quality, or compromise length of survival for the sake of greater comfort? It is not clear that one of these is right and the other wrong.

2. It tends to conflate factual claims and value judgements (see Chapter 1). The idea of something being 'medically, or clinically, indicated' sounds as though it is purely a factual issue, whereas it often includes values. Thus, in the case of Laura, her surgeon Ms S claims that mastectomy is 'clinically indicated'. However, this phrase conceals the values that go into making the decision.

3. It does not take into account values other than the patient's well-being, and in particular the valuing of patient autonomy (see Chapter 3). Even if Ms S is correct that mastectomy would best promote Laura's interests, we may feel that Laura's values are crucial. We will discuss termination of pregnancy more in Chapter 13, but in general it is completely inappropriate for doctors to decide for patients whether they should continue or terminate a pregnancy. It is simply not their place. That is, surely, up to Laura to decide.

The informative (consumer) model

At the opposite end of the spectrum is a model that sees the doctor's role as a provider of medical facts. The patient decides what she wants; then, the doctor carries out that part of the management plan that requires technical or clinical skills. According to this model, Ms S would simply provide Laura with facts about the various options (termination/continuation, mastectomy/lumpectomy, radiotherapy/chemotherapy), and Laura would pick whichever option she prefers (Fig. 5.1).

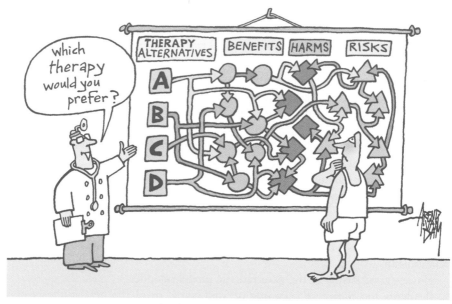

informed consent

Figure 5.1 The informative model of informed consent (© Arend van Dam, reproduced with permission)

The informative model derives from one view of the principle of respecting patient autonomy, whereas the paternalistic model emphasizes the principle of beneficence. The advantage of the model is that it allows patients to choose their own management on the basis of good information, but without the intrusion of the doctor's values or interests. In many other walks of life, this is the model that people usually prefer. In matters such as buying a house or arranging repair of a car, we expect the experts to provide the important information and to carry out the client's wishes. This model may be particularly applicable to some medical decisions. When it comes to decisions about continuing/terminating a pregnancy, including in clinical genetics, doctors are usually urged to be 'non-directive' – i.e. not providing any guidance either way. This appears to be in line with the informative model.

There are several criticisms of the informative model:

1. It does not provide sufficient support for the patient in coming to a decision about managing her condition.
2. More sophisticated views of respect for patient autonomy emphasize the value of discussion (see Chapter 3). Patients may not know what their values are, nor how to weigh up the options available to them.
3. Patients may come to bad decisions – bad even based on their own valuation – because they may make mistakes. For example, they may place too much weight on something that they are afraid of or have irrational beliefs (Savulescu and Momeyer 1997). Discussion with the doctor will help to minimize this

risk, particularly as doctors are likely to have experience of the longer-term issues that have been important to other patients in similar situations.

4. It treats the doctor as technician.

The interpretative model

The interpretative model and the deliberative model (see below) represent more 'shared' forms of shared decision-making. Shared decision-making emphasizes the role of the doctor, as well as the patient, in making decisions. When there is disagreement, there is negotiation, and the possibility of the doctor trying to persuade the patient. However, most models of shared decision-making would envisage, in the end, that the patient's view should prevail, as long as the patient has been properly informed and as long as the doctor has made clear why he or she disagrees with the patient's decision.

According to the interpretative model, it is often helpful for the patient to discuss decisions about management with the doctor. The doctor may enable the patient to clarify her values and help her make the decision that is most in keeping with those values. Furthermore, the facts that the patient may need to know cannot necessarily be determined unless the doctor knows something about the patient's values. The doctor may also play a useful role in helping the patient to understand the implications of the different possible management decisions.

According to the interpretative model, if Ms S, the surgeon in the above case example, believes that Laura is making the wrong decision, it would be appropriate for her to discuss this further. Such discussion would be aimed at ensuring that Laura had thought clearly about the implications of choosing breast-conserving surgery – in particular the implications of a reduced chance of long-term survival. Ms S might also, based on this model, challenge Laura's negative view of mastectomy and explain the potential benefits of reconstructive surgery. It might be appropriate, too, for Ms S to tell Laura what treatment she would advise, as long as she gave the reasons for such advice.

With the increasingly prominent nature of evidence-based medicine, some models of shared decision-making focus on the issue of how patients can be helped to understand, and make use of, good-quality information in coming to health care decisions. Evidence-based patient choice is one such model (Edwards and Elwyn 2001, Hope 1996).

The deliberative model

The deliberative model shares many properties with the interpretive model, but differs in one important respect. In the deliberative model the doctor not only helps the patient to clarify her values, but may also discuss, and challenge, those values. According to the deliberative model, the doctor should be prepared to try to persuade the patient to alter her values if the doctor thinks that these are not right, just as a teacher or friend might seek to challenge values. This model can be derived from a concept of respect for patient autonomy that sees an element of moral development as part of promoting autonomy.

According to the deliberative model, it might be right for the surgeon, Ms S, to challenge some of Laura's values. The doctor may believe that Laura is overemphasizing concern for her physical appearance and undervaluing the importance of maximizing her chance of survival. She may also believe that Laura would be likely to change her values were she to have lumpectomy and, 3 years later, develop metastases. For both of these reasons, Ms S might seek to change Laura's current values, using a procedure like reflective equilibrium (Savulescu 1997).

Values might also be at stake when the doctor believes that a patient or a relative is overvaluing or undervaluing aspects of health care that impinge on others. In refusing the treatment that gives her the best chance of long-term survival, Laura may not be doing what would be best for her children. The doctor may believe that her values are wrong, and based on the deliberative model it may be appropriate for her to challenge those values.

In either the deliberative or the interpretative model, the doctor should not be overbearing in challenging a patient's decisions or values. In the end, it is for the patient to decide. The doctor should also be cautious about allowing his or her own personal values to impact the consultation. It would be wrong for Ms S to try to persuade Laura against termination of pregnancy on the basis of Ms S's own religious views. (In a parallel case, it would be just a wrong for a pro-choice doctor to attempt to persuade a patient to have an abortion against her religious objections.) We will return shortly to the question of the doctor's values in consultations.

These different models of the doctor–patient relationship are not mutually exclusive. It is not that one of them is right and the others are wrong. It is not even that doctors need to choose their own preferred style. Rather, the style of the consultation should be adapted to the needs of the patient (do they prefer to be told what would be best, do they want to make up their own mind, do they want some advice?) and to the specific decision. For complex and fraught decisions (perhaps decisions about the medical care of a patient nearing the end of life), it may be important for doctors to be more directive, more deliberative, even paternalistic (Xafis et al. 2014). For other decisions (e.g. termination of pregnancy), an informative approach may be the right one.

RESPONSIBILITIES OF DOCTORS

Responsibilities to Professional Codes of Conduct

Sometimes when people talk about medical ethics, they think primarily about professional codes. They might refer to the Hippocratic oath, or to more contemporary professional guidance, such as that from the General Medical Council (GMC) or the AMA (American Medical Association). These professional codes cannot be all there is to say about ethics. For one thing, there is a question about what the codes should say – we need ethics to help us determine what professional guidelines should say. Professional codes also sometimes change over time. (The Hippocratic oath originally prohibited surgery – 'cutting for stone'). The fact that a professional code forbids an option or permits an option does not resolve the question of whether or not the option is ethical. We also need ethics to help in situations where guidance is unclear.

The GMC is the professional body for doctors in the UK. It has the duty to ensure that those who are allowed to practise medicine (registered medical practitioners) are fit to do so. As part of this duty, it provides guidelines for doctors as to what is good practice, and it has a quasi-judicial process to decide whether a doctor is in breach of those guidelines. The main power of the GMC is to determine who can and who cannot practise medicine in the UK. Its ultimate sanction is to strike a doctor off the register if he or she is found to be in breach of the Council's standards of practice, with the result that the doctor cannot practise medicine in the UK. This sanction can be temporary or permanent. In addition, the GMC stipulates (in general terms) the syllabus for medical training and carries out regular visits to medical schools to ensure that students are receiving the appropriate education and assessment. Medical ethics and law are part of the 'core curriculum' for medical student education.

Doctors need to take the GMC's guidelines seriously, for three reasons. First, the guidelines represent the considered opinion of the professional body on what it is ethically right for doctors to do in various situations with regard to their professional work. Second, the GMC has the power to prevent a doctor from continuing to practise medicine. Third, although the GMC is not part of the legal system, the courts take its standards into account.

Medical students, particularly once they are involved in seeing patients, would be expected to behave to the same standards as doctors, for example with regard to medical confidentiality. The standards of behaviour expected of medical students may be higher than those expected of students generally, because medical schools must ensure that their graduates behave in a way appropriate to the professional standards of the medical profession.

Responsibilities to personal ethical codes

Do doctors (or other health professionals) have obligations to other ethical codes? In Case 5.1, Ms S had an ethical concern about Laura terminating her pregnancy. That concern related to her ethical views about abortion. But to what extent should professionals' personal views influence their medical practice?

Case 5.2

Two senior midwives, who were practicing Catholics, did not wish to be involved in the medical care of women who were having an abortion. When they were in a senior role coordinating the labour ward of a public hospital, they also did not wish to be placed in a position of supervising more junior midwives who were caring for women having an abortion. They wrote to their employer expressing their conscientious objection. The hospital indicated that, as they were not providing direct abortion-related care to the women, they did not have a right to conscientious objection. The midwives sought judicial review.

Should midwives or other health professionals have a right to object to elements of their professional role that conflict with their conscience?

This case is based on Greater Glasgow Health Board v. Doogan and Wood [2014].

Conscientious objection is the clearest example of a doctor's personal ethical codes influencing their practice. It is often compared to conscientious objection to military service. Since the eighteenth century, some countries have allowed individuals with objections (usually religious) to be exempted from conscription to armies. In medicine, conscientious objection is often associated with particular decisions around reproduction (e.g. abortion) or the end of life (e.g. euthanasia).

Perhaps surprisingly, there is little concrete law on conscientious objection. Two general principles apply in cases where a doctor has an objection to medical treatment. First, a patient does not have a right to demand that a particular doctor give them a particular treatment. Second, a doctor must ensure a patient receives a reasonable standard of care. This means that if a doctor does not wish to provide the patient with the treatment themselves, they are not required in law to do so, but they must ensure a colleague provides that treatment. If no colleague is available, then they may well be found liable in negligence if their refusal to treat causes a patient harm; and they may potentially even be subject to a criminal charge of gross negligence manslaughter if, for example, the patient were to die. There is specific provision in the Abortion Act which states that a person cannot be under a legal obligation to participate in an abortion if they have conscientious objection to it. However, whatever their objection, a doctor must 'participate in treatment which is necessary to save the life or to prevent grave permanent injury to the physical or mental health of a pregnant woman'. Note that the Abortion Act provision only applies to a case where there is 'conscientious objection' to abortion, and would not apply to a doctor who simply did not like the idea of abortion, but did not have an objection based in conscience.

Up for Debate Box 5.1 summarizes some of the ethical arguments around conscientious objection.

Where conscientious objection is allowed, there are questions about how conscience should be assessed (should objectors have to provide evidence of their beliefs? Should religious and non-religious objections be given equal weight?). Is there a way to non-arbitrarily separate permissible from impermissible forms of conscientious objection? (For example, could a doctor refuse to examine patients of the opposite gender? Can doctors refuse to provide prescriptions for oral contraceptives?) Furthermore, there is a question about what might be required of objectors (do they need to refer to another health professional – or can they object to that too? What about emergency situations?). Finally, who can object? Is it just the doctor/nurse/midwife directly involved in a procedure? What about administrators, cleaners or caterers who work in a health setting? Even if conscientious objection is permitted, some argue that doctors should (in conscience) not object (Wilkinson 2017).

In the case of the midwives (Case 5.2), the Supreme Court concluded that the specific conscience clause in the Abortion Act had been intended to refer to the direct elements of care involved in providing a termination of pregnancy. The judges ruled that the clause should not be interpreted to allow conscientious objection on the part of the 'host of ancillary, administrative and managerial tasks

DOCTORS AND PATIENTS

In defence of conscientious objection

1. Freedom of conscience and freedom of religion are fundamental rights of all citizens. They apply to health professionals, as well as to patients.
2. Professionals' ethical views are often centrally important to their lives. It is important to allow them to reflect those values in their work.
3. All medical decisions involve values. It is, therefore, impossible to ask doctors to set aside their values. Moreover, we want our health professionals to be ethically sensitive practitioners. It would be potentially dangerous to the practice of medicine to ask doctors to be mere technicians.
4. Prohibiting conscientious objection would potentially mean that some members of the community will choose not to pursue medicine, or will be forced to leave the profession.
5. If a society decides to make a particular medical service legally available (e.g. abortion), it is then up to society to decide how to provide that service. It is not up to individual practitioners to fulfil that demand.
6. There is no need to force health professionals to act against their conscience. There are plenty of health professionals who are willing to offer services (e.g. abortion, contraception or end of life care). Societies can and should arrange for those who are willing to offer treatment to provide it.
7. In many circumstances, it would be bad for patients to be treated by a doctor who is opposed to that treatment. Such doctors may not provide that treatment well.
8. Conscientious objection represents a valuable compromise for treatment options that are politically divisive and ethically controversial. It allows patients to access treatment they desire, without forcing health professionals to provide services that they regard as unethical.

Against conscientious objection

1. Medicine is different from the military. Doctors (and nurses/pharmacists, etc.) are not conscripted. They choose to work in the health profession.
2. Health professionals do have freedom of conscience and of religion. They can express that freedom in their choice of work and in their personal lives. However, where they are employed in a public role, there are obligations that come with that role.
3. Publicly employed professionals in other fields are not free to object to basic conditions of their employment. (For example, a biology teacher in a government school cannot object to teaching sex education, or evolution – if those are part of the curriculum.) That is different from work in the private sector. When doctors take on the profession of medicine, they take on obligations to the public to provide services which are legal, desired by the patient and which are in the patient's interests and consistent with distributive justice.
4. Countries like Sweden and Finland have removed a legal right to conscience objection. Personal objections or values are considered under standard labour law. They are accommodated as the needs of the service allow. There is no apparent reduction in quality of applicants to medicine, medical care or patient experience.
5. Asking doctors to set aside their personal values does not reduce them to mere technicians. They can and should engage in discussion and deliberation with

Continued

patients about the patient's values and about treatment options (see consultative and deliberative decision-making above).

6. Conscientious objection amounts, in essence, to a conflict between the rights of patients and the rights of professionals. However, in such a conflict, the rights of the patient should take precedence – they are sick, vulnerable and disempowered.

7. Allowing conscientious objection has a serious negative impact on patients' access to services that they have a legal right to access. This is a particular problem in areas where there may be few health professionals, or in places where a large number of professionals express a conscientious objection. While some patients may be able to navigate health services and find a non-objecting practitioner, others (for example, the young, elderly, sick, non-English speaking) may find it very difficult or impossible to do this.

8. A right to conscientious objection places an unfair burden on other health professionals and on health systems.

9. For politically and ethically controversial treatment choices, health systems should provide reasonable accommodation to allow, where possible, dissenting health professionals to work in ways that do not conflict with their personal ethical views. However, that does not amount to a right to conscientious objection. It may require professionals to either provide some services that they do not agree with, or to move to a different area of their profession.

that might be associated with those acts' (Greater Glasgow Health Board v. Doogan and Wood [2014]).

For further reading around conscientious objection, see the end of this chapter.

RESPONSIBILITIES OF PATIENTS

Individual responsibility

Doctors clearly have ethical responsibilities that impact on the doctor–patient relationship. But perhaps patients do too?

The NHS constitution includes a long list of patient rights. However, it also includes a set of responsibilities – for example to register with a GP, provide accurate information about health, condition and status, follow an agreed course of treatment, keep appointments, treat NHS staff and other patients with respect, etc. (Department of Health and Social Care 2015).

What is the source of these responsibilities? One source might be a responsibility to oneself or to one's own health. The question of individual responsibility for health and the health consequences of decisions is sometimes raised in relation to resource allocation. For example, should a smoker or an alcoholic receive equal priority for treatment with someone whose lung or liver disease is unrelated to their lifestyle choices? We will discuss that question in more detail in Chapter 10. The issue there is about fairness – whether it is fair to prioritize treatment on the basis of responsibility. However, even if there is no question of resources, perhaps patients have a moral obligation to look after themselves?

The idea that patients have a duty to look after their own health seems to be potentially linked to an older, moralizing view of medicine. According to that view, some patients are 'bad' – smoking, drinking, ignoring medical advice, not visiting their GP. In contrast, 'good' patients follow their doctors' prescriptions, exercise regularly, avoid unhealthy food, etc. The moralizing view might have originated in the idea that the body belonged to a divine creator. However, that view does not make much sense in a more secular or pluralistic world. It also has fallen out of vogue for the same reasons as a paternalistic approach to the doctor–patient relationship has. Patients have a range of different values and priorities. There is not a single right way of living a life. What is more, as long as their decisions affect only themselves, what business is it of the doctor or of society to moralize?

It is of course reasonable for doctors to provide health advice and guidance, and for public health programs to encourage and incentivize healthy behaviour. It is much more worrying if that advice carries stern moral overtones.

Collective responsibility

One plausible reason that patients might have responsibilities to their health is because of the impact of their behaviour on the wider health system. In the NHS constitution, the list of responsibilities is prefaced by a comment that '[t]he NHS belongs to all of us. There are things that we can all do for ourselves and for one another to help it work effectively, and to ensure resources are used responsibly'. Providing accurate health information, keeping appointments and following agreed medical plans are all ways to maximize efficient use of GP and specialist consultations.

The responsibility to not waste limited health care resources is a form of 'collective responsibility'. This refers to an ethical duty that is shared by members of a group, and does not fall uniquely or particularly on individuals. However, such responsibilities also often have another feature – to be fulfilled, they depend on all or most of the group acting in a particular way.

Case 5.3

James and Rania are considering whether or not to immunize their child. They live in a part of the country where there are high immunization rates. The immunization would protect their daughter against a viral illness that used to be common, but is now very uncommon. When the illness occurs in otherwise well children, it is usually fairly mild, but rarely can be very serious. The vaccine is generally safe, but there are rare unpleasant reactions to the vaccine. James and Rania conclude that, for their child, the risk of a complication from the vaccine is higher than the risk of her contracting the virus and becoming seriously unwell. They decide not to vaccinate their daughter.

Do James and Rania have a responsibility to immunize their child, even if they are right that it might be worse for her as an individual?

The situation in Case 5.3 is sometimes called a 'collective action' problem. In collective action problems, individuals make decisions that, taken in isolation, are potentially rational and better for them, but, when taken as a group, are worse for everyone. In James and Rania's case, thinking purely about their situation, their decision might be better for their daughter. However, if everyone thinks that way, the immunization program will not generate sufficient herd immunity – rates of the viral illness will rise, and many patients will become seriously unwell. Other examples in medicine include antibiotic prescribing. If one patient is prescribed antibiotics unnecessarily for a cold, they will probably not be any worse off. However, if many patients are prescribed antibiotics, that will contribute to antibiotic resistance. We will discuss collective responsibility in more detail and return to some of these examples (including Case 5.3) in Chapter 20.

REVISION QUESTIONS

1. After outlining the various treatment options, a patient asks you 'Doctor, what would you do?' Explain different possible responses to this question, drawing on different models of the doctor–patient relationship.
2. Paternalism in medicine is always wrong. Do you agree?
3. Do doctors in the UK have a legal right to conscientiously object to abortion? Are there exceptions?
4. Is it morally wrong for a patient to smoke?

Extension case 5.4

A doctor is consulting with a patient who has had breast cancer and is very reluctant to start chemotherapy (a family member had very severe side effects from treatment for a different cancer). The doctor has been reading about influences on patient decision-making in the literature. He employs several strategies in counselling the patient. He positively frames the risk of side-effects from chemotherapy (explaining that there is an 85% chance of her not having serious side-effects). He mentions a recent patient in the clinic who had chemotherapy in a similar situation and had a very good response to the treatment (a 'social comparison'). The doctor also emphasizes the risk of not undertaking chemotherapy (negative framing).

Was this an acceptable way of counselling?

Health systems sometimes attempt to influence choices in ways that will encourage healthy behaviour. Read about 'nudging' in health care. Are nudges ethically acceptable in the doctor–patient relationship?

Read for example:

Thaler and Sunstein (2008), Levy (2017), Sunstein (2015), Avitzour et al. (2018), Ploug and Holm (2015).

REFERENCES

Avitzour, D., Barnea, R., Avitzour, E., Cohen, H. and Nissan-Rozen, I. 2018. "Nudging in the clinic: the ethical implications of differences in doctors' and patients' point of view." *Journal of Medical Ethics* doi: 10.1136/medethics-2018-104978.

Department of Health and Social Care. 2015. "The NHS Constitution for England." Accessed 1/11/18. https://www.gov.uk/government/publications/the-nhs-constitution-for-england/the-nhs-constitution-for-england-patients-and-the-public-your-rights-and-the-nhs-pledges-to-you.

Edwards, A. and Elwyn, G. 2001. *Evidence-based patient choice: inevitable or impossible?* Oxford: Oxford University Press.

Emanuel, E. J. and Emanuel, L. L. 1992. "Four models of the physician-patient relationship." *JAMA* 267 (16):2221-6.

Greater Glasgow Health Board v. Doogan and Wood [2014] UKSC 68

Hope, T. 1996. *Evidence-based patient choice*. King's Fund.

Levy, N. 2017. "Nudges in a post-truth world." *Journal of Medical Ethics* 43 (8):495-500. doi: 10.1136/medethics-2017-104153.

Ploug, T. and Holm, S. 2015. "Doctors, patients, and nudging in the clinical context – four views on nudging and informed consent." *American Journal of Bioethics* 15 (10):28-38. doi: 10.1080/15265161.2015.1074303.

Savulescu, J. and Momeyer, R W. 1997. "Should informed consent be based on rational beliefs?" *Journal of Medical Ethics* 23:282-88.

Savulescu, J. 1997. "Liberal rationalism and medical decision-making." *Bioethics* 11 (2):115-29. doi: 10.1111/1467-8519.00049.

Sunstein, C. R. 2015. "The ethics of nudging." *Yale Journal of Regulation* 32 (2).

Thaler, R. H. and Sunstein, C. R. 2008. *Nudge: improving decisions about health, wealth, and happiness*. New Haven, Conn.; London: Yale University Press.

Wilkinson, D. 2017. "Conscientious non-objection in intensive care." *Cambridge Quarterly of Healthcare Ethics* 26 (1):132-42. doi: 10.1017/S0963180116000700.

Xafis, V., Wilkinson, D., Gillam, L. and Sullivan, J. 2014. "Balancing obligations: should written information about life-sustaining treatment be neutral?" *Journal of Medical Ethics* doi: 10.1136/medethics-2013-101965.

FURTHER READING ON CONSCIENTIOUS OBJECTION

Brock, D. W. 2008. "Conscientious refusal by physicians and pharmacists: who is obligated to do what, and why?" *Theoretical Medicine and Bioethics* 29 (3):187-200. doi: 10.1007/s11017-008-9076-y.

Cowley, C. 2016. "A defence of conscientious objection in medicine: a reply to Schuklenk and Savulescu." *Bioethics* 30 (5):358-64. doi: 10.1111/bioe.12233.

Giubilini, A. 2017. "Objection to conscience: an argument against conscience exemptions in healthcare." *Bioethics* 31 (5):400-8. doi: 10.1111/bioe.12333.

Petropanagos, A. "Conscientious objection to medical assistance in dying (MAiD)." Royal College of Physicians and Surgeons of Canada. Accessed 1/11/18. http://www.royalcollege.ca/rcsite/bioethics/cases/section-5/conscientious-objection-medical-assistance-e.

Savulescu, J. 2006. "Conscientious objection in medicine." *BMJ* 332 (7536):294-7. doi: 10.1136/bmj.332.7536.294.

Savulescu, J. and Schuklenk, U. 2017. "Doctors have no right to refuse medical assistance in dying, abortion or contraception." *Bioethics* 31 (3):162-70. doi: 10.1111/bioe.12288.

Sulmasy, D. P. 2008. "What is conscience and why is respect for it so important?" *Theoretical Medicine and Bioethics* 29 (3):135-49. doi: 10.1007/s11017-008-9072-2.

Wicclair, M. R. 2011. *Conscientious objection in health care: an ethical analysis*. Cambridge: Cambridge University Press.

Part **2**

Core topics

Chapter 6

Consent

Case 6.1

A new junior doctor on a busy surgical unit is asked by her registrar to consent a patient for a colonoscopy. The doctor explains some of the risks of the procedure, but does not mention the risk of intestinal perforation. The patient signs the consent form and undergoes the colonoscopy. Unfortunately, the patient has a perforation and a prolonged hospital stay. He later sues the hospital and doctor for failing to obtain informed consent.

    Should the junior doctor have agreed to obtain informed consent? Does the patient have a legal claim?

INTRODUCTION

Medical students often become aware of the issue of consent during their first surgical attachment. They see junior doctors asking patients to sign a 'consent form'. 'Consenting' the patient can become, for the junior doctor, yet another thing to do to the patient, like taking blood and obtaining a chest X-ray.

But the idea of doctors 'consenting' patients seems to get consent back to front. It is the patient who 'consents' – not the doctor. From the legal point of view, consent is, effectively, a power of veto. A competent patient has the right to refuse any examination, investigation or treatment, but does not have the right to demand treatment. From the ethical point of view, the approach taken to consent is fundamental to the doctor–patient relationship (see Chapter 5), and a key test of the degree to which patient autonomy is respected (Fig. 6.1).

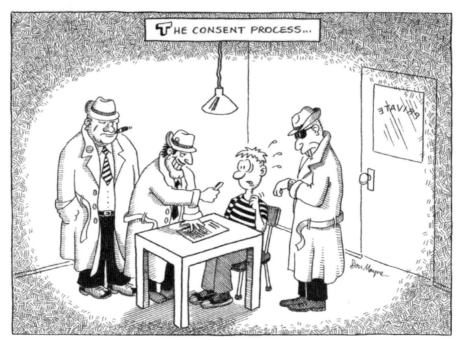

Figure 6.1 The consent process (© 2000, Don Mayne, used with permission)

THE CONCEPT OF INFORMED CONSENT

The philosophical basis of informed consent rests on the principle of patient autonomy (see Chapter 3). According to Lidz et al., for consent to be valid the doctor *discloses information* to a patient *who is competent*, the patient *understands* the information and the patient *voluntarily makes a decision* (Lidz 1984). The three main elements of valid consent ('informed', capacity and voluntariness) are incorporated into English law.

Faden & Beauchamp have criticized this analysis as being too centred on the provision of information (Faden, Beauchamp, and King 1986). It is too easy to provide extensive information and then claim that the doctor has carried out her duty to the patient (see Fig. 5.1). Such an approach may be legally safe, but is not ethically right. They propose that informed consent should be thought of as 'autonomous authorization'. According to this view, informed consent is a type of action. True informed consent requires that the patient does not merely assent, but specifically authorizes the doctor to initiate the medical plan. Some patients may not wish to be given a great deal of information and may wish the doctor to make the decisions and choose the plan of management. But this situation is to be clearly differentiated from the patient who passively assents to the doctor without autonomously engaging in the decision.

OVERVIEW OF THE LAW ON CONSENT

There are two main areas of law concerned with consent: battery and negligence. Both are part of the civil, common law (see Chapter 4). In addition, there are some statutes of relevance, in particular the Mental Capacity Act 2005, which is the major legislation governing those aged over 16 years who lack capacity (see Chapter 7); the Children Act 1989, which governs some aspects of consent with regard to children (see Chapter 11); the Family Law Reform Act 1969 (see Chapter 11), which governs some aspects of consent with regard to children (minors) aged 16 and 17 years; and the Mental Health Act 1983 (see Chapter 8), which regulates some aspects of consent with regard to mentally disordered patients.

We will return to capacity and its relevance to consent in the next chapter.

In order to understand the law on consent, it is necessary to consider both battery and negligence. These two are legally very different claims. In the case of a battery, the claim is that the patient did not consent. In the case of negligence, the claim is that the doctor failed to properly inform the patient about the procedure and its risk. In a case of negligence, therefore, as in Case 6.1 above, the patient may have given their consent to the procedure – the question is whether there was negligence in how that consent was obtained.

Battery

Case 6.2

A medical resident is attending surgery as part of her gynaecology rotation. Prior to the procedure (but while the patient is anaesthetized), the consultant surgeon asks the resident to perform an internal examination of the patient, though the patient has not consented for this specifically.

If the junior doctor performs an examination of the patient without her consent, would she be liable to a charge of battery?

A medical student attends surgery as part of her general surgery rotation. The consultant surgeon asks her to scrub in to assist during the surgery, though the patient has not consented to this specifically.

Is it ethical for students to assist in surgery without consent? Would that count as touching a patient, and hence battery?

In general, if one person touches another person without her consent, this constitutes a battery for which damages may be awarded (civil law) and for which, in extreme cases, a criminal prosecution might be brought. The key legal statement with regard to the clinical setting goes back to a judgement made in 1914 in the case of Schloendorff v Society of New York Hospital [1914]. The patient had given consent to an abdominal examination under anaesthetic, but had specifically requested no operation. The surgeon removed a fibroid. Although this is a US case, the statement concerning battery has been absorbed into English common law. The judge in that case (J Cardozo) said: 'every human being of adult years and sound mind has a right to determine what shall be done with his own body; and a surgeon who performed an operation without the patient's consent commits an assault' (i.e. battery). In marked contrast to negligence (see below), there is no need to prove that the person touched has suffered harm as a result of the touching in order for damages to be awarded. However, if there has been harm, this can lead to a higher level of damages being awarded than would be in a case where there was no harm. (As mentioned in the last chapter, in an unusual recent case, a consultant surgeon was fined £10,000 and sentenced to a community order after pleading guilty to writing his initials with an argon beam on livers that were transplanted into two anaesthetized patients.)

There are no legal cases involving medical students or junior doctors performing examinations or assisting without specific consent as in Case 6.2. It might be claimed that patients have implicitly consented to medical student or junior doctor involvement in their care (by attending a teaching hospital). It is also sometimes argued that student or resident involvement in procedures is a necessary part of their education (Gibson and Downie 2012, Kermode-Scott 2012, Shaw 2005). If that is the case, teaching hospitals should provide information to patients about the involvement of students and trainees in clinical care. Given the sensitivity of intimate physical examination, doctors and medical students should obtain specific consent prior to performing this (whether the patient is awake or anaesthetized). One important reason for this is that we might reasonably expect that some patients would object to this sort of examination being performed by students, with or without their knowledge. It would be a serious betrayal of patients' trust. However, it is not clear that specific consent is always required for the sort of assisting that medical students often provide in theatre (e.g. holding a retractor). It seems less likely that many patients would object to this, or that this would represent a breach of patient trust.

If the doctor has not obtained consent, the patient could successfully sue for battery. In practice, however, more legal cases concerning the question of consent focus on negligence, because the issue is usually about the appropriate amount of information that should have been given to the patient.

Negligence

The legal concept of negligence was discussed in Chapter 4. We will discuss negligence here as it relates to consent. Before providing treatment (for example, an operation) or undertaking a diagnostic test, the doctor has an obligation under the law of negligence to inform the patient about the nature of the procedure, the material risks attached to it and the alternative forms of treatment a patient may prefer. A patient could successfully sue a doctor on the grounds that the doctor was negligent in not providing certain key information. But, and this is a significant hurdle for anyone claiming in the law of negligence, it must be shown that the patient suffered a harm. There are two elements here. Consider the colonoscopy case (Case 6.1). First, no case would succeed unless it could show that the operation had caused harm (e.g. something went wrong during the operation). Of course, in many cases where a doctor has failed to mention a risk, the operation is still a success, and so no damages will be payable. Second, the claimant would need to persuade the court that, if they had been told of the risk, then they would not have consented to the procedure. Again, in many cases the judge will take some convincing that a sick patient would not have agreed to a procedure if they had been informed of a small risk. For example, in Case 6.1, it may be that, even if the junior doctor had informed Mr H of the risk of bowel perforation, Mr H would still have agreed to the colonoscopy.

Who can seek consent?

For the law, the key requirement is whether the patient consents or not. It does not matter who obtains the consent, although normally the health care professional who is performing an operation will want to make sure the patient has given effective consent. From an ethical point of view, the crucial issue is that the patient has access to the relevant information to make a decision.

General Medical Council guidance recommends that those undertaking a procedure may delegate the informed consent process to someone who is suitably trained, has relevant knowledge of the procedure and understands the risks involved (General Medical Council 2008). With the appropriate training and knowledge, consent for a procedure like endoscopy could be delegated to a junior doctor or nurse (Everett et al. 2016).

What information should be given?

The nature of the procedure

From the point of view of battery, the key statement was given by Justice Bristow in Chatterton v Gerson [1981]. Bristow said: 'in my judgement once the patient is informed in broad terms of the nature of the procedure which is intended, and gives her consent, that consent is real, and the cause of the action on which to base a claim for failure to go into risks and implications is negligence, not trespass' (i.e. negligence, not battery). Note that, for the purposes of battery (i.e. whether there was proper consent), the patient does not need to know of the risks of the procedure, but rather the general nature of the procedure. If the case involves failing to disclose risks or information about alternative procedures, then the claim should be brought in negligence.

Let us take an example. A surgeon recommends a partial colectomy (removal of part of the colon) for severe diverticulitis. In order for the patient's consent to be valid, from the point of view of battery, the surgeon would need to inform the patient that the operation involved an abdominal incision followed by removal of part of the colon with subsequent rejoining of the two ends of the colon. If a colostomy were also being considered, then the patient ought to be told of that possibility. From the point of view of battery, it would not be necessary for the doctor to give any information about the risks, benefits or alternative treatments. However, from the point of view of negligence this would be important.

Risks and benefits

Case 6.3

Mrs W had been almost blind in her right eye since childhood. At age 47, she had surgery on her right eye to improve its appearance and possibly improve her vision. Her surgeon did not inform Mrs W of a rare complication of surgery (1:14,000) – that she could develop inflammation in her good (left) eye (sympathetic ophthalmia). Unfortunately, Mrs W developed that complication and became completely blind.

(This case is based on the Australian High Court case of Rogers vs Whittaker [1992].)

In the recent important case of Montgomery v Lanarkshire Health Board [2015] (Herring et al. 2017), Mrs Montgomery had not been informed by her obstetrician of the risk of her baby becoming stuck during vaginal delivery (shoulder dystocia).

The Supreme Court, in that case, issued authoritative guidance on what risks needed to be disclosed to a patient by a doctor. All *material* risks need to be disclosed. A risk may be material for two reasons:

- A reasonable person in the patient's position would be likely to attach significance to the risk; or
- The doctor ought to reasonably be aware that the *particular patient* would attach significance to the risk.

Note that this does not require the doctor to disclose all risks. If the risk was so small that no-one would attach significance to it, it would not need to be disclosed. For example, extremely rarely, colonoscopy can be complicated by appendicitis. However, this has been reported in the medical literature only a handful of times, while an estimated 15 million colonoscopies occur each year in the US alone. It does not appear that doctors would be obliged to inform patients of this rare complication when obtaining consent for colonoscopy.

The significance of risks for a particular patient may be important. From the perspective of ethics, this reflects the fact that patients vary in their values, priorities, hopes and fears. In the case of Mrs W (Case 6.2), it may be that the average person would attach no significance to a 1:14,000 chance of inflammation in the other eye. If, however, the patient only had vision in one eye, then they may attach great significance to the risk, as appeared the be case for Mrs W. Similarly, where a patient asks about a particular risk (Mrs Montgomery asked her obstetrician if the baby's size was a potential problem), that indicates that it is a material one to the patient and so must be disclosed.

The Supreme Court did not want to give a precise statistic on when a risk becomes material, because whether it is material depends on the likelihood of the outcome and its severity. The more severe the possible outcome and the higher the risk, the more likely it is to be material. The more trivial the possible outcome and the lower the risk, the less likely it will be material. If doctors are unsure whether the risk is material, the safest course of action will often be to disclose it.

The Supreme Court applied the same principle to alternative forms of treatment. The doctor must offer the patient reasonable alternative or variant treatments. In the facts of Montgomery itself, the patient was in labour, and the doctor failed to offer Mrs Montgomery the option of a caesarean section. Even though the particular doctor would not have recommended a caesarean section, it was a reasonable alternative, and so should have been offered to the patient.

The Court also confirmed the existence of what is called the 'therapeutic exception'. If the doctor decides that telling the patient of risks would be seriously detrimental to the patient's health, they can decide not to inform the patient of the risk. As the Supreme Court noted, it will be very rare for this exception to apply. A case where the disclosure would induce a serious panic attack could be one case in which this exception would apply. Again, if a doctor is unsure if the 'therapeutic exception' applies, it is probably best to make the disclosure.

The legal status of the 'consent form'

It is routine for patients to be asked to sign a consent form before undergoing surgery. Does this mean that it would be illegal to perform surgery on a competent patient without a signed form? The answer is no. From the legal point of view, the key thing is that the patient has given valid consent (see Box 6.1). That consent can be given verbally. The purpose of a written consent form for surgical procedures is twofold: first, it provides a mechanism to ensure that consent is obtained and to communicate that fact to other members of the health care team; second, from the legal point of view it provides evidence that the patient has given consent. The consent form has no other legal force; in particular, it is not a contract. One important implication is that a patient may withdraw consent after signing the consent form. A patient with capacity can withdraw consent at any time, in which case it would normally be illegal (battery) to proceed with the operation.

When can consent be implied?

Because touching without consent can constitute battery, a patient's consent is needed even when taking the pulse or examining the chest. And yet doctors rarely obtain specific consent for such routine parts of the medical examination. Does this mean that patients could successfully sue doctors much of the

---

Box 6.1 Some key legal principles relating to consent

- Adults with capacity have a legal right to refuse medical treatment or demand withdrawal of treatment, even if this refusal results in death or permanent injury.
- Adults without capacity should be treated 'in their best interests' (Mental Capacity Act 2005).
- Under the Mental Capacity Act 2005, doctors (and other people) can make decisions on behalf of an adult who lacks capacity.
- A person is legally adult at age 18 years.
- Those aged 16–17 years can consent to treatment, but not necessarily refuse beneficial treatment (see Chapter 11).
- Those aged less than 16 years may, if they have capacity, consent to treatment (see Chapter 11).
- A parent or guardian can give proxy consent on behalf of a minor (aged less than 18 years).
- Parents and guardians are under a legal duty to act in the minor's best interests. If doctors and parents cannot agree on the minor's best interests, a court may need to decide either who should judge best interests or what those best interests are.
- The Mental Capacity Act defines an adult as a person of 16 years and over. There is thus an overlap between the Act and the common law in relation to young people aged 16 and 17 years (see Chapter 11).
- A medical professional who fails to disclose a material risk to a patient can be liable in negligence.
- A patient can only give effective consent if they understand, in broad terms, the nature of the procedure.

time? The answer is no, because the courts recognize the concept of 'implied consent'. If the doctor says, 'I would like to take your pulse' and the patient proffers her wrist and sits quietly while the doctor takes the pulse, then the patient's consent is taken to be implied by her behaviour. If, however, a competent patient were to say, 'There's no way you're going to take my pulse', it would constitute battery if the doctor went ahead and took the patient's pulse. The mere fact, however, that a person voluntarily comes to see a doctor or is admitted to hospital does not imply consent to any examination, investigation or treatment. A competent patient could come to the doctor and then refuse to be touched in any way.

Consent form disclaimers

In order to avoid being sued in battery, the surgeon must describe 'the general nature of the operation'. This would normally include the fact that an incision will be made, the rough site of the incision and what part or parts of the body will be removed. The surgeon may not know, until he is already carrying out the operation, exactly what needs to be done. What is the legal force of a consent form disclaimer to the effect that the surgeon will do whatever is necessary in the patient's best interests?

A doctor would normally be justified in proceeding without a patient's consent if a condition were discovered in an unconscious patient for which treatment was necessary (i.e. if it would be unreasonable to postpone treatment). In a Canadian case (Marshall v Curry [1933]), a grossly diseased testicle was discovered during a hernia operation. It was removed on the grounds that removal was necessary for the hernia repair and that the gangrene was thought to be a threat to the patient's life. The court upheld the surgeon's action. In another Canadian case (Murray v McMurchy [1949]), a doctor was successfully sued in battery when he tied the patient's fallopian tubes during a caesarean section because he discovered fibroids in the uterine wall and was concerned about the hazards of a future pregnancy. These Canadian cases are likely to reflect English law. In the English case of Devi v West Midlands Regional Health Authority [1980], a 29-year-old woman who had four children and hoped for more was admitted to hospital for a minor operation on her womb. In the course of the operation, her womb was found to be ruptured. She was sterilized, without her consent or knowledge, because it was feared that, if she were to become pregnant again, her womb would rupture. The patient won her claim.

Voluntariness

To be effective, consent must be given voluntarily. There is little case law on this. In one case, a woman refused to consent to a contraceptive injection. She was found to lack capacity to make the decision because she was utterly subservient to her husband and so could not voluntarily make the decision (A Local Authority v Mr and Mrs A [2010]). However, the courts have also made it clear that simply because a patient feels under pressure to consent to a treatment (that a medical professional is strongly recommending) does not mean that a patient is not acting voluntarily.

REVISION QUESTIONS

1. A patient has signed a consent form for surgery. Does that mean that surgery can proceed?
2. How much detail do surgeons need to provide when obtaining informed consent? How has the Montgomery case changed that?
3. Can consent be delegated? In what circumstances?
4. When does the 'therapeutic exception' permit a medical professional not to disclose a material risk?
5. When is a patient not able to make a voluntary decision to consent to treatment?

Extension case 6.4

The exploratory operation

Mr A has chronic abdominal pain. Investigations have not revealed a cause. A laparotomy (exploratory operation) is needed. It is explained to Mr A that the cause is not certain, and permission is sought to carry out whatever is considered necessary at operation. Mr A wishes this to be done, and so grants a carte blanche to the surgeon to remove whatever she thinks necessary. On laparotomy the surgeon discovers a bowel carcinoma. She removes the carcinoma and sufficient healthy bowel on either side to try to ensure that the entire tumour is removed.

As Mr A did not give explicit consent for the removal of the carcinoma and part of the bowel, could he successfully sue in battery on the grounds that the nature of the operation had not been sufficiently explained?

The additional finding

Mr A has intermittent abdominal pain. Investigations reveal gallstones, and the cause of the pain is thought to be due to this. Mr A gives consent for the operation involving removal of the gallbladder, and also for anything else to be done that is thought necessary. At operation, the surgeon finds that, although there are gallstones, the cause of the pain is probably a carcinoma, which he discovers at the head of the pancreas. The surgeon removes not only the gallbladder but also the pancreatic carcinoma.

Because Mr A did not give explicit permission for the removal of part of his pancreas, could he successfully sue in battery on the grounds that he did not give this consent?

The incidental finding

Mrs B has acute abdominal pain. A diagnosis of appendicitis is made, and Mrs B gives her consent for surgery, including removal of her appendix. At operation, the surgeon discovers that, in addition to an acutely inflamed appendix, Mrs B also has an ovarian tumour. This tumour is not likely to have contributed to her acute abdominal pain. The surgeon considers that it is in Mrs B's best interests for the ovary containing the tumour to be removed. She therefore removes it. Could the surgeon be successfully sued for battery on the grounds that Mrs B did not give explicit permission for her ovary and ovarian tumour to be removed? Would it make any difference if Mrs B had explicitly given her consent for any procedure that the surgeon deemed, at surgery, to be in her best interests?

REFERENCES

A Local Authority v Mr and Mrs A [2010] EWHC 1549 (Fam).

Chatterton v Gerson [1981] QB 432.

Devi v West Midlands Regional Health Authority [1980] CLY 687.

Everett, S. M., Griffiths, H., Nandasoma, U., Ayres, K., Bell, G., Cohen, M., Thomas-Gibson, S., Thomson, M. and Naylor, K. M. 2016. "Guideline for obtaining valid consent for gastrointestinal endoscopy procedures." *Gut* 65: 1585-601.

Faden, R. R., Beauchamp, T. L. and King, N. M. P. 1986. *A history and theory of informed consent*. New York; Oxford: Oxford University Press.

General Medical Council. 2008. "Consent: patients and doctors making decisions together." https://www.gmc-uk.org/ethical -guidance/ethical-guidance-for-doctors /consent/part-2-making-decisions-about -investigations-and-treatment.

Gibson, E. and Downie, J. 2012. "Consent requirements for pelvic examinations performed for training purposes." *CMAJ: Canadian Medical Association Journal = Journal de l'Association Medicale Canadienne* 184 (10): 1159-61. doi: 10.1503/cmaj.110725.

Herring, J., Fulford, K., Dunn, M. and Handa, A. 2017. "Elbow room for best practice? Montgomery, patients' values, and balanced decision-making in person-centred clinical care." *Medical Law Review* 25 (4): 582-603. doi: 10.1093/medlaw/fwx029.

Kermode-Scott, B. 2012. "Canadian trainees could be accused of "battery" for performing pelvic examinations under anaesthesia, say legal analysts." *BMJ* 344: e2426. doi: 10.1136/bmj.e2426.

Lidz, C. W. 1984. *Informed consent: a study of decision making in psychiatry*. New York, NY: Guilford Press.

Marshall v Curry [1933] 3 DLR 260.

Montgomery v Lanarkshire Health Board [2015] UKSC 11.

Murray v McMurchy [1949] 2 DLR 442.

Rogers vs Whittaker [1992] HCA 58; 175 CLR 479.

Schloendorff v Society of New York Hospital [1914] 105 NE 92.

Shaw, A. S. J. 2005. "Do we really know the law about students and patient consent?" *BMJ* 331: 522.

Chapter 7

Capacity

Case 7.1

Ms W was a 26 year-old who had a history of mental illness and repeated self-harm. She called an ambulance and was admitted to hospital after she took ethylene glycol (anti-freeze) with the aim of ending her life. On previous occasions, Ms W had accepted medical treatment; however, on this occasion she refused all treatment except comfort measures.

At the time of presenting to hospital, Ms W was conscious, alert and able to communicate her wishes, and persisted in her requests not to receive treatment for the ethylene glycol overdose (which would save her life). She also gave the doctors a signed 'advance directive', prepared three days beforehand, which set out her clear wish not to be treated.

Should the doctors respect Ms W's wishes?

This case is based on that of Kerrie Wooltorton (Szawarski 2013).

Capacity refers to the ability to give or withhold consent. (The term 'competence' is sometimes used interchangeably with capacity, but the latter term is used in the Mental Capacity Act and is the one that we will use in this book.) There is a fundamental difference between the way the law deals with patients with capacity and those without (Fig. 7.1).

Patients with capacity have the right to refuse treatment. It is generally unlawful for a doctor to treat a patient who has capacity without their consent,

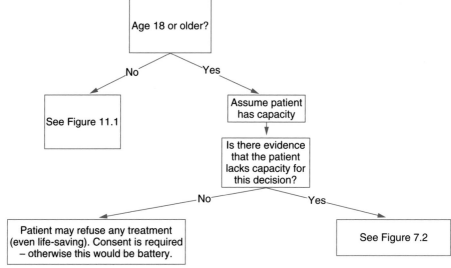

Figure 7.1 Capacity and decisions

even if, without that treatment, they will die, or even if the doctor believes the patient is making a mistake. Ms W's doctors received legal advice that, if she had capacity, it would not be lawful for them to treat her against her wishes. (Note that one question in cases like that of Ms W is whether the Mental Health Act rather than the Mental Capacity Act applies. See further discussion in Chapter 8).

The case of a patient who lacks capacity is more complex and needs more detailed consideration (see below). In brief, patients lacking capacity should be treated in their best interests. The legal concept of best interests, as we shall see, puts a great deal of weight on patients' previous views when they had capacity, including any advance decisions that they have made, and including the views of any proxy decision-makers that they have appointed.

In the first part of this chapter, we will discuss how to determine whether the patient lacks capacity. Then, in the second part, we will consider how decisions should be made for patients who lack capacity.

DOES THE PATIENT LACK CAPACITY?

A patient lacks capacity under the Mental Capacity Act if 'because of an impairment of, or a disturbance in the functioning of, the mind or brain' they are unable to understand the information relevant to the decision; weigh it and retain it; and use it to communicate their decision. Note that, under the Act, a person is presumed to have mental capacity. This means a doctor should treat a patient as though they have capacity unless there is clear evidence they do not (Fig. 7.1). Doctors should not assume a patient lacks capacity simply on the basis of advanced age or their appearance. The Act also says that it is wrong to conclude that a patient lacks capacity simply because they are making an unwise decision.

In English law, a person becomes an adult on his or her 18th birthday. The Mental Capacity Act, however, applies to anyone aged 16 years and over. This means that, in relation to 16- and 17-year-olds, there is an overlap between the Act and common law. The law on consent to medical treatment with regard to those aged under 18 years ('minors') is rather more complex than that for adults (see Chapter 11).

The approach to capacity endorsed by both law and most ethical analyses (see Buchanan and Brock 1989) is what is known as the 'functional' approach. This focuses on the process by which the person comes to the particular decision or carries out a particular task at a particular time. One implication of this approach is that capacity is not all or nothing. A person may, at the same point in time, have capacity to make some decisions (e.g. whether to take a particular medication) but not others (e.g. whether she is capable of living alone).

Elements of capacity

Buchanan and Brock distinguished three central elements to capacity:
1. Understanding and communication
2. Reasoning and deliberation
3. The person must have a 'set of values or conception of the good'.

The first element is needed to ensure that the person can become informed and express a choice. This in turn requires cognitive (intellectual) abilities. The understanding requires not only an 'intellectual' understanding but also 'the ability to appreciate the nature and meaning of potential alternatives – what it would be like and "feel" like to be in possible future states …' (Buchanan and Brock 1989, p. 24).

The second element requires sufficient short-term memory to retain the relevant information and allow the process of decision-making to take place.

The third element, the set of values, is necessary for someone to weigh up the pros and cons of different alternatives and reach a decision.

Assessing capacity

There are many situations in which doctors need to assess a patient's capacity. Some involve situations (as in Ms W's case) where it is important to know if the patient has capacity to consent to (or refuse) treatment. Other situations involve assessment outside the clinical context: for example, the doctor may be asked to assess a person's capacity to make a will.

The first two elements of Buchanan and Brock's analysis were effectively incorporated into English common law, eg Re C (Adult: Refusal of Treatment) [1994], and with slight amendment form the current four legal criteria for capacity specified in the Mental Capacity Act (see Box 7.1, which also summarizes other key legal principles relating to capacity).

Here are four steps to assessing capacity that incorporate the ethical and legal considerations discussed above.

Box 7.1 Some key legal principles relating to capacity

The legal criteria for capacity (Mental Capacity Act 2005)

A person lacks capacity if 'he is unable to make a decision for himself in relation to the matter in question because of an impairment of, or a disturbance in, the functioning of the mind or brain' (Section 2(1)).

A person is unable to make a decision (i.e. lacks capacity) if he or she is unable (Section 3(1)):

- to *understand* the information relevant to the decision
- to *retain* that information
- to *use or weigh* that information as part of the process of making the decision, or
- to *communicate* his or her decision (whether by talking, by using sign language or by any other means).

An imprudent decision is not, by itself, sufficient grounds for incapacity

A person should not be regarded as lacking capacity merely because she is making a decision that is unwise or against her best interests (see Section 1(4) of the Mental Capacity Act 2005). An unwise decision might alert a doctor to the need for assessment of capacity, but that assessment must be made by analyzing the way the decision is made (see text), not from the decision itself.

Capacity is 'issue-specific'

Capacity is not assessed 'globally'. One can only talk of capacity to do a particular thing. Thus, a patient may have capacity to make a will, but lack capacity to consent, or refuse consent to a particular operation (or vice versa). Indeed, a patient may have capacity to consent to one type of treatment, but not to another.

The standard of proof is the 'balance of probabilities'

The usual standard for proof in civil cases is 'balance of probabilities', as opposed to 'beyond reasonable doubt'. Thus, in assessing capacity, courts will be concerned with whether, on the balance of probabilities, the patient has or lacks capacity (see Section 2(4) of the Mental Capacity Act 2005).

The presumption of capacity

An adult is presumed capable of doing something until the contrary is proven by acceptable evidence. The onus of proof therefore lies with showing that someone does not have capacity (see Section 1(2) of the Mental Capacity Act 2005).

The presumption of continuance

Once incapacity has been established, it is presumed to continue until the contrary is proven by acceptable evidence.

Capacity is, ultimately, a legal, not a medical, decision

'... it is for the court to decide [*the question of capacity*], although the court must have the evidence of experts in the medical profession who can indicate the meaning of symptoms and give some idea of the mental deterioration which takes place in cases of this kind' (Mr Justice Neville in Richmond v Richmond [1914]).

In practice, courts usually take considerable notice of doctors' assessments of capacity.

> **Box 7.1** Some key legal principles relating to capacity — cont'd
>
> **Enhancing capacity**
>
> Under the Mental Capacity Act 2005, doctors (and other carers) have a duty to ensure that information is given in the most appropriate way (such as using simple language and visual aids, if helpful), and that steps are taken to try to enhance the patient's capacity (for example, by providing a quiet comfortable setting in which to talk with the patient).

Step 1: Identify the information relevant to the decision

Capacity is specific to a particular decision. The first step in assessing capacity is to clarify what information is critically relevant to making the decision. The critically relevant information includes the information that is needed to understand, in broad terms, what would be involved in carrying out a decision.

Step 2: Assess cognitive ability

a. Understanding and believing the relevant information

Does the person have sufficient intellectual ability to understand the various aspects of the critically relevant information? For example, did Ms W understand what would happen if she did not receive medical treatment for ethylene glycol poisoning? She had written in her advance directive:

'Please be assured that I am 100% aware of the consequences of this and the probable outcome of drinking anti-freeze, e.g. death in 95–99% of cases and if I survive then kidney failure, I understand and accept them and will take 100% responsibility for this decision.'

The standard should not be set too high. Most healthy people without learning disability have the capacity to make decisions about their own health care and to understand the main points at issue.

A person may understand the information presented but not be capable of believing it because, for example, of a relevant delusion or other mental disorder. If this is the case, then he or she might lack capacity. Patients should not, however, generally be judged as lacking capacity simply because they do not believe the information from the doctor, for example, through scepticism about professionally based knowledge or a strong belief in complementary therapies. The key question will be whether the delusion means they fail to understand the basic nature of the procedure. A patient whose mental disorder meant they did not believe they had cancer would not have capacity to refuse treatment for cancer. However, a patient who understood fully what the treatment was, but refused because of a religious belief that they would be healed by prayer, would have capacity.

b. Retain the information

Can the person *retain* the information long enough to use it to come to a decision? Severe memory impairment, even in the absence of other intellectual deficits, may mean that someone lacks capacity for a specific task. If Ms W had a reduced state of consciousness at the time of presenting to hospital, she might not have been able to remember information she was being told, and thus lack capacity (this didn't appear to be an issue in the actual case).

c. Use or weigh the information and make a choice

Does the person have *sufficient ability* to weigh up the relevant information? Again, the standard for this should not be set too high.

d. Is the person able to communicate the decision?

Many patients, for example following stroke, may have difficulty communicating their views and decisions, even though they have the capacity to make their own decisions. It is therefore important in assessing capacity to make every effort to ensure that difficulties in communication are overcome. This may involve a careful and patient approach to listening to the patient, or using writing if the problem is primarily one of speech difficulty. If, despite all reasonable attempts to enable the patient to communicate her decision, she is unable to do so, then, according the Mental Capacity Act, she should be regarded as lacking capacity.

Step 3: Assess other factors that may interfere with capacity

Cognitive impairment is only one factor that may interfere with the three elements of information processing. Other causes that need to be specifically addressed include:

Mental illness

Ms W had a history of depression and a personality disorder. Did this mean that she lacked capacity to refuse treatment?

As already, noted, a *delusion* may interfere with *believing* the information. However, the fact that a person has delusional beliefs, for example as part of schizophrenia, does not necessarily mean that person lacks capacity for a particular decision. The delusion would have to interfere with the understanding, believing or decision-making process specific to the particular decision.

An *affective illness* (depression or mania) may interfere with the weighing-up of information and coming to a decision. For example, a person suffering from a depressive disorder may refuse beneficial treatment because she does not feel herself to be worthy of treatment.

It can be difficult to assess the effect of mental illness on capacity to make a particular decision. When in doubt, it may be helpful to ask: is the decision likely to be different from what the person would decide if free from mental disorder? In Ms W's case, the on-call doctor believed that she did have capacity, and the coroner ultimately supported that assessment. (Treatment was withheld as requested, and she died the day after presenting to hospital.)

Step 4: Can capacity be enhanced?

A person's capacity to make a decision depends not only on the person, but also on the environment. The assessment of capacity must not be treated like a school exam. If patient autonomy is to be properly respected, doctors should try to enable patients to have the capacity to make decisions. This might be done in several ways:

- By treating any mental disorder that affects capacity and any physical disorder (such as a urinary tract disorder) that may be causing an acute confusional state.
- If capacity is likely to improve, wait, if possible, until it does improve to allow the patient to be properly involved in decisions.
- Be aware of the possibility that medication may adversely affect capacity.
- If capacity fluctuates (e.g. it depends on the time of day), assess capacity and discuss treatment, if appropriate, when the patient is at her best.
- If there is a need to assess capacity for different tasks or decisions, assess these separately.
- Choose the environment that maximizes the patient's capacity, including minimizing distractions such as excessive noise.
- Consider whether the person might be helped if a relative or friend is with her.
- Allow the person time to take in and process information.
- Make explanations simple, and use written information and diagrams where these are likely to be helpful.

The Mental Capacity Act 2005 places on health professionals a duty to enhance capacity if possible and to enable decision-making. These include the duty not to treat a person as unable to make a decision unless all practicable steps to help him to do so have been taken without success (Section 1(3)).

MAKING DECISIONS FOR PEOPLE WHO LACK CAPACITY

The ethical approach to people who lack capacity

There are four theoretically possible approaches to making decisions about the health care of patients who lack capacity (Buchanan & Brock 1989):

1. Best interests
2. Substituted judgement
3. Proxy
4. Advance directives.

Best interests

One approach for a doctor faced with a patient lacking capacity is to ask which plan of management serves the patient's best interests. In Chapter 3 we outlined different approaches to the question of what is in a person's best interests. These different approaches will give different answers to the question of what is in a person's best interests in some clinical situations (see Case 3.1). Sometimes different people will have different views about what would be in the patient's best interests (Wilkinson and Savulescu 2018).

Substituted judgement

The criterion of substituted judgement asks the following hypothetical question: if the patient were (magically) able to gain capacity, what decision would he or she make? In order to try to answer this question, the doctor could use a range of evidence, such as reports of what the patient has said about this kind of situation in the past; the kind of general values the patient held; and experience with other patients.

Proxy

An alternative approach is for someone else (a proxy) to be appointed to make decisions on behalf of the patient. For example, the patient could ask someone they trust to make decisions for them when the time comes. Such an approach of course leaves the proxy with the question: how should they decide?

Advance directives

Finally, in some circumstances, it is possible to know exactly what the patient would have wanted (without having to exercise our imagination, or without having someone stand in for them) because they have made it clear in advance. Advance directives are statements made by people, at a time when they have capacity, about how they would want to be treated in the future if they were to lose the capacity (Fig. 7.2). Such directives might be more or less explicit. There are various synonyms for advance directives, for example: living wills, advance decisions and advance statements. See Up for Debate Box 7.1 for arguments in support of and against advance directives.

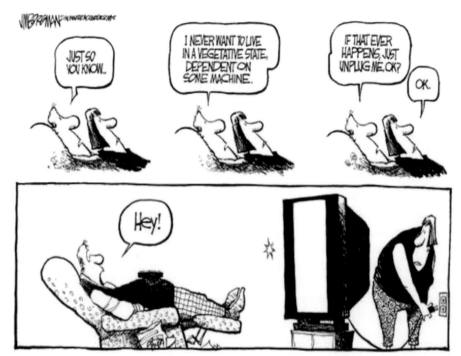

Figure 7.2 Advance directive (© Jim Bergman, reproduced with permission)

Up for Debate Box 7.1 Should advance directives be respected?

For

1. Modern medical ethics places strong emphasis on patient autonomy. We normally think that patients' wishes about treatment should be respected, if possible. Advance directives respect and extend patient autonomy. They provide the strongest and clearest evidence of the patient's wishes.

2. People often worry about what will happen to them if they become unwell and are unable to express their wishes. Evidence from the US suggests that many patients become less anxious about the possibility of unwanted treatments if they have an advance directive, and doctors who have had experience with advance directives have usually found them helpful.

3. Advance directives may lower health care costs, because in many circumstances they indicate that patients would want less aggressive treatment than they would otherwise receive.

Against

1. Patients may not be able to imagine what life would be like if they were (for example) to become unwell or disabled and lose capacity. They may have overly negative (or positive) impressions about future illness, and thus their advance directive may not be fully informed.

2. Advance directives are sometimes either too vague or too specific. The statements made in the directive will need to be interpreted when applied to the specific situation. The patient's actual condition may be different from that implied by any of the statements in the advance directive. (For example, a patient may indicate that they do not wish for certain treatments if they develop dementia. But what if they have a stroke? Does their statement apply to that?)

3. The person might have changed her mind since making the decision (and while still having capacity), without altering the directive.

4. The person themself may have changed substantially since the advance directive was written. Does the old advance directive apply to the new (changed) person (see Case 2.2)?

THE LEGAL APPROACH TO ADULTS WHO LACK CAPACITY

As we have seen, a procedure can be undertaken on a patient with capacity only with that patient's consent.

With regard to adults lacking capacity, current law uses elements from all four of the approaches outlined above (Fig. 7.3).

For people aged 16 years and over, the main relevant statute is the Mental Capacity Act 2005 (MCA; Box 7.2). If there is no *Lasting Power of Attorney* (see below), and the patient has not made an *advance decision* (see below), then doctors have the duty to assess what is in a patient's best interests (see Chapter 3).

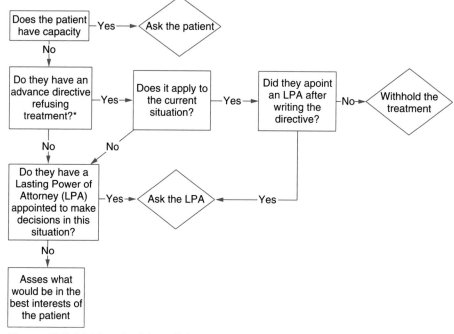

Figure 7.3 Making decisions if the patient lacks capacity

Box 7.2 Overview of the Mental Capacity Act 2005

1. The Act came into force in 2007.
2. It applies to people aged 16 years and over.
3. The Act applies primarily to those who lack capacity. It states, however, that 'a person is not to be treated as unable to make a decision unless all practicable steps to help him to do so have been taken without success'. The Act also states that '[a] person is not to be treated as unable to make a decision merely because he makes an unwise decision'.
4. The Act covers the following areas:
   - It provides the legal criteria for *lack of capacity* (see Box 7.1).
   - It provides the legal definition of *best interests* (see Chapter 3).
   - It states that doctors have a *duty to consult friends and relatives* of a patient in order to help determine the patient's best interests, if this is practicable and appropriate. The doctor must also consult a person named in any Lasting Power of Attorney, or any Deputy appointed by the court.
   - It provides for a person, when competent, to appoint a *Lasting Power of Attorney.*
   - It provides for a person, when competent, to create an *advance decision to refuse treatment.*
   - It gives some *legal protection* to doctors and other carers in their determination of a patient's best interests.
   - It created the Court of Protection to make decisions relating to the MCA, if necessary.

Case 7.2

Mr B was a 73-year-old man who lived alone and had no significant family or friends. He had long-standing schizophrenia, as well as diabetes. He had a diabetic foot ulcer and had been an inpatient in acute and rehabilitation hospitals for over a year. Mr B was refusing all treatment for the foot ulcer apart from dressings, and had developed gangrene of his foot. His doctors wished to perform a below-knee amputation, and believed that without this he would soon develop septicaemia and die. Mr B expressed that he was not afraid of dying and was strongly opposed to surgery. He had been assessed to lack capacity.

This case is based on that of Wye Valley NHS Trust v B (Rev 1) [2015].

Best interests assessment for a patient lacking capacity

When making a decision about someone's best interest, the law requires the issues to be considered from the perspective of the patient. As Lady Hale in Aintree University Hospital NHS Foundation Trust v. James [2013] put it:

'The purpose of the best interests test is to consider matters from the patient's point of view. That is not to say that his wishes must prevail, any more than those of a fully capable patient must prevail. We cannot always have what we want. Nor will it always be possible to ascertain what an incapable patient's wishes are. … But in so far as it is possible to ascertain the patient's wishes and feelings, his beliefs and values or the things which were important to him, it is those which should be taken into account because they are a component in making the choice which is right for him as an individual human being.'

The MCA lists factors that should be taken into account in deciding what is in a person's best interests:
- The person's current wishes and feelings
- Their past wishes and feelings
- Beliefs, values and other matters that would have influenced them if they had capacity.

In assessing best interests, the MCA gives a great deal of weight to what the person would have wanted (i.e. this is a substituted judgement) and to any statements made by the person, when competent, about how they wish to be treated. These could take the form of specific written refusals of treatment (i.e. advance directives – see below), or expressions of the patient's views, preferences and wishes (these are referred to as advance statements).

If the person lacking capacity is able to express their views, these will be taken into account too, although they do not have the right to refuse treatment. In Mr B's case, the judge, Justice Peter Jackson, was heavily influenced by Mr B's views about treatment. He also took into account his long-standing fierce independence and strong desire not to go into a nursing home (which appeared inevitable if he had an amputation). The judge concluded that it would not be in Mr B's interests to perform the amputation.

It is, of course, frequently the case that the patient never considered and never spoke about what she would have wanted in the circumstances that have arisen. It is therefore often not possible for doctors, or for relatives and friends, to judge best interests on the basis of what the person would have wanted. In such cases, some judgement has to be made on the basis of external judgements about what is in the person's best interests. Such judgement might, for example, be based on the 'mental state theory' of best interests (see Chapter 3) and be a judgement about the patient's likely quality of life, given different management options.

The Act recognizes the difficulties in judging the best interests of an incompetent patient and provides protection (s.4(9)) to a person (e.g. a doctor) who acts or makes a decision in the reasonable belief that he is doing so in the best interests of the person who lacks capacity. A doctor must be able to point to objective reasons to demonstrate why he believed he was acting in the person's best interests, and, even if it is subsequently shown that a doctor was mistaken in his opinion of best interests, he will still receive the protection of the Act, providing that it was a reasonable decision.

There are special elements of the MCA that apply if a patient lacking capacity needs to be restrained or prevented from leaving a place of treatment (see Box 7.3).

Box 7.3 Restraint and deprivation of liberty

Restraint

There are circumstances when doctors, or other carers, believe that it would be in the best interests of a patient who lacks capacity to use threats or force in order to impose treatment on them. Such use of threats or force is called *restraint*. Restraint could be physical (e.g. being held down or shackled), chemical (e.g. medication), mechanical (a locked door) or psychological. For such restraint to be lawful, two conditions must be satisfied (Section 6 of the MCA): first, the doctor reasonably believes it to be necessary *in order to prevent harm* to the patient; and second, the use of restraint must be *proportionate* (it should be the least restrictive way of avoiding that harm).

Deprivation of liberty

In other circumstances, health professionals or carers believe that it is in the best interests of a patient to prevent them leaving a health care (or other) environment. A deprivation of liberty is defined as a situation where a patient is under continuous supervision and control by staff and is not free to leave. A deprivation of liberty must be approved either by a court order or under the Deprivation of Liberty Safeguards (DOLS) procedures in Schedule A1 of the 2005 Act. Under Schedule A1 of the 2005 Act, a supervisory body can authorize the deprivation of a resident's liberty only if it is in the best interests of the individual concerned, and if the detention is a proportionate response to any harm, given its likelihood and severity. The difference between 'restraint' and 'deprivation of liberty' is one of degree or intensity. While the ethical justification for deprivation of liberty is the same as restraint, there are additional safeguards built in. For example, patients (or their representatives) can appeal against a deprivation of their liberty.

The law in Scotland is different from that in England and Wales with regard to incompetent patients aged 16 years and over and with regard to children (see Chapter 11). The Mental Health (Care and Treatment) Act 2003 governs some aspects of consent in Scotland (see Chapter 8).

The role of the family

> **Case 7.3**
>
> Mrs R is a 71-year-old woman who sustained a severe hypoxic brain injury following an out-of-hospital cardiac arrest. She has been on the medical ward for more than three months, and it is believed that she is in a minimally conscious state. The medical team have been communicating with her family, but there are different opinions. Her partner believes that she would not wish to be kept alive in her current condition. Her estranged husband (they never divorced, but have been separated for more than 10 years) wishes for treatment to continue. Several siblings have strong religious views that life-prolonging treatment should be provided for Mrs R. (Mrs R was religious in the past, but no longer attended church.)
> Should the family's wishes be followed? Which ones?

When patients are not capable of making decisions for themselves, clinicians usually involve families or close friends. The MCA imposes a legal duty on doctors to consult a range of people when determining the best interests of a person who lacks capacity. Section 4(7) states that the decision-makers (e.g. doctors and other health professionals) must take into account, if it is practicable and appropriate to consult them, the views of:

- anyone named by the person as someone to be consulted on the matter in question or on matters of that kind
- anyone engaged in caring for the person or interested in his or her welfare
- any person appointed as a Lasting Power of Attorney
- any deputy appointed by the court.

There are five different types of information that patients' relatives might provide:
1. Explicit instructions that the patient had given to the family.
2. A general view of the patient's values.
3. Information about the patient's quality of life and likely quality of life. Relatives are often in a better position than doctors to judge these issues.
4. The relatives' opinion of what is best for the patient.
5. The relatives' opinion as to what is best for themselves.

The MCA cites the importance of consultation and, in particular, gathering evidence of the person's past and present wishes and feelings, beliefs and values, to help assess what would be in the person's best interests. Elements 1–3 in the above list are obviously relevant. In Case 7.3, the various family members might be providing evidence of Mrs R's wishes. Those who had been closest to her (particularly in recent times) might be expected to have most relevant information relating to that.

The views of family members (element 4) as to what would be in the patient's best interests can be considered, though they would not necessarily have great weight in the assessment of an adult's best interests. It would seem a mistake, for example, to include the religious values of family members in an assessment of Mrs R's interests if she no longer shared those values. The interests of family members themselves (element 5) are not usually considered to be part of an assessment of the patient's best interests.

Having said that, if a particular management decision will go strongly against the interests of the relatives, it is less likely in the long run to be in the best interests of the patient. Furthermore, it is important to many people that they should not become a burden to their families (Lindemann and Nelson 1995). So there may be a degree of overlap between the interests of the patient and that of the family.

For patients who lack capacity and who do not have any family members or friends to consult, and where there are serious treatment decisions to be made, an 'Independent Mental Capacity Advocate' should be appointed and consulted.

Lasting Power of Attorney (LPA)

Section 9 of the MCA introduces the provision for a Lasting Power of Attorney (LPA). This allows people to appoint someone (or more than one person) to act as a proxy decision-maker for them if they lose capacity. There are two different types of LPA that can be appointed: an LPA for property and financial affairs, and an LPA for Health and Welfare. As the names suggest, these cover different types of decisions, and only a Health and Welfare LPA can make health care decisions.

An LPA for Health and Welfare can consent to (or decline consent for) medical treatment. If they have been specifically authorized by the patient, that can include decisions about life-sustaining treatment.

Doctors may, in some circumstances, choose not to follow the LPA's decision. They could do this if they believe that the LPA is not acting in the patient's best interests.

If a patient has not appointed an LPA, the Court of Protection can appoint a Deputy to make health care decisions on behalf of the patient (family members can apply to be appointed a deputy).

In Scotland, there is also provision for proxy consent for incompetent adults.

Advance decisions

Sections 24–26 of the MCA set out the provisions that enable competent adults aged 18 years and over to make advance decisions to refuse treatment. An advance decision must specify the treatment that is to be refused, and will apply only at a time when the patient lacks capacity. Note that advance decisions do not empower patients to demand a particular treatment, but only to refuse treatment. (This is the same as the situation for patients with capacity - they can refuse, but not demand, treatment.)

Except in the case of life-sustaining treatment, advance decisions can be oral or written.

The formalities required for an advance decision to refuse life-sustaining treatment under the MCA are that:

1. the advance decision must be in writing
2. it must be signed
3. the signature must be witnessed
4. the document must be verified by a specific statement expressly stating that the advance decision is to apply 'even if life is at risk'
5. the specific statement must also be signed by the maker and witnessed.

(In the case of Ms W. (case 7.1), her advance decision did not take the above form, so would not have legal force under statutory law, though it might be included as relevant within a best interests assessment.)

An advance decision may be invalid in certain circumstances (Section 25), including: if the patient has withdrawn the decision (while she had capacity to do so), if the patient has overridden the advance decision by subsequently creating an LPA that covers the decision in question or if the patient has done something inconsistent with the advance decision.

It is likely that many advance decisions will be relevant to the circumstances that actually arise, but their application is not always straightforward. Doctors will need to exercise considerable judgement in interpreting advance decisions that are ambiguous in their application to the situation that arises. An advance decision may not be applicable if the circumstances are different than those specified, or if there are reasonable grounds for believing that the patient's circumstances have changed in ways that would have affected their advance decision (Section 25(4)). There are further issues that are not explicitly stated in the Act but that must, in our view, be relevant to the question of the validity of the advance decision. These are:

- Is the advance decision (whether written or reported by a friend or relative) genuinely that of the patient?
- Did the patient have capacity to make the decision at the time it was made?
- Was the patient in possession of the relevant facts at the time of making the decision?

The position in law, at least since the MCA, appears to be that, if a valid advance decision exists that covers the circumstances that have arisen, then it must be followed. The Code of Practice to the MCA states (clause 9.52): 'If healthcare professionals are satisfied that an advance decision to refuse treatment exists, is valid and applicable, they must follow it and not provide the treatment refused in the advance decision'. The difficulty for doctors will be to judge whether an advance directive is valid. As we have seen, the Act says (Section 25(4)) that the advance decision does not apply if there are 'reasonable grounds for believing that circumstances exist which [the patient] did not anticipate at the time of the advance decision and which would have affected his decision had he anticipated them' then.

As regards Scotland, the position is less clear, mainly because the Adults with Incapacity (Scotland) Act 2000 does not deal directly with the issue of advance decisions to refuse treatment. The Act does, however, state that account shall be taken of the present and past wishes of the adult when interventionist activity is being taken (Section 1(4)). This provision presumably allows for a valid advance decision to refuse treatment to be determinative.

REVISION QUESTIONS

1. What does 'capacity' refer to? Why does it matter?
2. You have been asked to assess whether an elderly patient is able to consent for surgery. How would you go about doing that?
3. A patient has a history of mental illness and is refusing treatment. Should their refusal be respected?
4. An adult patient lacks capacity. Can their next of kin consent for surgery on their behalf?
5. A patient both has an advance directive and has appointed a Lasting Power of Attorney. Which should you follow?
6. A patient has an advance decision stating that, in the event of a cardiac arrest, they would want full resuscitation, including intensive care admission. Should their doctor follow that instruction?

Extension case 7.4

In an elderly care home, some patients with dementia have electronic tags attached to them so that nurses can be notified if they leave the care home, and they can then be located and brought back. Some staff members are concerned that this tagging is similar to electronic monitoring of prisoners or those on probation.

Does this represent a deprivation of liberty? Is it ethically justified?

Read about restraint and ethics in dementia:

Hughes and Louw (2002), Foster, Herring, and Doron (2014), Robinson et al. (2007).

REFERENECES

Aintree University Hospital NHS Foundation Trust v. James [2013] UKSC 67.

Buchanan, A. E. and Brock, D. W. 1989. *Deciding for others: the ethics of surrogate decision making, Studies in philosophy and health policy*. Cambridge: Cambridge University Press.

Foster, C., Herring, J. and Doron I. (Eds). 2014. *Law and ethics of dementia*. Oxford: Hart.

Hughes, J. C. and Louw, S. J. 2002. "Electronic tagging of people with dementia who wander." *BMJ* 325: 847-8.

Lindemann, H. and Lindemann Nelson, J. 1995. *The patient in the family: an ethics of medicine and families*. New York; London: Routledge.

Re C (Adult: Refusal of Treatment) [1994] 1 WLR 290.

Richmond v Richmond [1914] III LT 273.

Robinson, L., Hutchings, D., Corner, L., Finch, T., Hughes, J., Brittain, K. and Bond, J. 2007. "Balancing rights and risks: Conflicting perspectives in the management of wandering in dementia." *Health, Risk & Society* 9 (4): 389-406. doi: 10.1080/13698570701612774.

Szawarski, P. 2013. "Classic cases revisited: the suicide of Kerrie Wooltorton." *Journal of Intensive Care Society* 14 (3): 211-4.

Wilkinson, D. and Savulescu, J. 2018. *Ethics, conflict and medical treatment for children: from disagreement to dissensus*. Elsevier.

Wye Valley NHS Trust v B [2015] EWCOP 60.

Chapter **8**

Mental health

Case 8.1 (this is an extension of Case 7.1)

Ms W was a 26-year-old who had a history of mental illness and repeated self-harm. She was admitted to hospital after she took ethylene glycol (anti-freeze) with the aim of ending her life. Ms W refused all treatment except comfort measures.

Ms W was judged to have capacity, and thus could legally refuse treatment; however, it was anticipated that this posed a serious risk of harm to her (she would potentially die).

Should her doctors have provided involuntary treatment for Ms W on the basis of mental illness?

This case is based on that of Kerrie Wooltorton (Szawarski 2013).

Most countries have legal mechanisms that are designed specifically for people with mental disorder (Koch, Reiter-Theil, and Helmchen 1996). In England and Wales the major statute is the Mental Health Act 1983 (amended by the Mental Health Act 2007), and in Scotland it is the Mental Health (Care and Treatment) (Scotland) Act 2003. These Acts have two main functions: they enable the state to enforce hospital admission for the assessment and treatment of patients with mental disorder that go beyond the powers of common law; and they provide mechanisms, including appeal mechanisms, designed to ensure that such powers are not misused. Could mental health legislation be invoked to treat Ms W in Case 8.1?

One first question is why there is separate legislation for patients with mental illness. Under common law (see Chapters 6 and 7) a patient with mental capacity can refuse treatment. This provides legal protection for individual patient autonomy. If a patient lacks capacity, they cannot refuse treatment, and the Mental Capacity Act (MCA) supports treatment of the patient in his best interests.

Why is anything more needed for patients with mental disorder? If, despite the mental disorder, the patient has capacity, should he or she not have the same right to refuse treatment as any other patient? On the other hand, if the patient lacks capacity, then he can be treated under common law in his best interests. Some may feel that a special legal regime for those with mental illness is a form of disability discrimination.

JUSTIFYING A MENTAL HEALTH ACT

The major problem with relying on the MCA alone is that a medical professional may wish to provide treatment for a person with a mental disorder who is posing a threat to themselves or others. However, the MCA only allows treatment without consent in cases where the patient lacks mental capacity. So, it cannot be used in cases where a person has a mental disorder, but has mental capacity. As is discussed in Chapter 7, the legal concept of capacity (to consent to or refuse treatment) has focused on whether a patient has the cognitive ability to understand and weigh up the key issues relevant to the decision. Mental illness can affect the process of decision-making other than through its effect on cognitive ability. A person suffering from moderate depressive illness may have good cognitive abilities. For example, she may be able to understand, believe and retain all the issues relevant to a decision about treatment. However, the illness may affect her ability to weigh up the issues, or may distort her values. She may refuse treatment because she thinks herself worthless. Once treated, and no longer suffering from depressive illness, her values may change such that she is then pleased that her refusal was overridden. It would be unacceptably paternalistic for a doctor to override a patient's choice merely because she disagreed with the patient's decision. However, if the patient's decision appears to be the result of a treatable mental illness, there is a potentially good reason to override their choice. Fig. 8.1 displays the different approaches to treatment refusal.

English law takes the approach that it is right to override a patient's refusal on the combined grounds that it is in her best interests to do so and that she is suffering from a mental illness (at least with regard to the treatment of the mental illness itself). A person can be treated for the mental disorder under the Mental Health Act (MHA) even though she has capacity.

The problem with this approach is that it discriminates between those who are mentally ill and those who are physically ill (Dickenson and Savulescu 1998). One alternative would be to allow a patient's refusal of treatment to be overridden only if the patient lacks the capacity to refuse. This would ensure consistency between the Mental Health Act and the MCA. But, as the example of moderate depressive illness suggests, it would require a more sophisticated account to be given of how people might lack capacity than the common law currently uses.

In Ms W's case, she was assessed through the lens of mental capacity, and treatment was withheld because she was judged to have capacity. However, some

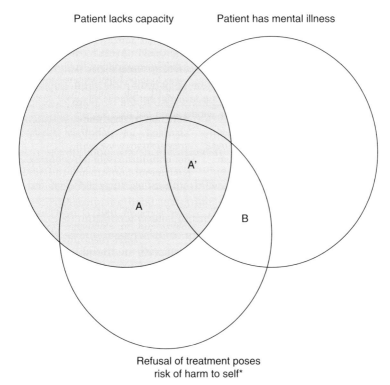

Patient lacks capacity   Patient has mental illness

A'

A

B

Refusal of treatment poses
risk of harm to self*

Figure 8.1 Refusal of treatment – two different justifications for doctors enforcing treatment. If the patient lacks capacity and treatment refusal would risk harm to the patient (i.e. treatment would be in their best interests), treatment may be provided (this corresponds to regions A and A' in the figure). If the patient has a mental illness, there is the possibility that treatment may be enforced (if refusal would risk harm to self) even if the patient has capacity (region B). Note, though, that the treatment would need to relate to the patient's mental disorder (and not an unrelated medical condition). (NB: It is not shown in this figure, but treatment can also be enforced because of risk of harm to others. See main text.)

commentators on the case have pointed out that, if she had been formally assessed by a psychiatrist, she might have been judged to have a treatable mental illness (David et al. 2010; Muzaffar 2011).

THE PROTECTION OF THE PATIENT OR THE PROTECTION OF OTHERS

There are two principal reasons for enforcing hospital treatment on a mentally disordered person. The first is for the sake of the person himself. The second is for the protection of others. The MHA tries, in one piece of legislation, to address these two quite distinct issues as though they can be approached in the same way. One justification for this is that, in practice, a mentally disordered person may pose a risk to both himself and others. A problem, however, is that the grounds that justify enforced hospital admission in the two situations are rather different.

If a doctor is overriding a patient's refusal of treatment for the sake of the patient himself, the ethical justification is paternalistic, and (often) based on reduced capacity. In contrast, if individuals pose a risk of harm to others, that is usually the business of the criminal law, and not of medicine. It may not seem appropriate to use the criminal law in the case of some mentally ill people, because, as a result of their mental illness, they are not responsible for their dangerous acts. The central ethical justification for invoking mental health involvement in the case of mental illness and risk to others is *responsibility*, rather than capacity.

Perhaps because of the mixed justification for intervention, the MHA makes little use of the concepts of either capacity or responsibility. The result is that it can be argued that the MHA discriminates against the mentally ill in two ways. In the first place, as we have seen, it enables a mentally disordered patient's refusal of treatment to be overridden, even though they might have capacity. In the second place, it gives society much wider powers to forcibly restrain, for the protection of others, mentally disordered people compared with those without mental disorder. For example, mentally disordered people, if they are considered to be dangerous, may be kept in a secure place for an indefinite period. Those without mental disorder cannot be kept in a secure place, however dangerous they are thought to be, if they have either not yet committed a crime, or have committed a crime and have served their prison sentence. For these reasons, it has sometimes been suggested that the MHA is inconsistent with the United National Convention on the Rights of Persons with Disability, which specifically prohibits discrimination against people on the basis of mental disorder (Szmukler and Weich 2017).

Of relevance, Northern Ireland passed a piece of legislation in 2016 that fuses the two pieces of legislation present in England and Wales. The Mental Capacity Act (Northern Ireland) justifies intervention on the basis only of impairment of decision-making capacity and best interests (Lynch, Taggart, and Campbell 2017).

THE MENTAL HEALTH ACT 1983

The most important aspects of the MHA are concerned with the issue of compulsory detention in hospital. There are three key facts about the MHA:

1. The Act is relevant only for a person with a mental disorder.
2. The Act is concerned only with the treatment (or assessment) of the mental disorder, and not with the treatment of an independent physical disorder (see Case 8.2).
3. The Act does not have to be used in cases where the patient lacks mental capacity. Such patients should be dealt with under the MCA 2005 (see Chapter 7).

Ms H was a 41-year-old woman with a history of paranoid schizophrenia. She was pregnant, and her fetus was growing poorly. She lacked capacity because of her schizophrenia. At week 37 of her pregnancy, Ms H's obstetrician wished to induce labour, but there was a concern that the fetus might become distressed, and an urgent caesarean section would then be required to save the fetus. Her psychiatrist believed that, if the fetus were to die, this would have a deleterious effect on Ms H's mental health.

Would restraint and treatment (including caesarean section if necessary) be justified?

This case is based on Tameside & Glossop Acute Services Unit v CH (a patient) [1996].

In the case of Ms H, the interests of her fetus did not have legal force (see Chapter 13). She lacked capacity, and thus treatment might be provided in her best interests. However, would caesarean section be regarded as treatment of an independent condition, or as something 'ancillary' to her mental illness? The court in this case concluded that caesarean section would be ancillary (i.e. related) to treatment for her mental illness. This is the same justification for treating self-inflicted injuries or overdoses in patients who have attempted self-harm.

(However, critics of the decision in the real case felt that the inclusion of obstetric treatment as 'ancillary treatment' was a distortion of the MHA; see, for example, Dolan and Parker 1997. See Chapter 13 for further discussion of forced caesarean section.)

Mental disorder

A key term in the MHA is 'mental disorder' (Box 8.1). There are four things to note:

1. The term 'mental illness' is not defined in the MHA, although its scope has been clarified to some extent by use and by subsequent guidelines. In practice, it would rarely be considered appropriate to detain a person suffering from a 'neurotic' disorder alone (e.g. agoraphobia or obsessive–compulsive disorder).

2. There are three important exclusions from mental disorder (see Box 8.1).

3. Learning disability (mental impairment) and psychopathic disorder meet the legal definition of mental disorder only when 'associated with abnormally aggressive or seriously irresponsible conduct'.

4. The final category ('any other disorder or disability of mind') allows considerable scope for invoking the MHA. However, a patient whose mental disorder fitted this category alone could only be admitted for assessment (section 2, up to 28 days), and not treatment (section 3). Furthermore, the three listed exclusions still apply (e.g. a person could not be committed on the grounds of substance use or paedophilia), and it cannot be used to justify compulsory admission simply on the grounds that a person is making a bad decision.

Box 8.1 The key term 'mental disorder' in the Mental Health Act

Five 'types' of mental disorder are distinguished in the MHA. One purpose in distinguishing these is that different types feature separately in some parts of the Act.

1. Mental illness

   This is not defined further in the Act, although there are guidelines (from the Department of Health) suggesting that this is either sustained cognitive impairment or, essentially, psychosis (delusions, hallucinations, disordered thinking).

2/3. Mental impairment/Severe mental impairment

   This is severe learning disability coupled with behavioural problems. The behavioural problems need not be caused by the 'mental impairment' (they need only be associated with it).

4. Psychopathic disorder

   'A persistent disorder or disability of mind (whether or not including significant impairment of intelligence) which results in abnormally aggressive or seriously irresponsible conduct on the part of the person concerned'.

5. 'Any other disorder or disability of mind'

   Something of a catch-all.

Three important exclusions (which, by themselves, would not count as a mental disorder):

1. Dependence on drugs and alcohol
2. Promiscuity (included because some people used to be detained in hospital because of sexually promiscuous behaviour)
3. Sexual deviancy

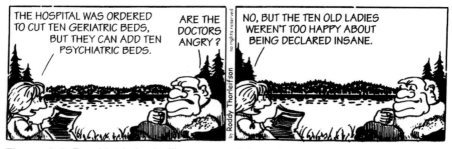

Figure 8.2 Psychiatric beds (From mooselakecartoons.com https://mooselakecartoons.com/medical/)

Compulsory detention in hospital (Fig. 8.2)

There are three necessary conditions for compulsory detention in hospital (although the precise details of these depend on which section of the Act is relevant):

1. The patient is suffering from a mental disorder.
2. The nature and degree of the mental disorder make it appropriate to receive treatment in a hospital for that disorder.
3. It is necessary, either for the health or safety of the patient or for the protection of others, that she be detained in hospital.

All three of these conditions are needed to justify admission. The powers under the MHA relevant to compulsory detention and treatment are summarized in Box 8.2. Sections 2, 3, 4 and 5 are particularly important.

A current presumption that is central to mental health legislation is that it aims to enable people to benefit from medical (psychiatric) care. Thus, if a person who suffers from a mental disorder (within the meaning of the MHA) is not treatable (for example because the person has an intractable severe personality disorder), then under the current MHA that person cannot be kept secure against his will.

There is some nuance to the definition of 'treatable'. A person might have a personality disorder of a type for which some psychological treatment is appropriate, but which in this person's case is not effective. Under the original 1983 Act, such a person could not be detained, because he did not pass the treatability test. A subtle change was made in the 2007 Act to allow compulsory detention in these circumstances. The political purpose was to increase the number of people who

---

Box 8.2 Summary of the powers under the Mental Health Act (MHA) to detain and treat patients in hospital without consent

Section 2: Admission for assessment

Provides for patients to be admitted to hospital for a period of up to 28 days. It usually applies to patients for whom the diagnosis is uncertain and a period of assessment is required (otherwise Section 3 would be used). However, assessment can probably also cover assessment of response to treatment. Deterioration in a patient's mental health is sufficient grounds – danger to self or others is not the only criterion.

An application for admission must be made by the patient's nearest relative or an approved social worker and supported by a recommendation by two registered medical practitioners. In practice, one of the doctors is normally the general practitioner and one a psychiatrist of specialist registrar or consultant status.

Section 3: Admission for treatment

This allows for longer periods of treatment (up to 6 months, and renewable). It is based on a diagnosis of a mental disorder as set out in the Act (see Box 8.1), but does not include the category 'any other disorder of mind'. Authorization is the same as for Section 2.

Section 4: Emergency admission

The purpose of this section is to arrange emergency compulsory admission (up to 72 hours) when there is no senior psychiatrist available within the time needed. It needs the approval of only the general practitioner (and applicant, e.g. social worker) to be applied. The use of this section should be kept to a minimum.

Section 5: Subsection 2: Detention of a patient already in hospital

A person may be a voluntary patient in hospital (usually in a psychiatric hospital) when her condition changes so that it is thought that she should stay in hospital (and she is no longer willing to do so). In this case, the patient may be detained in hospital (for up to 72 hours). This can be done quickly without a second medical opinion (i.e. this does not need the general practitioner's approval).

can be detained, particularly those who are thought to be dangerous and have a personality disorder. Such patients might pass the new test because there is an 'appropriate treatment', i.e. a treatment is available that is appropriate to the patient's mental disorder, even if it is not likely to work for the individual patient.

Applications under the MHA are made either by the nearest relative or by an approved social worker (approved under Section 13 of the MHA as having particular expertise in the area of mental health). In general, the latter is preferred, to protect the longer-term relationship of the relative with the patient.

The MHA places some restrictions on specific types of treatment. Thus, psychosurgery can be undertaken only with the valid consent of the patient and a second medical opinion. Drug treatment for mental disorder for longer than 3 months, and electroconvulsive therapy, can be imposed without consent only if supported by a second medical opinion.

Enforcing treatment outside hospital

The focus of the MHA is on hospital treatment. However, over the past two decades there has been a substantial move towards the treatment of psychiatric disorder in the community. Guardianship orders (Sections 7–10 of the MHA) enable the appointed guardian to require a patient to reside at a specified place; to attend a specified place for medical treatment; and to allow, for example, a doctor access to the patient. However, most of the guardian's powers are not enforceable, and rely on the cooperation of the patient. There has been much debate over the issue of whether, and how, treatment of mental disorder can be enforced outside hospital. This has been partly in response to the perceived need to protect the public from dangerous attacks by mentally disordered people in the community who have stopped taking their medication.

The MHA 2007 created community treatment orders for suitable patients following an initial period of detention and treatment in hospital. This allows professionals to enforce treatment on patients after they have been discharged from hospital, and makes it easier to readmit such patients involuntarily to hospital.

Further issues covered by the Mental Health Act

In addition to the areas already described, the MHA covers many other aspects of the care of people with mental disorder. These include the powers of police to take a person who appears to be mentally disordered to a place of safety and the admission to hospital of mentally disordered people who come before the court.

The MHA Commission is set up to give second opinions under the MHA, to examine complaints, to check the working of the Act and to make recommendations (to the Secretary of State) as to what should be put into the Code of Practice. Mental Health Review Tribunals review the justification for individual patients being detained under the MHA. Patients may appeal against their detention to the tribunal. There is one tribunal for each health region.

The Mental Health (Care and Treatment) (Scotland) Act 2003 is the key statute in Scotland relating to the management of people with mental disorder.

REVISION QUESTIONS

1. What is the difference between mental capacity and mental illness?
2. If a patient with mental illness refuses treatment, should this be respected?
3. What is the ethical justification for compulsory detention of patients with mental illness who pose a risk of harm to others?
4. What is the difference between emergency admission, admission for assessment and admission for treatment under the Mental Health Act?
5. Northern Ireland has a single law relating to mental capacity and mental health. Is this a good idea? Why? Why not?

Extension case 8.3

A 20-year-old, Mr L, is admitted to hospital having lost a lot of blood after cutting himself.

1. Mr L refuses a blood transfusion on the grounds that he is a Jehovah's Witness. Should the doctor transfuse Mr L against his wishes?

   If he were not a Jehovah's witness, would his request (not to be transfused) be respected? (If you are recommending different treatment depending on the patient's religion, is that discriminatory?)

2. Mr L refuses a blood transfusion on the grounds that he is a member of a religious sect that believes that the second coming of their prophet is imminent and is seeking to leave his earthly body to journey to the next world together with other followers of his religious leader.

   What is the difference between a genuine religious belief and a religious delusion? How should health professionals (and the law) respond to idiosyncratic religious views?

   Read Fulford (2004).

REFERENCES

David, A. S., Hotopf, M., Moran, P., Owen, G., Szmukler, G. and Richardson, G. 2010. "Mentally disordered or lacking capacity? Lessons for management of serious deliberate self harm." *BMJ* 341: c4489.

Dickenson, D. and Savulescu, J. 1998. "The time frame of preferences, dispositions, and the validity of advance directives for the mentally ill." *Philosophy, Psychiatry, & Psychology* 5 (3): 225-46.

Dolan, B. and Parker, C. 1997. "Caesarean section: a treatment for mental disorder? Tameside & Glossop Acute Services Unit v

CH (a patient) [1996] 1 FLR 762." *BMJ* 314: 1183.

Fulford, K. W. M. 2004. "Neuro-ethics or neuro-values? Delusion and religious experience as a case study in values-based medicine." *Poiesis & Praxis* 2 (4): 297-313. doi: 10.1007/s10202-004-0061-x.

Koch, H.-G., Reiter-Theil, S. and Helmchen, H. 1996. *Informed consent in psychiatry: European perspectives of ethics, law and clinical practice.* Baden-Baden: Nomos.

Lynch, G., Taggart, C. and Campbell, P. 2017. "Mental Capacity Act (Northern Ireland)

2016." *BJPsych Bulletin* 41 (6): 353-7. doi: 10.1192/pb.bp.117.056945.

Muzaffar, S. 2011. "'To treat or not to treat'. Kerrie Wooltorton, lessons to learn." *Emergency Medicine Journal* 28: 741-4.

Szawarski, P. 2013. "Classic cases revisited: the suicide of Kerrie Wooltorton." *Journal of Intensive Care Society* 14 (3): 211-4.

Szmukler, G. and Weich, S. 2017. "Has the Mental Health Act had its day?" *BMJ* 359: j5248.

Tameside & Glossop Acute Services Unit v CH (a patient) [1996] 1 FLR 762.

Chapter 9

Confidentiality

Case 9.1

Dr M was a trainee GP who participated in an anonymous online educational forum set up by the GP deanery. She regularly posted clinical scenarios on the forum and benefited from the feedback and discussion posted by other trainees.

Dr M had seen a patient in her clinic, Mr X, who had previously had a stroke and currently was experiencing sexual difficulties and low mood. Dr M later posted an anonymous description of the case on the online forum. However, Mr X subsequently found the case online and recognized himself from the description. He was upset at the breach of his confidentiality.

This case is based on one reported to the Medical Protection Society (Birch 2013).

Confidentiality is one of the cornerstones of trust that enables patients to be open with doctors about their symptoms and problems, and to undergo physical examination (Fig. 9.1). From the moment that medical students start their clinical training, they have access to confidential information. They will be expected to have the same standards of confidentiality as qualified doctors.

If a patient, like Mr X, is concerned that a doctor has wrongly breached confidentiality, he can pursue his grievance in several ways: by complaining to the

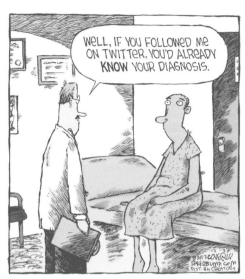

Figure 9.1 Confidentiality in the age of social media (© Dave Coverly/www. speedbump.com, used with permission)

doctor (or, in the case of a junior doctor, to the doctor's consultant); by taking the complaint to the doctor's employer or to the General Medical Council (GMC); or by taking the case to court.

THE ETHICAL BASIS FOR MEDICAL CONFIDENTIALITY

Much of the information a patient gives a doctor, and which a doctor gains about a patient in her professional duties, is confidential. This means that the doctor should not divulge that information to another person without the agreement (possibly implied) of the patient.

Four ethical grounds for the importance of confidentiality
Respect for patient autonomy

An important principle in medical ethics is respect for patient autonomy (see Chapters 1 and 3). This principle emphasizes the patient's right to have control over his own life. It implies that a person has the right, by and large, to decide who should have access to personal information about himself. It is this principle that, in this view, underpins the importance of medical confidentiality. In Case 9.1, given that Mr X did not give permission for his medical details to be discussed with other doctors, posting of the case details was a violation of his autonomy.

Can there be a serious breach of confidentiality if the patient never knows about the breach? If respect for patient autonomy is a key justification for preserving confidentiality, the answer is yes. If Mr X did not wish for his personal details to be discussed with others, his autonomy has not been respected, whether or not

Mr X knows this. (For similar reasons, you could be wronged if someone says something hurtful about you behind your back – even if you never find out about it.)

However, an autonomy-based justification would not necessarily see anything wrong with breaches of confidentiality in other cases – for example if the patient lacked capacity or awareness (and so had no desire for information to be kept confidential).

Implied promise

Some views of the doctor–patient relationship (see Chapter 5) see it as having elements of an implied contract. Such a contract potentially includes a promise to keep information about patients confidential. Patients generally expect doctors to treat information confidentially, and professional guidelines emphasize the importance of high standards of confidentiality. Thus, patients may reasonably believe that, when they come to their doctor, what they say will be kept confidential. If the doctor subsequently breaches confidentiality, the patient may feel that the doctor has broken an implied promise.

This view of confidentiality is different from that of patient autonomy. It does not ultimately depend on what the patient would want or believes. It depends on a concept of the doctor–patient relationship.

Virtue ethics

Virtue ethics (see Chapter 2) focuses on the question of what makes a virtuous person, rather than what it is right to do in particular circumstances. One of the characteristics of a virtuous doctor, it might be argued, is that she is trustworthy and respects her patients' confidences. According to this view, in posting Mr X's case online Dr M might have acted contrary to what is expected of a virtuous doctor. How serious this breach of confidentiality is regarded might depend on the specific account of the virtuous physician and the role of other (possibly conflicting) virtues. For example, a different virtue for doctors might be that of self-education and reflective practice, including learning through sharing experience with other doctors.

Consequentialism

According to this view, it is the consequences of the breach of confidentiality that determine the seriousness of the breach, and, indeed, underlie whether breaching confidentiality is wrong in the first place. There are several different types of consequence that could be relevant here, and the analysis of the situation depends in part on how these are viewed.

As in Case 9.1, the particular patient might discover the breach in confidentiality, with several possible consequences: he is angry or upset; he loses trust in that particular doctor; his loss of trust results in him receiving poorer health care because of a reluctance to see the doctor; he loses trust in doctors in general – and this might lead to poorer health care. However, according to a consequentialist view, if Mr X never learned of the breach of his confidentiality, there would have been no harm in Dr M posting the case online.

There may be an effect on others. Mr X may, for example, make a complaint that becomes more widely known, leading to other people losing trust in Dr M or in doctors more generally, with a deleterious effect on health care. From the point of view of rule consequentialism (see Chapter 2), if the profession does not set a very high standard of confidentiality, then patients may have insufficient trust in doctors, avoid attending doctors or avoid disclosing important personal details, with resulting poor health. The issue is not just about ill-health: there are other consequences of untreated illness. For example, if people with uncontrolled epilepsy drive, they may kill other road users. There is a public interest in ensuring that such people receive good health care in order to maximize control of the epilepsy.

However, there may in some circumstances be positive consequences of breaching confidentiality. There are obviously important educational benefits in doctors being able to learn and gain feedback from their own and other doctors' clinical experience. There may be particular circumstances where breaching confidentiality would avoid serious harm to the patient or others. As we will see, English law places significant weight on the consequences of confidentiality. This is reflected in the 'public interest' (i.e. wider consequences) justification for both respecting and (sometimes) violating patient confidences.

What should Dr M have done? Up for Debate Box 9.1 outlines two different views. GMC guidance on disclosing personal information for education or training stipulates that publishing patient details in a seminar, conference or journal would require explicit patient consent if 'you consider that the patient could be identified'. Merely omitting a patient's name may be insufficient. Some illnesses or situations may be sufficiently uncommon that the patient (or others) could identify them. Alternatively, the combination of several different characteristics could allow triangulation and identification (e.g. age, illness, profession) (General Medical Council 2017a).

THE LEGAL APPROACH TO CONFIDENTIALITY: THE BALANCING OF PUBLIC INTERESTS

There is now extensive GMC guidance on patient confidentiality. Although not legally binding, the GMC guidelines (Box 9.1 lists the main principles) are particularly important for three reasons:

1. A patient with a serious grievance is more likely to complain to the GMC than to sue.
2. The courts take a great deal of notice of the GMC guidelines.
3. The guidelines represent the medical profession's self-imposed standards and amount to a public statement of what standards patients can expect from their doctor.

The guidelines allow patient information to be shared with other health professionals as long as that is part of the 'direct care' of the patient. Usually patients will be aware that this is likely to occur, and can be regarded as having implicitly consented to the sharing of this information. However, hospitals or medical practices should provide patients with information about how their data or medical details

Up for Debate Box 9.1 Should doctors report or discuss case histories without patient consent?

Con: Strict (deontological) view of confidentiality

Patients expect doctors to respect their confidential information, and the public expects doctors to respect patient confidentiality absolutely (with some very rare exceptions where this would prevent harm to others).

Doctors should seek explicit patient consent to discuss the patient's details with others (who are not directly involved in the patient's medical care).

Patient consent should be sought even if it is unlikely that the patient will ever learn of the discussion (for example, in a closed medical conference).

Patient consent should be sought for publication of a case history (for example, in a journal or textbook), whether or not the doctor believes that the patient could identify themselves. Removal (or changing) of identifying details is not sufficient.

Pro: A minimal risk (consequentialist) approach

Doctors and other patients benefit from discussion and publication of clinical cases and clinical experience.

Reporting and discussing of cases (outside of a patient's clinical care) should seek to minimize the risks of:

Self-identification – the patient identifies themselves and feels that their trust has been betrayed.

Identification by others – other people identify the patient, and therefore learn confidential medical information about them.

While both of these harms should be avoided wherever possible, the latter is the more serious harm.

Doctors may only discuss or report 'other identifiable' cases with patient consent. This is particularly important where case reports will be published online or in a journal.

Doctors may report cases that are 'self-identifiable' (but not 'other identifiable') without patient consent, if there is good reason to not obtain consent. However, it will often be preferable and possible to avoid the possibility of self-identification (for example, through publishing fictionalized or composite cases that contain details from multiple different patients).

For further discussion see Isaacs et al. (2008), Wilkinson and Savulescu (2015).

will be used and shared. Patients should be able to object to disclosure of personal information (and this should be respected in most circumstances).

Box 9.2 summarizes the key legal aspects of confidentiality. There is, however, important statute law that covers specific situations, as summarized in Box 9.3.

In a legal case involving confidentiality, the court tends to focus on two questions. The first (and generally more straightforward) is whether the disclosure of information was indeed a breach of confidence, or whether the patient had consented to the disclosure or the information was public knowledge. Most information given to a doctor in a clinical setting will be of a private or intimate nature, but perhaps some information may not be. If information is already in the public domain, the information may not be regarded as confidential. It should be noted that rights

> **Box 9.1** Confidentiality and the GMC: key principles (General Medical Council 2017b)
>
> 1. To avoid inadvertent breaches of confidentiality, doctors should use the minimum necessary personal information and use anonymized information if it is practicable to do so and if it will serve the purpose.
> 2. Health professionals have a duty to manage and protect information against improper access, disclosure or loss.
> 3. Doctors should be aware of their responsibilities in managing and protecting information.
> 4. Doctors should ensure that they are handling personal information lawfully.
> 5. Doctors may share relevant information for direct medical care (in accordance with other principles of confidentiality), unless the patient has objected.
> 6. Explicit consent should be sought to disclose identifiable information about patients for purposes other than their care or local clinical audit. (Consent may not be required if the disclosure is required by law or can be justified as being in the public interest.)
> 7. Doctors should, wherever possible, tell patients about disclosures of personal information that they would not reasonably expect. They should keep a record of decisions to disclose, or not to disclose, information.
> 8. Doctors should support patients to access their information, for example by enabling them to have access to, or copies of, their health records.

of confidentiality continue even after a patient has died. The second question is whether the breach can be justified. This is normally done by claiming it was in the public interest to make the disclosure (see below).

The balancing of public interests

The legal basis for confidentiality is not as clear as one might expect (Herring 2018). However, it is clear that the obligation of confidentiality is not absolute. There are circumstances in which doctors can justifiably breach confidentiality. Some of these arise from legislation (see below). The most problematic justification is, however, the public interest criterion: that a breach is justified if the public interest in breaching confidentiality outweighs the public interest in maintaining confidentiality. It is problematic because there is little guidance from the courts as to the meaning of public interest.

Case 9.2

Mr W was confined in a secure hospital after he was convicted of killing five people. A psychiatrist was asked by Mr W's lawyers to prepare a confidential report, which they hoped would support his release from hospital. However, the psychiatrist, Dr E, concluded that Mr W was still dangerous. W's application was withdrawn, and the psychiatrist became aware that his report would not be included in Mr W's medical notes. He sent his report to the medical director of the hospital and to the home office.

Was Dr E justified in breaching confidentiality?

This is based on the case of W v Edgell [1990].

Box 9.2 Key legal aspects of confidentiality

There is a general legal obligation for doctors to keep confidential what patients tell them. This obligation is not absolute:

There are situations when the law obliges doctors to breach confidentiality and others where the law permits doctors to breach confidentiality.

In both of these situations, it is important that the doctor breaches confidentiality only to the relevant person(s) or authority(ies).

From the legal perspective, what is important is the public interest for patients to be able to trust their doctors to maintain confidentiality. Therefore, the issue of when it is lawful, and when it is not lawful, for a doctor to breach confidentiality is often a question of balancing public interests.

The General Medical Council (GMC) provides professional guidelines on the issue of confidentiality. Although these do not have the force of law, they are taken seriously by the courts. No breach of confidentiality has occurred if: a patient gives consent, or the patient cannot be identified.

Sharing information about patients with other members of the health care team for the purpose of providing the best treatment is not generally viewed by the law as a breach of confidentiality.

A doctor must take reasonable precautions to prevent confidential information from falling into the wrong hands (i.e. confidential medical information must be kept reasonably secure).

The NHS Confidentiality Code of Practice for NHS staff (Department of Health and Social Care 2003) is a lengthy and detailed document that describes what a confidential service looks like, provides a description of the main legal requirements, recommends a generic decision support tool for sharing/disclosing information and lists examples of particular situations for sharing information.

Box 9.3 Statutes relevant to medical confidentiality

NB: Most legal aspects of confidentiality are governed by common law. The following statues govern the law in restricted circumstances.

Public Health (Control of Diseases) Act 1984 (Notifiable Diseases), amended by the Health Protection (Notification) Regulations 2010

A doctor must notify the relevant local authority officer (usually a public health consultant) if he or she suspects a patient of having a notifiable disease or food poisoning. The following information must be provided (by completing a specific certificate): patient's name, age, sex, address, suspected disease, approximate date of onset and date of admission to hospital (if appropriate). An up-to-date list of notifiable diseases can be obtained from NHS Direct at http://www.nhsdirect.nhs.uk.

Abortion Act 1967

A doctor carrying out a termination of pregnancy must notify the relevant Chief Medical Officer, including giving the name and address of the woman concerned.

Notification of births and deaths – Births and Deaths Registration Act 1953

Parents have a legal duty to register the details (child's name, sex, date and place of birth; parents' names, places of birth, address; and father's occupation) of a birth with the local registrar within 42 days. The doctor or midwife normally has a duty to inform the district medical officer of the birth within 6 hours.

Continued

Box 9.3 Statutes relevant to medical confidentiality—cont'd

Stillbirths (a baby born dead after the 24th week of pregnancy) must also be registered. Doctors attending patients during their last illness must sign a death certificate giving cause of death (to their best knowledge). The certificate must be sent to the registrar. The registrar must inform the coroner of deaths that occur without attendance of a doctor at the last illness, or during an operation or while the effects of an anaesthetic persist.

Road Traffic Act 1988

All citizens, including doctors, must provide the police, on request, with information (name, address) that might identify a driver alleged to have committed a traffic offence. This would not normally justify providing clinical information without the patient's consent or a court order.

Human Fertilization and Embryology Act 1990, amended by the Human Fertilization and Embryology (Disclosure of Information) Act 1992 and Human Fertilization and Embryology Act 2008

This Act regulates assisted reproduction and research on human embryos outside the human body. Relevant to confidentiality are the following:

The Human Fertilization and Embryology Authority keeps a register recording the names of all those for whom infertility treatments under the Act were provided, and of all those born, or probably born, as a result of such treatments. The doctors providing such treatments must therefore provide the names of the relevant patients to the register.

Individuals aged over 18 years are entitled to find out whether they are on the register, whether the register shows that their parents may not be their genetic parents and whether they are related to a person they propose to marry.

The confidentiality of gamete donors is strictly protected.

The patient's consent is normally needed before information (e.g. that the patient has undergone treatment for infertility) is passed to someone else – even to the patient's own general practitioner (GP).

NHS Venereal Diseases Regulations 1974

This requires health authorities to take all necessary steps to ensure that information capable of identifying patients with sexually transmitted diseases should not be disclosed, except for the purpose of treating the disease and preventing its spread. Such disclosure, furthermore, can be made only to a doctor, or to someone working on a doctor's instruction in connection with treatment or prevention. This allows contact tracing. However, it does not allow those working in a genitourinary clinic to inform an insurance company of a patient's sexually transmitted disease – even with the patient's consent. Case notes from genitourinary clinics are kept separate from other hospital records. GPs are not routinely informed of the patient's attendance at such clinics, although the patient may request that the GP be informed.

The Children Act 1989

See Chapter 11.

Terrorism Act 2000 and 2006 and Counter-Terrorism and Security Act 2015

The Act imposes a duty on health professionals to report their suspicions that a person has been involved in terrorist activities. This duty of disclosure applies even if the health professional has not specifically been asked for information.

The Human Rights Act 1998

Article 8 of the Convention on Human Rights states: 'Everyone has the right to respect for his private … life' (see main text for impact on medical confidentiality).

In Mr W's case, the court concluded that the public interest in preventing dangerous criminal acts justified release of the confidential information. (This is the UK equivalent of a much earlier US court case – Tarasoff [1976]. In that case, a psychologist was found to be liable for not warning someone that they were at risk of harm from a patient with paranoid schizophrenia.) The UK court concluded that, in order for the disclosure to be justified, the risk must be 'real, immediate and serious'. In other words, the public interest in maintaining medical confidentiality is strong. It seems likely that a doctor who breached medical confidentiality in order to help the police with regard to a crime against property could be found liable. Disclosure should be limited to those with a legitimate interest in knowing the information. Finally, only the minimum information necessary to protect the public should be disclosed.

The impact of the Human Rights Act 1998 (HRA) on confidentiality

Prior to the Human Rights Act 1998 (HRA), medical confidentiality was seen as a *public* interest. The HRA, and the case of Campbell v MGN [(2004)] (see below), established more clearly than before that, in English law, people have a *private* right to confidentiality. However, because this is not absolute, and as the public interest in medical confidentiality is considered to be strong, the HRA has had relatively little impact on medical confidentiality. Its impact has been greater in other settings, such as confidentiality and the media, where the private right to confidentiality has given greater protection to individual privacy than previously.

The leading case on the impact of the HRA on confidentiality is Campbell v MGN [2004]. Although no medical practitioner was involved in disclosing medical information (the case was about the publication of details of a famous model's drug therapy), several important points were made by the judges. These are worth noting, as they would undoubtedly influence a court's approach should a case alleging breach of medical confidentiality arise.

First, the case marked a shift in language, away from the idea of balancing public interests to a balance of Article rights. The relevant articles are 8 (right to respect for private life) and 10 (right to freedom of expression). This means that, although the balancing exercise is basically the same as balancing public interests, it must be more 'carefully focused and penetrating'. Second, by emphasizing the values underpinning respect for private life, namely privacy and personal autonomy, the need for a confidential relationship becomes less important. In other words, the right to privacy attaches to private information, irrespective of the circumstances in which that information was disclosed.

Confidentiality and genetic information

Some confidential information has implications for other people as well as the patient. That is particularly the case for genetic diagnoses that may imply that other family members are at risk of significant illness.

Patients will, in most cases, agree to share information about a genetic diagnosis with family members. GMC guidance recommends that patients should be encouraged to share relevant information, and that their consent should be sought before sharing a genetic diagnosis with other family members. If the patient refuses consent, it might still be justified to disclose information (in the 'public interest') if there is a risk of death or serious harm (General Medical Council 2017b).

Case 9.3

In 2007, Mr C was convicted of manslaughter for shooting and killing his wife. However, he was also found to have an altered mental state and diminished responsibility, and was detained under the Mental Health Act (see Chapter 8). Two years later, he was diagnosed with Huntington's disease (a late-onset inherited neurodegenerative disorder).

Doctors at the hospital where the diagnosis was made had considered whether Mr C's daughters should be told about the diagnosis (they had a 50:50 chance of inheriting the disorder). Mr C refused permission for the information to be shared, as he expressed a concern that they might become upset or have an abortion. On the same day, one of Mr C's daughters told him that she was pregnant.

Subsequently (after giving birth), Mr C's daughter learned by accident of her father's diagnosis, and she was herself diagnosed with Huntington's disease.

Should Mr C's doctors have breached his confidentiality to pass information on to his daughters?

This is based on the case of ABC v St. George's Healthcare NHS Trust and others [2017].

Some ethicists have pointed out that the shared nature of a genetic diagnosis (a diagnosis in one family member will often generate information or risk for others) means that such diagnoses should not be regarded as unique information for the individual (Lucassen and Gilbar 2018) (see also Chapter 18). There may also be ways of communicating risk of a heritable illness without breaking a patient's confidence. For example, Mr C's daughter might have been informed that she had a family history of early-onset dementia, and that she had various options for further testing (Lucassen and Gilbar 2018).

In the case of Mr C's daughter, the first judge struck the case out as unarguable, but the Court of Appeal subsequently found that the daughter had a plausible claim in negligence against the doctors (and thus the case should be heard in court). The court held that doctors could have a duty of care towards family members. The case did not resolve the question of whether there was definitely a duty; it simply accepted that this was arguable. At the time of writing, the case has not been heard again in court (it is listed to be heard in November 2019). One issue the case left open was how to deal with the fact that some children, in cases of this kind, would not want to know that they had Huntington's disease.

Confidentiality and sexually transmitted diseases

As with diagnosis of an inherited genetic disorder, diagnosis of a sexually transmitted disease may have implications for others – primarily sexual contacts of the patient.

Case 9.4

Mr H has recently been diagnosed with HIV and commenced on treatment. He tells his GP that he wishes the diagnosis to be kept strictly confidential. His wife attends the same practice, and he does not wish her to learn of the diagnosis, as he fears that his marriage would end. She is pregnant and expecting to deliver soon.

Should the GP inform Mr H's wife?

GMC guidance recommends that doctors seek consent of the patient to inform contacts. Mr H's doctor should encourage him to inform his wife, as she may also have HIV and would benefit from diagnosis and treatment, and as this would also potentially benefit their newborn (HIV prophylaxis would reduce the risk of acquiring HIV). If the patient refuses consent, the doctor may consider that they have a duty to inform Mr H's wife to prevent serious harm to her and her newborn (Chan 2013).

Confidentiality, the police and driving

Case 9.5

A patient, J, presents to the emergency department with a knife injury to his abdomen. He states that he injured himself by accident, and does not wish to involve the police. J's doctor believes that this is unlikely. Should she notify the police?

This is based on a case example discussed on the GMC website (General Medical Council).

Doctors must disclose information to satisfy a specific statutory requirement, such as notification of a known or suspected communicable disease, and if ordered to do so by a judge or presiding officer of a court.

Doctors should not disclose personal information to a third party such as a solicitor, police officer or officer of a court without the patient's express consent, except in unusual circumstances, such as to prevent serious harm to another person.

According to the NHS Confidentiality Code of Practice, staff are permitted to disclose personal information:

> 'in order to prevent and support detection, investigation and punishment of serious crime and/or to prevent abuse or serious harm to others where they judge, on a case by case basis, that the public good that would be achieved by the disclosure outweighs both the obligation of confidentiality to the individual patient concerned and the broader public interest in the provision of a confidential service'. (Department of Health and Social Care 2003)

The Code acknowledges that, although the concept of 'serious crime' is unclear, it does include rape, murder, manslaughter, treason, kidnapping and child abuse, but would not include theft, fraud or damage to property. As to the risk of harm, the Code states that this would include disclosures to prevent child abuse, neglect, assault, traffic accidents and the spread of infectious diseases.

GMC guidance on reporting gunshot and knife wounds recommends that, in Case 9.5, the doctor should promptly inform the police that a patient has been admitted to the emergency department with a knife wound (General Medical Council 2018). J should be encouraged to speak to the police; however, if he refuses to do so, disclosure of some confidential information may be warranted in the public interest.

What of patients who have medical conditions that may affect their ability to drive? Drivers have a legal duty to inform the DVLA if they have a condition that may affect their safety as a driver, either now or in the future. It is not currently mandatory for doctors to notify the DVLA; however, GMC guidance makes clear that doctors have a duty to ensure that patients understand if their medical condition may impair their ability to drive, and explain that the patient should inform the DVLA about the condition (General Medical Council 2017c).

If patients continue to drive when they are not fit to do so, doctors should endeavour to persuade them to stop. If the patient is continuing to drive, and if doctors believe that this poses a serious risk of death or serious harm to others, doctors should disclose relevant medical information immediately, in confidence, to the medical adviser at the DVLA. Before giving information to the DVLA, doctors should try to inform the patient of their decision to do so. If a patient is incapable of understanding medical advice, for example because of dementia, doctors should inform the DVLA immediately.

CONFIDENTIALITY AND MEDICAL STUDENTS

The position of medical students raises two issues: first, the question of students' access to confidential information; and second, their legal responsibilities with regard to maintaining confidentiality. If they are to be properly educated, students need to have access to confidential information about patients. Although in practice clinical students are often part of the health care team, the prime reason for their access to confidential information is for the purpose of their own education. The GMC states: 'Patients' consent to disclosure of information for teaching and audit must be obtained unless the data have been effectively anonymized'.

There is little doubt from the legal point of view that patients have the right to refuse to see medical students, and to refuse to allow medical students access to their notes. It might be argued that patients should not normally exercise such a right; that a patient cannot expect, on the one hand, to be looked after by well-trained doctors and, on the other hand, to not enable medical students to receive training.

Medical students, just like doctors, have a duty to keep information about patients that they learn in the course of their clinical studies confidential. It seems unlikely that courts would sanction breaches of confidentiality in students that they would not allow in doctors. Furthermore, students would be expected, when they introduce themselves, to make it clear to patients that they are students and not doctors.

Occasionally a patient may tell a student something and ask the student not to tell anyone else – not even the doctors and nurses. The student will have to use some judgement in such circumstances. It is probably safer for the student to share the information with the relevant consultant, rather than withhold information that may be important, either for the sake of the patient or in the public interest. It is unwise for students to promise to keep information confidential from the consultant in advance of knowing what that information is.

CONFIDENTIALITY AND THE PATIENT LACKING CAPACITY

The patient lacking capacity cannot, by definition, give consent for information to be passed on to someone else. The general legal criterion, in the case of patients without capacity, is for doctors to act in the patient's best interests (as defined by the Mental Capacity Act; see Chapters 3 and 7). Sharing information about diagnosis, treatment and prognosis with close relatives or key carers would normally be seen as being in a patient's best interests. However, a patient who lacks capacity has the same legal protection from casual breaches of confidentiality as a competent patient, and the same protection from being harmed through a breach of confidentiality.

CONFIDENTIALITY AND CHILDREN

The key legal issue is whether the child has capacity to give or withhold permission for information to be shared (see Chapter 11). A child aged 16 years and above is assumed to have capacity to make this decision, unless there are specific grounds (such as learning disability) for doubting this. The doctor owes the obligation of confidentiality to the child, and not to the parents. Thus, the doctor must generally seek the child's permission, either explicitly or by inferring from the child's conduct, in order to discuss the case with the parents. This is also the case for a child aged less than 16 years who is 'Gillick competent'. In R (Axon) v Secretary of State for Health [2006] (a case concerning under-16s seeking access to abortion), the court said that children who are 'Gillick competent' have the same rights to confidentiality as an adult. The doctor could encourage the child to allow him to discuss the matter with her parents, but the doctor would still ultimately need the child's consent to do this. In the case of a child under 16 who is not 'Gillick competent', the doctor would normally be acting lawfully in discussing her medical treatment with the parents; and indeed, parental consent for treatment would normally be necessary (see Chapter 11).

Whether the child has capacity or not, breach of confidentiality is permitted according to the GMC (2013) guidelines where the child is at risk of death or serious harm. The guidance gives examples of where there is 'risk of neglect or sexual, physical or emotional abuse' or 'a child or young person is involved in behaviour that might put them or others at risk of serious harm, such as serious addiction, self-harm or joy-riding'.

The legal position in Scotland is different. The Age of Legal Capacity (Scotland) Act 1991 gives various legal rights to children under 16 years old, including the right to confidentiality if the child has the capacity to understand the relevant issues.

Court proceedings, medical records and the doctor

Doctors may be asked to show the medical records of a patient to, for example, a solicitor, because they are relevant evidence in court proceedings. The general principle is that records (or copies of the records) may be released only with the permission of the patient, or in response to a court order (in which case the order must be complied with). The procedure is slightly different in different settings.

The police have no right to inspect a person's medical records – although a doctor may consider it right to breach a patient's confidentiality to the police in some circumstances (see above). A circuit judge (but not a magistrate), however, can order the medical records to be released to the police.

If a coroner asks to see the medical records of a dead patient, this should be complied with. On the other hand, if a life insurance company requests the medical records of a dead patient, this should be complied with only with the consent of a personal representative of the dead person's estate.

See Box 9.4 for a summary of when doctors should and should not breach confidentiality.

Box 9.4 Summary of when doctors should or should not breach confidentiality

When doctors should not breach confidentiality (unless with consent of patient)

'Casual breaches', e.g. for amusement, or carelessly.

Simply to satisfy another person's curiosity.

To prevent minor crime, or to help conviction in the case of minor crime. Most crime against property would probably count as minor crimes in this context.

To prevent minor harm to someone else.

In the case of doctors working in a genitourinary clinic, no information that might identify a patient examined or treated for any sexually transmitted disease should be provided to a third party, except to prevent serious harm to others.

A doctor should not write a report or fill in a form disclosing confidential information (e.g. for an insurance company) without the patient's consent (preferably written).

NB: It would be unwise for a doctor to lie in order to protect patient confidentiality, for example to write on an insurance form that the patient has not had an HIV test when in fact she has. If the patient subsequently made an insurance claim and the lie was discovered, not only might the insurance company refuse to pay, but the patient might successfully sue the doctor because the doctor's actions had led to her not being insured.

Box 9.4 Summary of when doctors should or should not breach confidentiality—cont'd

When doctors must breach confidentiality (to specific authorities only)

Notifiable diseases

Termination of pregnancy

Births

Deaths

To police, on request: name and address of driver of vehicle who is alleged to be guilty of offence under Road Traffic Act 1988

Search warrant signed by circuit judge

Under court orders

When doctors have discretion (see main text)

Sharing information with other members of the health care team in the interests of the patient

Patient continuing to drive who is not medically fit to do so (NB: The GMC advises doctors to inform a DVLA medical officer)

When a third party is at significant risk of harm (e.g. spouse of HIV-positive person)

The detection or prevention of serious crime.

REVISION QUESTIONS

1. Do doctors have absolute duty to protect patient confidentiality?
2. After a long and tiring day at work, a junior doctor describes to his partner one of the difficult cases that he faced during the day. He does not provide any identifying details of the patient. Is this a breach of confidentiality? Is it wrong? Does it make any difference if his partner is also a doctor (at a different hospital)?
3. During a consultation for palliative care, an elderly man with a terminal illness (and not long to live) discloses to a junior doctor that, many years earlier, he had killed several people but had never been caught.
   Does public interest justify breaching confidentiality for a death bed confession?
   (This is based on Tincknell et al. 2018.)
4. A police officer rings the emergency department asking for information about a road traffic accident that took place earlier that evening. What should the casualty officer do?
5. A patient is seriously ill in hospital and lacks capacity. Is it a breach of confidentiality for her doctor to discuss her medical condition with her children? What about her ex-husband? Her neighbour and close friend?

Extension case 9.6

Dr Y has been the GP for a family for several years. He has treated the eldest son, A, for asthma since childhood. A's mother presents to the surgery. She mentions that she is concerned about A's behaviour. She describes him spending large periods of time alone on his computer and becoming increasingly withdrawn. She mentions that he has been mixing with the wrong people and describes him as expressing 'extreme' religious and political views.

Dr Y is concerned that A might have become radicalized and may be at risk of engaging in terrorist activities. However, when he raises this with A's mother, she becomes distressed and asks him to forget about it. Dr Y is also concerned that perhaps he is prejudging A because of his ethnic and religious background. He has no proof of A's risk. He has not seen A in the surgery for some time.

Should Dr Y breach confidentiality to notify authorities of his concerns?

The 'Prevent Duty' is a statutory duty to take actions to prevent people from being drawn into terrorism. It only applies to health authorities, not to doctors. Is that justified?

See Medical Defence Union (2018) and Agnew (2015).

REFERENCES

ABC v St. George's Healthcare NHS Trust and others [2017] EWCA Civ 336.

Agnew, M. 2015. "Confidentiality and disclosing information to protect others." General Medical Council, accessed 8/11/18. https://gmcuk.wordpress.com/2015/09/02/confidentiality-and-disclosing-information-to-protect-others/.

Birch, R. 2013. "From the case files." Medical Protection Society, accessed 08/11/2018. https://www.medicalprotection.org/uk/articles/practice-matters-june-2013-from-the-case-files.

Campbell v MGN [2004] UKHL 22.

Chan, T. K. 2013. "Doctors have a duty to breach patient confidentiality to protect others at risk of HIV infection." *BMJ* 346:f1471.

Department of Health and Social Care. 2003. "Confidentiality: NHS Code of Practice." Accessed 8/11/2018. https://www.gov.uk/government/publications/confidentiality-nhs-code-of-practice.

General Medical Council. "GMP in action. Case studies: Dr McDonald." Accessed 8/11/2018. https://www.gmc-uk.org/gmpinaction/case-studies/dr-macdonald/scenario-02/.

General Medical Council. 2017a. "Confidentiality: disclosing information for education and training purposes." Accessed 08/11/2018. https://www.gmc-uk.org/-/media/documents/confidentiality—disclosing-information-for-education-and-training-purposes_pdf-70063667.pdf.

General Medical Council. 2017b. "Confidentiality: good practice in handling patient information." Accessed 08/11/18. https://www.gmc-uk.org/ethical-guidance/ethical-guidance-for-doctors/confidentiality.

General Medical Council. 2017c. "Confidentiality: patients' fitness to drive and reporting concerns to the DVLA or DVA." Accessed 8/11/18. https://www.gmc-uk.org/ethical-guidance/ethical-guidance-for-doctors/confidentiality—patients-fitness-to-drive-and-reporting-concerns-to-the-dvla-or-dva.

General Medical Council. 2018. "Confidentiality: reporting gunshot and knife wounds." Accessed 8/11/2018. https://www.gmc-uk.org/ethical-guidance/ethical-guidance-for-doctors/confidentiality—reporting-gunshot-and-knife-wounds.

Herring, J. 2018. *Medical law and ethics.* 7th ed. Oxford: Oxford University Press.

Isaacs, D., Kilham, H. A., Jacobe, S., Ryan, M. M. and Tobin, B. 2008. "Gaining consent for publication in difficult cases involving children." *BMJ* 337:a1231.

Lucassen, A. and Gilbar, R. 2018. "Alerting relatives about heritable risks: the limits of confidentiality." *BMJ* 361:k1409.

Medical Defence Union. 2018. "Counter-terrorism and confidentiality." Accessed 8/11/18. https://www.themdu.com/guidance-and-advice/guides/counter-terrorism-and-confidentiality.

R (Axon) v Secretary of State for Health [2006] EWHC 37 (Admin).

Tarasoff v. Regents of University of California [1976] 17 Cal.3d 425.

Tincknell, L., O'Callaghan, A., Manning, J. and Malpas, P. 2018. "Deathbed confession: when a dying patient confesses to murder: clinical, ethical, and legal implications." *Journal of Clinical Ethics* 29 (3): 179-84.

W v Edgell [1990] 1 ALL ER 835.

Wilkinson, D. and Savulescu, J. 2015. "A case of consent." *Journal of Medical Ethics* 41 (2): 143-4. doi: 10.1136/medethics-2014-102406.

Chapter **10**

Resource allocation

Health care systems throughout the world face enormous challenges in determining how resources should be allocated. No system has sufficient funds to provide the best possible treatment for all patients in all situations. Several dozen new pharmaceuticals are licensed each year in the UK. Almost all have some benefit over existing drugs. Many are expensive. When is the extra benefit worth the extra cost? Both publicly funded systems such as the British National Health Service (NHS) and private insurers face this fundamental question.

Whenever there are difficult questions about rationing or restricting treatment because of limited resources, one temptation is to suggest that more funding should be devoted to health care. The question of how much countries should spend on health is a political issue of great importance. Fig. 10.1 shows the relationship between health care spending and life expectancy in different countries.

In this chapter, we focus on ethical and legal questions relating to allocation of available resources. We will have to leave the question of how much to spend on health care to another day.

Case 10.1

Mr C was a 62-year-old man with morbid obesity (body mass index 43, 140 kg) and multiple medical complications (e.g. diabetes, arthritis), whose doctors had recommended

Continued

Case 10.1—cont'd

bariatric surgery. The local primary care trust, however, had a policy of only funding surgery for patients with a body mass index of more than 50. Mr C applied to an 'Individual Funding Request' (IFR) panel, arguing that exceptional circumstances applied, and surgery should be funded. His request was denied, and Mr C embarked on a legal appeal.

(This is based on the case of R (Condliff) v North Staffordshire Primary Care Trust [2011].)

Should treatment be rationed?

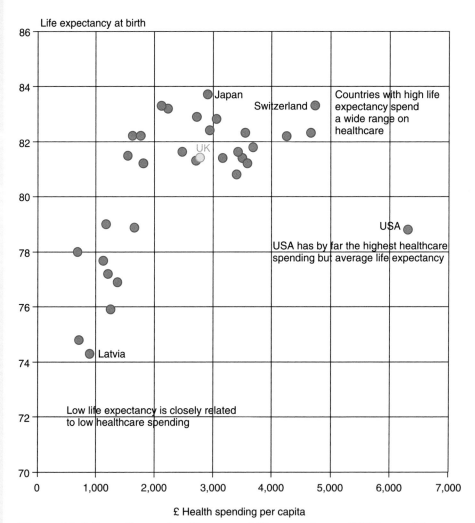

Life expectancy at birth and current healthcare expenditure, per person for OECD member-states (current PPPs), 2014

Figure 10.1 Spending on healthcare and life expectancy. OECD countries 2014. (From Office for National Statistics 'How does UK healthcare spending compare internationally?' ONS, 2016, used with permission.)

Faced with cases like Mr C's, we can separate out ethical questions – whether treatment should be rationed, or on what basis – from legal questions. We will address the ethical questions first.

RATIONING AND ETHICS

Should treatment be rationed? 'We shouldn't put a price on life'

Discussion of resource allocation, distributive justice and 'rationing' in cases like that of Mr C is often met with the rebuke that we should not put a price on life.

This is an example of a motherhood statement that appears attractive, but is nevertheless deeply ethically mistaken. Imagine that there is a health budget of £100,000. There are many people with life-threatening diseases. It costs £20,000 to treat disease A. It costs £100,000 to treat disease B. We are faced with a choice: save five lives of people with disease A, or one life of a person with disease B.

In general, people strongly believe that we should save the greatest number of lives (other things being equal). A famous philosophical thought experiment asks people to imagine a parallel case to the one above. Imagine you are manning the sole coastguard boat on duty. Two boats have been overturned some distance from each other. There are five people on one life raft 50 miles due north, and one person on another life raft 50 miles due south. A storm is brewing, and it is highly likely you will only be able to reach one life raft before the storm overturns them and the people drown. In a survey of the general population, almost everyone chose to save five lives rather than only one (Arora et al. 2016). Philosopher John Taurek has famously denied this (Taurek 1977). He argues that to treat everyone equally is to give each an equal chance of what matters most – their life. This involves tossing a coin.

What is clear is that, given finite resources, decisions about how much to spend on life-saving treatment equate to differences in numbers of people saved. Indeed, they also equate to differences in how long people will live and the quality of their lives. There are different ethical theories about how to allocate resources. However, there is no way to avoid these problems and avoid the need to ration treatment.

Maximizing benefit: Cost-effectiveness analysis, QALYs and utilitarianism

One widely used way of deciding between different priorities for funding in a publicly funded health care system is to compare their cost-effectiveness. In a cost-effectiveness analysis, the costs of an intervention are divided by its benefits, generating a cost-effectiveness ratio. Interventions with a lower cost-effectiveness ratio are preferred.

Cost-effectiveness analysis takes into consideration two factors that are ethically important. The cost of treatment will have direct implications for the number of individuals who are able to benefit from health systems with a fixed budget. As the hypothetical budget above illustrates, choosing a less expensive (but equally effective) treatment simply means that more patients are able to be treated (e.g.

choosing a cheaper life-saving treatment will mean that more lives are saved). The *effect* of treatment has implications for the amount of health benefit that can be promoted or improved for a given health budget. Choosing more effective treatments means that it is possible to have a greater impact.

There are different ways of comparing the effectiveness of treatments (Table 10.1).

Table 10.1 Different ways of evaluating the effectiveness of treatments.		
Quality-adjusted life years (QALYs)	Combines a measure of longevity (life years saved by treatment) with quality of life (based on surveys of preferences for different health states). A year of healthy life is judged to have a value of 1.	Regards full health as equally valuable at any point in the lifespan. Widely used in public policy (e.g. by NICE in the UK).
Saved young life equivalents (SAVEs) (Nord 1992)	Interventions are compared with a reference intervention that would save a young person from dying and restore them to full health. Allows evaluations to include distribution (e.g. priority for the worse off).	Assumes that the maximum benefit of intervention is saving life of young person. Enables direct and intuitive comparison of interventions.
Healthy-years equivalents (HYEs) (Mehrez and Gafni 1989)	Expresses the number of years of life in full health that are regarded as equivalent to actual numbers of years spent in a state of imperfect health. Does not assume equal weight for quality of life at different age.	Complex to assess in practice. Unclear how much difference there is from QALYs.
Disability-adjusted life years (DALYs) (Anand and Hanson 1997)	Sum of years of life lost due to disability, and years of life lived with disability. (Full health has a value of 0, and death is represented by 1). Incorporates age-weighting (young or middle-aged adults receive more weight than the elderly or young children).	Used to measure burden of disease. Inverted judgement compared with QALY (higher DALY = greater burden of disease).
Willingness to pay	Asks individuals how much they would be willing to pay for health gains.	Used in cost–benefit frameworks for public policy. Potentially disadvantages those on lower incomes (since those who are wealthy may be willing to pay more for a health gain).

We will focus our discussion below on QALYs, as these are most widely used. Some of the same issues apply to other methods of assessing effectiveness.

The central argument in favour of QALYs is as follows: the purpose of health care in general is to increase both the quantity and the quality of life. Both quantity and quality are important to us, and if choices have to be made, we trade these two factors against each other. If we call the combination of quantity and quality the overall welfare of a patient then, in allocating resources within health care, we should maximize the amount of welfare. If, therefore, we have a specified amount of money to spend on health care, it should be so allocated as to buy the maximum amount of welfare. QALYs are, in effect, units of welfare. QALY theory is a direct descendant of utilitarianism (see Chapter 2).

Some examples of the cost per QALY of different kinds of health care are given in Table 10.2.

Table 10.2 Some estimates of cost per QALY for various health care interventions.

Intervention	Approximate Cost/QALY
Treating rheumatoid arthritis with drugs that slow disease progression	* (Saves money and improves health)
Warfarin compared to aspirin for 70-year-olds with atrial fibrillation	£2400/QALY
Diabetes education for newly diagnosed patients with type 2 diabetes	£3200/QALY
Implantable defibrillator to prevent sudden cardiac death in high-risk groups	£30,000/QALY
Screening heavy smokers with annual CT scans	£112,000/QALY
Annual HIV screening for people at low-moderate risk	* (Costs money and makes health worse)

From Cost-Effectiveness Analysis Registry, https://cevr.tuftsmedicalcenter.org/databases/cea-registry. Approximate costs converted to GBP and adjusted for inflation to 2018 value.

Case 10.2

A clinical commissioning group is charged with managing the budget for a local primary care trust.

They are considering a set of applications for funding that are of approximately equal cost:

- Community program – healthy exercise promotion. To prevent obesity and heart disease.
- Community nursing program for patients with terminal illness, in conjunction with a hospice. To improve quality of life in dying patients.
- Installing automatic defibrillators in community halls/sporting venues. To prevent death in patients experiencing a cardiac arrhythmia.
- Day care program for elderly. To improve quality of life and reduce loneliness in older members of the community.
- Expansion of GP practice. To reduce waiting times for appointments.
  Which of these should receive priority?

What is wrong with QALYs?

The main criticisms of QALYs boil down to three concerns:

That *welfare* is not the only value to be put into the equation.

That QALYs are *unjust* because they do not take into account who is experiencing them.

That the *calculation of quality is problematic*. Either such calculation is not possible, or it is so subjective and dependent on the way in which it is calculated that it renders the theory unworkable.

Welfare is not the only value

Many believe that it is more important to help people who are sicker – who have a greater health care *need* – even if this might generate less benefit. (See below for further discussion of prioritarianism.)

Secondly, people do not always value welfare equally at different points in the lifespan. For example, many people feel that the manner in which a person's life ends is of considerable importance. Seen from this perspective, the nursing program for patients with terminal illness mentioned in Case 10.2 might be important even if it does not generate many QALYs (because patients survive for only a short time).

Third, many people place more value on preventing death than on improving health. In the example, the defibrillators might prevent very few deaths, but some might still wish to give them a higher priority than a day care program or reducing GP waiting times (even if those would benefit many more people).

QALYs are unjust

The second main criticism is that QALYs take no account of justice. Life-saving treatment for patients who have a chronic illness or disability will generate fewer QALYs than a life-saving treatment for patients in full health. This leads to what John Harris has called 'double jeopardy' (Harris 1985). First of all, a person has some handicap. Then she becomes in further need of medical help. Because she has the first handicap, she appears less entitled, from the QALY perspective, to further medical help.

A separate issue of justice is what is known as the distribution problem. The QALY approach maximizes total welfare without regard to how such welfare is distributed. Should resources be used preferentially to give a great benefit to relatively few people, or relatively little benefit to a large number of people? For example, reducing waiting times for appointments might benefit a large number of people in the community (by a small amount). Is the QALY answer (to do whatever maximizes welfare overall) the right one?

The problem with calculating quality of life

If QALYs are to be used in practice, then there has to be a method for calculating quality of life. That is not always straightforward (Nord, Daniels, and Kamlet 2009). Some benefits might be easier to quantify, and may therefore be more likely to be funded. (For example, it may not be easy to measure the impact of GP waiting times, or of a community day care program.) Because the whole purpose

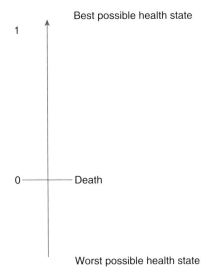

Figure 10.2 Putting a value on quality of life. Health utility is based on preferences in surveys for different health states. The best possible health state is given a value of 1, while the worst possible health state (if judged to be worse than death) has a negative value. For example, people might be asked to weigh up survival for different lengths of time. Imagine that you have a health condition (e.g. hemiplegia) and will survive for a year. Treatment A would restore you to full health, but you would survive for only 9 months. Would you take the treatment? By working out how short a survival would not be worth taking treatment A, it is possible to generate a value for health utility (e.g. if 9 months is the tipping point, that would give a health utility of 0.75). If someone would take the treatment even if they would only survive for 1 month, utility would be 0.08 (1/12). If someone would take treatment A even if it would lead to instant death, that implies that the health state has a negative utility (i.e. is worse than dying).

of QALYs is to help choose between different ways of spending health care money, quality of life cannot be just one person's view of quality of life. In practice, the kind of question that has to be answered is: what is the quality of life of being unable to walk and confined to a wheelchair? Or, what is the quality of life of having severe facial scarring? There is no single answer to these questions, as the answer will depend both on how the question is asked and on who answers it. With regard to the first issue, there are several different ways of approaching this question. Fig. 10.2 shows one way this is sometimes done. With regard to the second issue, there is a difference between the answers given by healthy people and those with a disability or illness (Sinclair 2012). People with serious health problems tend to rate their quality of life surprisingly highly. Furthermore, the correlation between quality of life and disease severity is not very strong (Fitzpatrick 1996).

Age and QALYs
Because QALYs are the product of quality and length of life, the cost per QALY will rise in inverse proportion to life expectancy. In practice, QALYs will tend to

disadvantage the elderly because they have a shorter life expectancy in general than do younger people. Some will be concerned that this mean that QALYs are *ageist*, i.e. that they unjustly discriminate against the elderly (Bognar and Hirose 2014, Rivlin 1995, Shaw 1994).

Egalitarianism and fair allocation

A different approach to allocating limited resources is based on the importance of fairness and equality. The idea that resources should be shared out equally is highly plausible. We are all familiar with the idea that, in dividing something like a cake, everyone should receive equal shares. However, there are different ways of allocating resources fairly or equally.

Equal shares. Everyone gets an equal share of the cake. But some people may not need or want treatment, while others need it much more. As Fig. 10.3 shows, equal treatment may be unfair if people have different starting points. Also, it may not be possible to give everyone equal shares if there is only a finite amount of a given resource.

Equal access to treatment. Treatment is made equally available to all (then only those who desire treatment will be seeking a slice of the cake). However, it may be that some will need treatment or benefit from treatment more than others. It may not be possible to give everyone equal access if there is only a finite amount of a given resource.

Equal chance of receiving treatment. For a finite (non-divisible) resource like organs for transplantation, it may not be possible for everyone to access treatment. Instead, everyone might be given an equal chance of receiving it. For example,

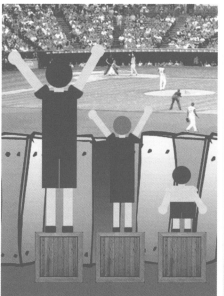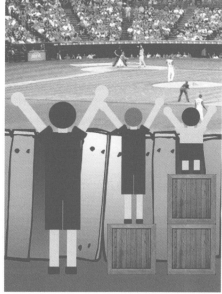

Figure 10.3 Two different forms of equality (© Professor Craig Froehle, used with permission)

organs might be allocated through a lottery, or provided on a first come, first served basis. However, again it may be that some will need treatment or benefit from treatment more than others (for example, should someone in a persistent vegetative state be put on the waiting list for a kidney transplant?).

Equal outcome from treatment. The baseball diagram indicates a desire to achieve an equitable outcome and points out that different levels of support may be needed to achieve that. However, in health care there is no conceivable way that everyone could achieve an equal outcome. Patients will still die, some will be sicker than others – regardless of how resources are distributed.

Equal consideration of interests. A health system might decide to allocate treatment in a way that considers equally every patient's potential to benefit from treatment (see above) and health needs (see below). It gives every patient's interest in treatment equal weight, and does not unfairly allocate based on factors that are not relevant (e.g. gender, race, political views, sexuality). However, that will inevitably mean that treatment is distributed unequally.

Case 10.3

Mr A has an advanced form of leukaemia that has not responded to treatment. He is an inpatient in a public hospital. There is a new treatment overseas, 'Lixira', that looks promising in early trials; however, it is not currently available in the public health system. There are no research trials that Mr A could enrol in to access the drug, and he is too unwell to travel overseas for the treatment. He asks his doctor if he can pay for the treatment. Mr A's doctor replies that hospital policy does not allow patients to pay for treatments that are not available to public patients.

Is this hospital policy justified?

(This is a fictional case and drug – though based on real examples that we have encountered.)

The hospital policy in Mr A's case is concerned about inequality. The idea that some patients could receive better treatment because they are wealthy seems to conflict with the basic idea that health care should be distributed fairly, not based on ability to pay.

However, in cases like this there are two different (related) ethical concerns. One is the concern that poorer patients are badly off – they are denied something that they deserve. The second concern is that richer patients are too well off – they are receiving more than they deserve. Our response to these two concerns is different.

If we are facing the first problem, the solution is to make Lixira available to all within the public health system. This improves the situation of those who are worse off. This approach to inequality is sometimes called 'levelling up equality'. However, sometimes that will simply not be an option. The cost of Lixira may be too great, or the evidence may be too slim to justify providing it in the public health care system.

If we are facing the second problem, one solution would be to prevent Mr A from paying for Lixira. That appears to be the hospital policy in his case.

This negatively affects the situation of those who are better off. It brings the wealthy down to the level of those who are poor (at least in terms of their access to health care). This approach is sometimes called 'levelling down equality' (Norheim 2009).

However, 'levelling down' in health care seems also to be problematic. It makes Mr A worse off (since he cannot access the treatment he wants and that might help him), but nobody else benefits. It seems to infringe his personal freedom to spend his money on whatever he chooses. (He could spend £100,000 on a flashy car, or in a casino, but not on a possibly life-extending drug.) What is more, it seems to discriminate against Mr A because he is seriously ill. If he were well enough, he could travel overseas to access Lixira. But because he is too sick to do this, the hospital denies him the opportunity to receive treatment.

Case 10.4

Julia is a 40-year-old woman who has smoked heavily for 20 years. She strongly desires to give up smoking, and has made many previous unsuccessful attempts to do so. Julia has gone to her GP to request a drug to help her give up smoking. The GP offers her a prescription for Varenicline, a nicotine partial agonist that has been shown to be effective. However, Julia has heard about a naturally derived medicine (Cytisine). She strongly prefers natural remedies, and is worried about side-effects from Varenicline. Cytisine is not currently funded in the public health system (because of relatively lack of evidence).

Should public health systems fund sub-optimal treatment?

As well as deciding what to do when patients request treatment that is not publicly available, health systems need to decide how to respond to requests for treatments that are available but might be less effective, or more expensive. Should patients be able to access sub-optimal treatment?

One response by a public health care system might be to provide funding only for the most effective (evidence-based) affordable treatment. For example, the NHS currently will provide Varenicline for people who wish to stop smoking, but not Cytisine. However, this appears to ignore the role of values in medical decision-making and the importance of patient autonomy.

A different response to these situations is the principle that we have elsewhere called Cost-Equivalence:

The Cost-Equivalence Principle: As well as providing the most effective, available treatment for a given condition, publicly funded health care systems should provide reasonable sub-optimal medical treatments that are equivalent in cost to (or cheaper than) the optimal treatment (Wilkinson and Savulescu 2017).

If the NHS allowed Julia access to Cytisine (instead of Varenicline), that would not cost the public health care system any more (it may actually cost less). It would treat her needs (and values) equally with someone else who wished to stop smoking but was happy to take Varenicline.

Responding to patient need and prioritarianism

As noted above, one problem with providing equal amounts of health care is that people have different needs for treatment. A different approach to allocating resources would aim to respond preferentially to those with the greatest need for treatment. For example, triage in an emergency department aims to respond to patients in order of urgency, not in order of when they arrived.

Rawls' approach

US philosopher John Rawls proposed a general theory of distributive justice, i.e. of how money and other goods should be distributed within a society (Rawls 1999). Rawls' approach has been applied to health care by Daniels (2008). He favoured developing a theory of social justice based on what rational individuals would choose. In order to ensure impartiality, Rawls constructed a device: the veil of ignorance.

Veil of ignorance

The veil of ignorance is a kind of thought experiment. Imagine that you are situated in some ethereal place, looking down on a vast array of different societies. Each of these societies distributes wealth among its citizens in a different way. In some societies, there are enormous differences between rich and poor. In others, goods are distributed almost equally. Some societies are, overall, well off; others are badly off. Imagine that you can choose to join one of these societies without knowing who, in that society, you will be. You might be among the richest, among the poorest or at any point in between. You also do not know what attributes you will have. You may have high or low intelligence. You may have one kind of personality or another. You may be male or female. The question is: which society would you choose to join?

Rawls argued that it would rational to choose to join the society in those who are worst-off are in the best position possible. This means that if you end up unfortunate, and being the most disadvantaged person in your new society, you will still do OK. The idea that justice is best achieved by the worst-off groups being maximally well off is known as the 'difference principle'. Applied to resource allocation, it gives rise to a later theory known as 'prioritarianism', whereby benefits matter more if they accrue to people who are worse off (Parfit 1997). Recall our priority-setting example in Case 10.2. Applying prioritarianism to that example might mean that nursing care for patients with terminal illness is funded first (even if it were clear that this would not generate the most QALYs).

Problems with prioritarianism

There are several problems with this approach to resource allocation. One problem is that it is often not clear who is worse off. Is it the sickest patient, the person who has most to lose without treatment or the person who has had the worst life so far?

Furthermore, it might appear that prioritarianism would face a 'bottomless pit' – very large amounts of resources might be expended on people who are very badly off, though they will in fact benefit very little from treatment. We asked earlier whether a patient in a persistent vegetative state should be listed for organ transplantation. They appear to be very badly off (with severe neurological impairment and organ failure), but it seems highly implausible that they should be given access to a limited resource like a kidney.

RESPONSIBILITY FOR BRINGING CONDITION ON ONESELF

If a patient's behaviour or lifestyle has contributed to her ill health, should she, therefore, be at a lower priority for health care?

Case 10.5

A local clinical commissioning group draws up a rule that patients who are obese or who are smokers will not be listed for elective surgery. Patients would be referred to weight loss programs or smoking cessation programs. In ordinary circumstances, they would only be eligible for surgery if they had stopped smoking for at least eight weeks, or lost weight. The group justified the restrictions as encouraging patients 'to take more responsibility for their own health and wellbeing, wherever possible, freeing up limited NHS resources for priority treatment'.

Is this policy justified?

This case is based on the Hertfordshire CCG Fitness for surgery policy (Donnelley 2017).

There are two different ways of considering responsibility in health care (Feiring 2008).

Backward-looking responsibility seeks to identify patients whose health conditions are partly or wholly the result of their own choices. Patients who have been responsible for their condition would have a lower priority for treatment.

Forward-looking responsibility aims to make patients take responsibility for their health care by imposing conditions on their treatment (Savulescu 2018).

Up for Debate Box 10.1 presents arguments in favour of and against taking into consideration responsibility in allocation of treatment.

The policy in Case 10.5 appears to have elements of both backward- and forward-looking responsibility. It imposes restrictions on access to surgery for people who are obese or smoke (that do not apply to other patients), presumably, in part, because they are considered responsible. However, the way in which restrictions apply is then exerted through conditions on future behaviour.

SOCIAL FACTORS, DEPENDANTS AND PRIORITY

If a patient's responsibility for illness would possibly reduce his priority for treatment, there are other factors that might increase someone's priority. For example, should someone with dependants (for example, children or frail elderly parents)

Up for Debate Box 10.1 Should responsibility for illness be taken into account when allocating treatment?

Arguments in favour

Autonomous adults make decisions. They then bear responsibility for the consequences of those decisions. Although there may be many situations in which it is difficult to assess responsibility, that is by no means always the case. The fully informed person who elects for sterilization (and then wants the procedure reversed) and the sportsperson who knows of the risk of soft tissue injury make choices in knowledge of the risks to their health.

Just as it is unfair for people to demand a larger share of limited health care resources, it is unfair for people to make choices and then expect the public health care system to pay the costs of those choices.

In many other walks of life, we expect people to accept the consequences of the choices they make. For example, someone who chooses to study hard will be rewarded, whereas someone who breaks the law will be punished. Why should medicine be any different?

It is unfair for patients who have taken care of their health to be denied treatment because another, who is responsible for his ill health, took priority (perhaps on the grounds of being more ill). At the very least, if resources are scarce, the issue of responsibility should be given some weight, even if the weight is small compared with other factors such as clinical need or ability to benefit.

Arguments against

Although we are free to choose different things in life, people have little effective choice over most of the factors that affect health, or at any rate cannot reasonably be blamed for what they have done. Consider a smoker. Upbringing, peer group pressure and perhaps genetic factors predisposing to addictive behaviour may combine to make her vulnerable to smoke. Furthermore, she may have become addicted to smoking when a teenager. Would it be right to hold her responsible for the health consequences of her smoking as an adult, 20 years later? More generally, attributing responsibility is too imprecise. Many people will be responsible to some degree for their health condition, but how would we work out whether or how much they are responsible?

Even if a person is responsible, this should have no influence over priority. Access to health care, and priority, should depend on factors such as clinical need, not responsibility. The central importance of health to our lives justifies health care being different from the other areas of life where we do expect people to accept the consequences of their own behaviour.

have a higher priority for health care? What about someone with wider value to society more generally? For example, in the setting of a health emergency (like a pandemic), it has sometimes been suggested that health care workers should have first access to treatment or vaccines. Is that justified (Rothstein 2010)?

According to the consequentialist perspective (see Chapter 2), we should consider all the consequences of our actions. If treating person A results in better overall consequences than treating person B, that provides a good reason in favour of treating person A. These overall consequences include those contributions to society that person A or person B would make.

However, many would argue that doctors, or health managers, should not make judgements about patients' 'social worth'. There are other ways in which society rewards people for what they contribute (e.g. by the level of income or through various honours). The provision of health care should not be one of these ways. Even if it is not wrong in principle to give higher priority to those of higher 'social worth', it is too difficult in practice to judge such worth. For example, we may not know of the good that one patient does in supporting other people.

FAIR PROCEDURE FOR MAKING ALLOCATION DECISIONS

Each theory of resource allocation that we have discussed highlights some relevant values, and each has some strengths and some weaknesses. There seems to be no one theory that should determine the use of resources. For these reasons, much recent work has focused, not on the theories, but on the process by which decisions should be made. Daniels and Sabin specify four conditions in order to implement what they call 'accountability for reasonableness' in allocation decisions (Daniels and Sabin 1997):

Publicity: Decisions regarding coverage for new technologies (and other limit-setting decisions) and their rationales must be publicly accessible.

Reasonableness: The rationales for coverage decisions should aim to provide a *reasonable* construal of how the organization should provide 'value for money' in meeting the varied health needs of a defined population under reasonable resource constraints.

Appeals: There is a mechanism for challenge and dispute resolution regarding limit-setting decisions, including the opportunity for revising decisions in light of further evidence or arguments.

Enforcement: There is either voluntary or public regulation of the process to ensure that the first three conditions are met.

In practice, such procedures usually involve setting up a group of people from a variety of backgrounds to decide issues of resource allocation (Hope et al. 1998), and this raises the question of who should be involved in this process and how should they be chosen. Such a group, even when provided with good evidence concerning both the cost and the effectiveness of a health care intervention, frequently faces problematic ethical choices. If the group is to behave in a responsible way, it needs to provide reasons for its decisions. It cannot avoid considering the values highlighted by the theories of allocation discussed above.

RATIONING AND THE LAW

If a health authority or health care provider were challenged in the courts on a decision about the allocation of resources (as in the case of Mr C – Case 10.1), then it would need to be able to explain its decision in two ways:

Was the *procedure* for making the decision reasonable?
Were the *grounds* for making the decision reasonable?

Legal challenges to resource allocation decisions

Decisions about the allocation of resources can be legally challenged through actions in either public or private law. The legal framework of the NHS imposes a number of specific legal obligations on the Secretary of State for Health. The NHS Act 2006 (which came into force in March 2007) primarily covers the structure and operation of the NHS. The obligations in the NHS Act 2006 include the promotion of a comprehensive health service designed to secure an improvement (a) in the physical and mental health of the people, and (b) in the prevention, diagnosis and treatment of illness.

One potential way of involving the courts in decisions of resource allocation is to claim that, in not funding a particular treatment or service, the NHS has failed in its statutory duty. The procedure involved is a part of public law, and is known as judicial review. If the claim succeeds, the court will strike down the decision to refuse treatment and require the decision to reconsidered. The court does not have the power to compel the NHS body to provide treatment.

The second (private action) approach is to use civil law to claim that some person or institution has been negligent in making the decision. If such a claim were to succeed, the claimant (e.g. patient) would be compensated for the loss suffered. The decision, however, would not be reversed.

From an analysis of the relevant cases, Montgomery concluded: '... judicial review is unlikely to be successful if it is based on an attack on the substance of the decision. Applications will be stronger if they allege that the process by which the decision was taken was flawed'. However, that too may be hard to prove to a court's satisfaction (Montgomery 2003). Charles Foster has argued that courts will only interfere with a resource allocation decision by an NHS body if that decision was 'frankly irrational' (Foster 2007). The most common ground for a successful judicial review is that the body has not followed its own guidance or procedures.

In the case of Mr C, the court rejected his appeal on the basis that his circumstances were not 'exceptional', and so the trust had followed its guidance in only granting funding in cases like his where they were exceptional. The court also rejected Mr C's argument that the IFR panel should have taken into account non-clinical factors in assessing his situation. (See below for discussion of including social factors in allocation decisions.)

[Mr C did eventually have surgery after the primary care trust later agreed to pay for the operation.]

In general, the courts have not been sympathetic to private claims either, and in particular to negligence claims. One of the reasons, Montgomery believes, why courts have been reluctant to become involved in rationing decisions is to ensure that authorities make decisions based on the best use of resources, rather than on satisfying those most likely to complain.

Although the general principle that the courts will not intervene in issues of resource allocation in the NHS seems to hold, there have been cases where health authorities have been held to be liable for failure to provide services.

One case involved β-interferon for sufferers of multiple sclerosis. A sufferer challenged the decision by a health authority to refuse to pay for the drug, and the challenge was successful on the grounds that the authority had failed to follow guidance issued by the Department of Health (R v North Derbyshire Health Authority [1997]).

A second case concerned three transsexuals who wanted gender reassignment surgery. Such surgery had been given a low priority by the authority and was not funded. The Court of Appeal found that the health authority's policy was flawed. In particular, the authority had failed to assess the effectiveness of various forms of treatment accurately (North West Lancashire Health Authority v A, D and G [1999]).

In a third case, a patient successfully appealed against the finding of an IFR panel (like the case of Mr C) (Ann Marie Rogers v Swindon NHS Trust [2006]). The court was critical of the apparent poor reasoning demonstrated by the panel. It would have been acceptable for a panel to decide only to provide treatment in 'exceptional cases' – 'provided that it is possible to envisage, and the decision-maker does envisage, what such exceptional circumstances might be'. (In the case, the court concluded that the IFR panel's assessment of exceptionality had been 'meaningless'.)

As to the impact of the Human Rights Act 1998 on access to treatment, several articles could be invoked by patients refused treatment (especially life-saving treatment). These include Article 2 (right to life), Article 3 (protection from torture or inhuman or degrading treatment), Article 8 (right to private life) and Article 14 (protection from discrimination). Article 14 is potentially the most promising approach if used by a patient alleging discrimination on the basis of, for example, age or disability (Herring 2018).

REVISION QUESTIONS

1. A clinical commissioning group draws up a list of criteria for accessing in-vitro fertilization. This includes an age cut-off for accessing treatment. Is this ageist?
2. A woman who is unable to access IVF because she is too old decides to take the clinical commissioning group to court. What are her legal options? Is she likely to succeed?
3. What is a QALY? What is its role in making decisions about allocating treatment?
4. Two patients with organ failure are potential matches for an organ that has come up for transplant. One of the patients is sicker. The other patient is currently less sick, but has a lower chance of complications from the transplant and would be likely to live longer post-transplant. What different ethical values are at stake in choosing which patient to transplant?
5. The NHS does not usually fund reversal of vasectomy (male sterilization). What do you think the ethical rationale for this policy would be? Is it justified?

Mrs W, a 75-year-old woman with severe arthritis of her hip, was put on a waiting list for a hip replacement. She was in considerable pain and had difficulty walking, but the local trust waiting list was 1 year. Mrs W applied for permission to travel to France for her treatment (where she could have the operation much sooner). If advance authorization is granted, the NHS will cover the costs of treatment in another country. However, the trust refused to authorize treatment. When Mrs W's hip pain deteriorated, and she still had another 3 or 4 months to wait for surgery, she went to France anyway and had her treatment. She then applied to the court to request that the cost of treatment (£3,900) be refunded. She argued that the refusal to authorize her overseas treatment infringed her right to freedom of movement.

Do patients have a right to travel overseas for medical treatment?

Should (or when should) public health systems pay for patients to travel overseas? Should they cover the equivalent costs of treatment in the home country, or the whole cost of treatment if more expensive?

This is based on the case of R (on the application of Watts v Bedford PCT and Secretary of State for Health [2004]). (In Mrs W's case, the English Court of Appeal referred a number of questions to the European Court of Justice. The European court decision in this case suggests that a patient would succeed in such a claim if the waiting time in the UK amounted to 'undue delay'.)

See for example Davies (2007) and Wilkinson and Savulescu (2018).

REFERENCES

Anand, S. and Hanson, K. 1997. "Disability-adjusted life years: a critical review." *Journal of Health Economics* 16 (6): 685-702.

Arora, C., Savulescu, J., Maslen, H., Selgelid, M. and Wilkinson, D. 2016. "The Intensive Care Lifeboat: a survey of lay attitudes to rationing dilemmas in neonatal intensive care." *BMC Medical Ethics* 17 (1): 69. doi: 10.1186/s12910-016-0152-y.

Bognar, G. and Hirose, I. 2014. *The ethics of health care rationing: an introduction.* London: Routledge.

Daniels, N. 2008. *Just health: meeting health needs fairly.* Cambridge: Cambridge University Press.

Daniels, N. and Sabin, J. 1997. "Limits to health care: fair procedures, democratic deliberation, and the legitimacy problem for insurers." *Philosophy & Public Affairs* 26 (4): 303-50.

Davies, G. 2007. "The effect of Mrs Watts' trip to France on the National Health Service." *King's Law Journal* 18 (1): 158-67. doi: 10.1080/09615768.2007.11427668.

Donnelley, L. 2017. "NHS provokes fury with indefinite surgery ban for smokers and obese." The Telegraph, 17 October 2017. Accessed 9/11/18. https://www.telegraph.co.uk/news/2017/10/17/nhs-provokes-fury-indefinite-surgery-ban-smokers-obese/.

Feiring, E. 2008. "Lifestyle, responsibility and justice." *Journal of Medical Ethics* 34: 33-6.

Fitzpatrick, R. 1996. "Patient-centred approaches to the evaluation of health care." In *Essential practice in patient-centred care,* edited by S. Ersser, R. A. Hope and K. W. M. Fulford. Oxford: Blackwell Science: 229-40.

Foster, C. 2007. "Simple rationality? The law of healthcare resource allocation in England." *Journal of Medical Ethics* 33 (7): 404-7. doi: 10.1136/jme.2006.017905.

Harris, J. 1985. *Value of life: an introduction to medical ethics.* Routledge & Kegan Paul.

Herring, J. 2018. *Medical law and ethics.* 7th ed. Oxford: Oxford University Press.

Hope, T., Hicks, N., Reynolds, D. J., Crisp, R. and Griffiths, S. 1998. "Rationing and the health authority." *BMJ (Clinical research ed.)* 317 (7165): 1067-9.

Mehrez, A. and Gafni, A. 1989. "Quality-adjusted life years, utility theory, and healthy-years equivalents." *Medical Decision Making* 9 (2): 142-9. doi: 10.1177/0272989X8900900209.

Montgomery, J. 2003. *Health care law*. 2nd ed. Oxford: Oxford University Press.

Nord, E. 1992. "An alternative to QALYs: the saved young life equivalent (SAVE)." *BMJ* 305: 875-7.

Nord, E., Daniels, N. and Kamlet, M. 2009. "QALYs: some challenges." *Value in Health* 12 (Suppl. 1): S10-5. doi: 10.1111/j.1524-4733 .2009.00516.x.

Norheim, O. F. 2009. "A note on Brock: prioritarianism, egalitarianism and the distribution of life years." *Journal of Medical Ethics* 35: 565-9.

North West Lancashire Health Authority v A, D and G [1999] EWCA Civ 2022.

Office for National Statistics. 2016. "How does UK healthcare spending compare internationally?". ONS, accessed 29/11/18. https://www. ons.gov.uk/peoplepopulationandcommunity/ healthandsocialcare/healthcaresystem/articles/ howdoesukhealthcarespendingcompareinternationally/2016-11-01.

Parfit, D. 1997. "Equality and priority." *Ratio* 10 (3): 202-21. doi: 10.1111/1467-9329. 00041.

R (Condliff) v North Staffordshire Primary Care Trust [2011] EWCA Civ 910.

R (on the application of Ann Marie Rogers v Swindon NHS Trust [2006] EWCA 392.

R (on the application of Watts v Bedford PCT and Secretary of State for Health [2004] EWCA Civ 166.

R v North Derbyshire Health Authority [1997] Med LR 327.

Rawls, J. 1999. *A theory of justice*. Rev. ed. Oxford: Oxford University Press.

Rivlin, M. M. 1995. "Protecting elderly people: flaws in ageist arguments." *BMJ* 310 (6988): 1179-82.

Rothstein, M. A. 2010. "Currents in contemporary ethics. Should health care providers get treatment priority in an influenza pandemic?" *The Journal of Law, Medicine & Ethics* 38 (2): 412-9. doi: 10.1111/j.1748-720X.2010.00499.x.

Savulescu, J. 2018. "Golden opportunity, reasonable risk and personal responsibility for health." *Journal of Medical Ethics* 44 (1): 59-61. doi: 10.1136/medethics-2017-104428.

Shaw, A. B. 1994. "In defence of ageism." *Journal of Medical Ethics* 20 (3): 188-91, 194.

Sinclair, S. 2012. "How to avoid unfair discrimination against disabled patients in healthcare resource allocation." *Journal of Medical Ethics* 38 (3): 158-62. doi: 10.1136/medethics-2011-100093.

Taurek, J. 1977. "Should the numbers count?" *Philosophy & Public Affairs* 6 (4): 293-316.

Wilkinson, D. and Savulescu, J. 2018. *Ethics, conflict and medical treatment for children: from disagreement to dissensus*. Elsevier.

Wilkinson, D. and Savulescu, J. 2017. "Cost-equivalence and pluralism in publicly-funded health-care systems." *Health Care Analysis* doi: 10.1007/s10728-016-0337-z.

FURTHER READING

The Journal of Medical Ethics published an interesting and lively debate between Harris on the one hand and Singer and colleagues on the other.

Harris, J. 1987. "QALYfying the value of human life." *Journal of Medical Ethics* 13: 117-23, *Harris argues against QALY theory*.

Harris, J. 1995. "Double jeopardy and the veil of ignorance – a reply." *Journal of Medical Ethics* 21: 151-7, *Harris defends his original position*.

Harris, J. 1996. "Would Aristotle have played Russian roulette?" *Journal of Medical Ethics* 22: 209-15.

Hope, T. 1996. "QALYs, lotteries and veils: the story so far." *Journal of Medical Ethics* 22: 195-6, *Summary of the debate*.

McKie, J., Kuhse, H., Richardson, J. and Singer, P. 1996. "Another peep behind the veil." *Journal of Medical Ethics* 22: 216-21.

McKie, J., Kuhse, H., Richardson, J. and Singer, P. 1996. "Double jeopardy, the equal value of lives and the veil of ignorance: a rejoinder to Harris." *Journal of Medical Ethics* 22: 204-8.

Singer, P., McKie, J., Kuhse, H. and Richardson, J. 1996. "Double jeopardy and the use of QALYs in health care allocation." *Journal of Medical Ethics* 21: 144-50, *Singer and colleagues reply to Harris*.

Chapter 11

Children and young people

Case 11.1

A 13-year-old, H, has developed severe heart failure as a complication of medical treatment earlier in childhood for leukaemia. Doctors have told H that she is likely to deteriorate and die if she does not have a heart transplant; they believe that this would be in her best interests. However, H has indicated that she does not wish to undergo this procedure. She feels that the risks of treatment are too great, and that she would rather spend time with friends and family. Her parents support H's wishes and do not consent to surgery.

Can parents refuse consent for treatment that would be in a child or young person's best interests?

Can a young person consent or refuse consent for a medical procedure on their own?

(This is based on the case of Hannah Jones (Verkaik 2008).)

Ethical issues in the medical care of children and young people overlap with those for other patients who lack or may lack capacity (see Chapter 7). However, there are differences. These include when capacity is assumed or not assumed to be present, the role of the patient's own values and the distinctive role of a particular group of surrogate decision-makers: parents. The way we think about children is fraught with tensions. On the one hand, we want to be protective, and on the other we want to encourage the young person's increasing autonomy. We value family relationships, wanting to give parents the right to make decisions about the care of their children without state interference. However, we also want to protect children from harm if their parents do not act in their best interests.

THE LAW

There are four key pieces of legislation relating to medical treatment and children/young people in the UK. Although there are some subtle differences between jurisdictions, the principles around treatment and consent are the same across the UK. The Mental Capacity Act (MCA) does not apply to children (it can apply to 16–17-year-olds who lack capacity).

1. The Children Act 1989 is the principal statute concerning children in England, Wales and Northern Ireland. It articulates a number of general principles (Box 11.1), as well as providing specific legal procedures. It also provides a 'welfare checklist' (Box 11.2) to help guide the courts. This is a list of factors that should be considered by the court in coming to a decision. (A subsequent act, the Children Act 2004, deals mainly with the system of children's services, with the intention of providing a better integrated service for the protection of children.)

Box 11.1 Some general principles of the Children Act 1989

The child's welfare is paramount.
The child is a person, not an object of concern: children of sufficient maturity should be listened to (although their wishes will not necessarily be followed).
Children should be brought up by parents or wider family, without the interference of the State, unless placed at risk.
Family links should be maintained if a child is placed out of the home.
Cooperation, negotiation and partnership should be the aim if conflicts arise.
Avoid delay when legal processes are required.

Box 11.2 The Children Act 1989: welfare checklist

The following should be taken into account by courts in guiding their decisions:
- The wishes and feelings of the child
- The child's physical, emotional and educational needs
- The likely effect on the child of a change in circumstances
- The age, sex and background of the child, and any characteristics the court considers relevant
- Any harm the child has suffered or is at risk of suffering
- The capability of parents and others to meet the child's needs
- The range of powers open to the courts

2. The Children (Scotland) Act 1995 applies to Scotland. This Act has similar general principles to the Children Act 1989; however, it makes more explicit reference to children's views. A young person aged 12 years and over is presumed to form a view, and their views should be taken into account where practicable. It also defines parental responsibilities and rights in more detail than the English Act.

3. The Family Law Reform Act 1969 is relevant to consent to treatment for patients aged 16 and 17 years in England and Wales. The Family Law Reform Act 1969 states: '...the consent of a minor who has attained the age of sixteen years to any surgical, medical or dental treatment ... shall be as effective as it would be if he were of full age [i.e. aged 18 years or above]; and ... it shall not be necessary to obtain any consent for it from his parent or guardian'. The Age of Majority Act (Northern Ireland) 1969 states similar principles for Northern Ireland.

4. The Age of Legal Capacity (Scotland) Act 1991 gives statutory power to mature minors under the age of 16 years to consent to treatment. The Act states (Section 2(4)): 'A person under the age of 16 years shall have legal capacity to consent on his own behalf to any surgical, medical or dental procedure or treatment where, in the opinion of a qualified medical practitioner attending him, he is capable of understanding the nature and possible consequences of the procedures or treatment'. This is the equivalent (in Scotland) of Gillick competence (see below). There is no statute that sets out principles relating to consent for young people aged 16 or 17 in Scotland; however, under common law, a person aged 16 years and above is presumed to have the ability to make medical decisions and consent to procedures.

Case 11.2

A newborn infant, Adam, is born extremely prematurely and transferred to another hospital for treatment. Adam's mother, Ellie, is also unwell and remains in intensive care at the first hospital. Adam is visited in hospital by Suzanna. Suzanna is in a long-standing relationship with Ellie, though they are not married. Suzanna was the egg donor for Adam (with donor sperm).

The doctors wish to perform urgent surgery for Adam, but are unsure if they can obtain consent from Suzanna.

Who can consent for a child?

Can a parent consent to a medical procedure? (which parent?)

The question of who can give consent for medical assessment and treatment of a child not yet old enough and mature enough to give his or her own consent depends on who has 'parental responsibility'. This is a key concept in the Children Act.

There are some general points about parental responsibility (PR):

- More than one person may have PR for a child (typically both parents will have PR).
- Many actions or decisions, including consent to medical examination or treatment, can be carried out by just one person with PR. There is no requirement for that person to consult anyone else with PR before acting (or giving consent to treatment).
- PR cannot normally be transferred or surrendered (except by adoption).

Those with PR have a duty to ensure that the child receives essential medical assistance and adequate full-time education, among other things. They have the right to make decisions on major issues such as day-to-day care and schooling. The law relating to who has PR is summarized in Box 11.3. If someone has PR, they may provide consent to a medical procedure until the young person reaches their 18th birthday.

In Case 11.2, Suzanna does not have legal PR for Adam. (She may gain this subsequently, e.g. if she is named on the birth certificate.) However, if treatment is urgently required to avoid harm to Adam, health professionals could provide that treatment without consent. As a matter of ethics rather than law, it would be important for the surgeons to discuss Adam's treatment with Suzanna and to obtain her agreement to proceed with surgery. The Children Act also specifically allows someone who 'has care of a child' but who does not have PR to do 'what is reasonable in all the circumstances of the case for the purpose of safeguarding or promoting the child's welfare'. This would potentially allow Suzanna (or, in other circumstances, teachers, child minders, other family members) in an emergency to consent to treatment.

If there were sufficient time (and no one else with PR were able to participate in decisions), doctors could apply to the court, either for a specific decision or for a care order (giving a local authority temporary PR).

There are limits to what parents can consent to. Parents can only consent to treatment that is in a child's best interests. If parents disagree, the consent of one person with PR is usually sufficient. However, the courts have specifically indicated that, for 'important issues', parents should consult; if parents are unable to agree, health professionals should apply to the court to determine the issue. This includes procedures that might be regarded as elective, in particular circumcision (Re J (child's religious upbringing and circumcision) [2000]) and immunization. In cases of disagreement, courts have been focused on the best interests of the child. Past court decisions where parents have disagreed have tended not to allow non-medical circumcision, but have allowed immunization (Re SL (Permission to Vaccinate) [2017], B (A Child: Immunisation) [2018]).

Can parents refuse consent to a medical procedure?

If parents (with PR) refuse consent to medical treatment that would be in a child's best interests to receive, then a court can authorize the treatment. (See section below on Disputes and the zone of parental discretion.) The most commonly cited example of this is where parents who are Jehovah's Witnesses decline consent for a blood transfusion for a child. In an emergency (for example, if a child had been

Box 11.3   Who has parental responsibility?

1. The birth mother of the child.
2. The father of the child, if he is married to the mother at the time of the birth of the child. (Parents do not lose parental responsibility if they divorce.)
3. A second female parent who is married to or in a civil partnership with the biological mother at the time of conception.
4. An unmarried father or an unmarried second female parent can gain parental responsibility if:
   - they are named on the birth certificate
   - they marry (or, for a second female parent, enter into a civil partnership with) the mother
   - they complete (together with the mother of the child) a legal 'parental responsibility agreement'
   - they are named by the court in a child arrangements order.

Where a husband does not deny paternity, and no other man asserts that he is the father, the husband is considered in law to be the father (whatever the biological fact).

Other people than parents may acquire parental responsibility:

1. Adoption – in which case the original parent(s) cease to have parental responsibility.
2. Guardian – parents with parental responsibility may (without involving a court) appoint a guardian to acquire parental responsibility for their child on their death.
3. A person obtaining a residence order (a court order specifying who a child will live with) normally acquires parental responsibility – this might be when a child is effectively given over to the care of a grandparent. The parent(s), however, do not lose parental responsibility.
4. A local authority named in a care order (again, the parent(s) do not lose parental responsibility).
5. An applicant granted an emergency protection order, but only for the duration of the care order.

Step-parents (by marriage or civil partnership) do not automatically have parental responsibility. They may acquire it by making a parental responsibility agreement, by an order from the court (e.g. a parental responsibility order, a special guardianship order or a residence order) or by adopting the child.

A person (e.g. an unmarried father) may be a parent without having parental responsibility. There are some legal consequences that arise from the status of being a parent (e.g. responsibility for child support). However, in the context of consent to medical treatment, the key legal issue is that of parental responsibility.

In the case of couples undergoing fertility treatment (licensed under the Human Fertilisation and Embryology Act) and involving donated gametes, the legal parents of the child are normally the birth couple and not the gamete donors.

In a case of surrogacy, the surrogate (birth) mother and her husband (or civic partner) will be regarded as legal parents at the time of birth and have parental responsibility. If the surrogate is not married or in a civic partnership, the biological father can be named on the birth certificate (and have parental responsibility). Subsequently, the intended parents can apply for a parental order, which will result in a new birth certificate and establish them as having parental responsibility.

involved in a road accident and had suffered massive blood loss), doctors should provide the medical treatment necessary to prevent harm to the child. In less time-critical situations, doctors should apply to the court for authorization to provide treatment in the child's best interests. The courts have almost always authorized such treatment (Re S [1993], An NHS Trust v Child B and Others [2014]).

Can a child or young person consent to a medical procedure?

Case 11.3

Department of Health guidance was published indicating that doctors could prescribe contraception to young people under the age of 16 without parental consent. Mrs G was a campaigner who was opposed to this circular. She had four daughters under the age of 16 years. She wrote to her health authority seeking assurance that none of her daughters would be given contraception, or abortion advice or treatment, without her knowledge and consent until they reached the age of 16 years. The health authority gave no such assurance. Mrs G went to the High Court.

Can young people under the age of 16 consent to medical treatment?

(This is based on the case of Gillick v West Norfolk & Wisbeck Area Health Authority [1986].)

As noted above, a young person aged 16 or 17 years may consent to medical treatment on their own in the same way as an adult. There is no requirement to seek separate consent from their parents, and a medical procedure could proceed even if parents refused consent. For example, a 16-year-old could consent to a termination of pregnancy against the wishes of her parents. (Health professionals would not be permitted to ask the young person's parents without her consent, since this would breach her confidentiality – see Chapter 9.)

A young person below the age of 16 may consent to medical treatment *if* they are deemed to be able to fully understand the decision. In Scotland, this is set out in the Age of Capacity (Scotland) Act. In the rest of the UK, this is based on a case known as 'Gillick' (Case 11.2). In the real case, the House of Lords decided, by three to two, against Mrs Gillick. Lord Scarman said: '... the parental right yields to the child's right to make his own decisions when he reaches a sufficient understanding and intelligence to be capable of making up his own mind on the matter requiring decision' (see Brazier 2003). Lord Fraser gave specific guidance on when doctors would be justified in providing contraception without parents' consent. The doctor would be justified if:

'...he is satisfied on the following matters:

1. that the girl (although under 16 years of age) will understand his advice;
2. that he cannot persuade her to inform her parents or to allow him to inform the parents that she is seeking contraceptive advice;

3. that she is very likely to begin or to continue having sexual intercourse with or without contraceptive treatment;
4. that unless she receives contraceptive advice or treatment her physical or mental health or both are likely to suffer;
5. that her best interests require him to give her contraceptive advice, treatment or both without the parental consent.' (Gillick v West Norfolk & Wisbeck Area Health Authority [1986])

A child is said to be 'Gillick competent' if they have sufficient maturity and intelligence to understand and consider the nature and risks of the proposed treatment, as well as any alternatives available (Gilmore and Herring 2011, Larcher and Hutchinson 2010).

In another case, Lord Donaldson used the analogy of consent as a key; both parents and the Gillick competent child hold keys that would unlock (permit) a procedure Re R (a minor) (Wardship: Medical Treatment) [1992]. For a young person under the age of 16, consent could be obtained *either* from the young person (if they are Gillick competent), or from a parent (with PR) or from a court.

For children who are not Gillick competent, it is still often important to give them the opportunity to express their view about treatment, and this should be taken into account in assessment of their best interests.

If a young person aged 16 or 17 lacks capacity, the MCA (see Chapter 7) applies. The doctor can treat either with the consent of a person with PR or under the protection of Section 5 of the MCA.

Can a child or young person refuse a medical procedure?

In contrast to the above, case law indicates that a young person aged 16 or 17 in England and Wales cannot refuse a life-saving treatment or one necessary to prevent serious harm. (In Scotland, more weight is given to respecting the minor's autonomy. There is uncertainty as to the extent to which Scottish law allows those under 18 years the absolute right to refuse medical treatment.) This also applies to a child or young person younger than 16, *even if* they are Gillick competent. In such cases, the consent of someone with PR would suffice to make treatment lawful, notwithstanding the young person's lack of agreement. One relevant case concerned a 16-year-old, W, with anorexia nervosa. The Court of Appeal authorized treatment against her wishes. This was partly on the basis that W lacked capacity as a consequence of her illness. However, the court was also clear about refusal of treatment by a minor, saying: 'No minor of whatever age has power by refusing consent to treatment to override a consent to treatment by someone who has PR for the minor' Re W [1992].

Cases of Jehovah's Witness teenagers (including those aged 16 or 17) who wish to decline a blood transfusion have, in almost all cases, seen the courts give permission to transfuse (see e.g. Re P (Medical Treatment: Best Interests) [2003]).

This would appear to mean that, in Case 11.1, H's refusal to consent to a heart transplant could be overridden. However, even if health professionals *could* legally override a young person's refusal of treatment, that does not mean that they must do so. In the real version of the case, the young person managed to convince child protection officers of her point of view. The hospital elected not to proceed with the court order. (She later changed her mind and had the heart transplant at age 14 (Retter 2013).)

Fig. 11.1 provides a flow-sheet to guide consent in children.

ETHICAL CONSIDERATIONS

How much weight should we give to the wishes of young people?

The legal framework described above contains a paradox. Adolescents who are judged to have capacity and to understand the nature and significance of medical decisions can *consent* to medical treatment, but cannot refuse treatment. However, normally we think that it would be wrong to impose treatment against the wishes of a patient with capacity. The right to refuse treatment appears to derive implicitly from respect for patient autonomy. How can we make sense of this paradox?

One way of defending the current legal approach would be to point out that capacity exists on a *spectrum*. Capacity is not all or nothing. Decisions also vary in their complexity and ramifications. Patients may have the capacity to make some decisions, but not others. The level of capacity needed to consent to some decisions (e.g. a decision to use contraception in a sexually active teenager) may be different from the capacity needed to consent to other decisions (e.g. a decision not to receive a life-saving medical treatment). However, *if* we understand decisions in that way, that would imply a more complex picture about decisions. Some decisions to undertake medical treatment might be very complex and challenging. One possible example is gender reassignment surgery. Another might be a decision to undergo risky experimental treatment. Some 16–17-year-olds (or younger adolescents) who would have capacity to make some medical decisions should not make *these* decisions on their own. On the other hand, some decisions to refuse medical treatment may be within a young person's capacity to decide. For example, in H's case (from the start of the chapter), it appeared that she could have had a very clear understanding about the nature and significance of the decision because of her previous experience of illness and medical treatment. It seems potentially the right answer to respect her decision. Most doctors would be reluctant to enforce treatment on a 16–17-year-old with capacity, even with consent from someone with PR, except in emergency situations to prevent death or serious harm.

A different rationale for not allowing teenagers to refuse medical treatment is based, not on autonomy, but rather on paternalism and best interests. It is in the best interests of some young people to receive access to contraception if they are sexually active. Requiring their parents to be involved in decisions may not be their best interests (e.g. it may mean that they do not use effective contraception). However, allowing teenagers to refuse medical treatment that would prevent serious harm or would save their life would, in many circumstances, be *contrary* to their best interests. Although this is paternalistic, paternalism is not always bad. Parents and wider society make decisions all the time for children, for the sake of their future well-being, that they do not like (Fig. 11.2). The law draws an arbitrary

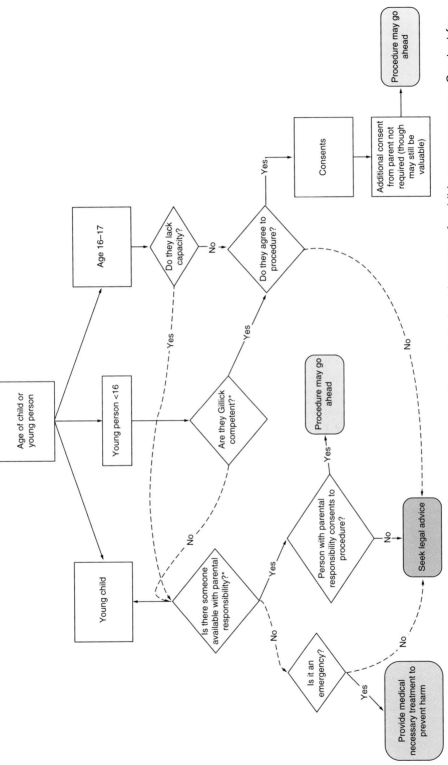

Figure 11.1 Summary of consent for medical procedures judged to be in the best interests of a child or young person. See text for discussion and more details.

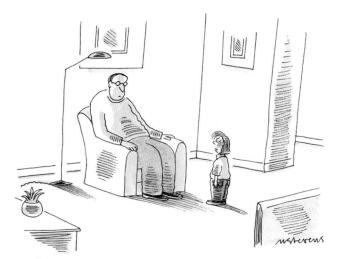

"Why do you always have to be so paternalistic?"

Figure 11.2 Paternalism (© Mick Stevens, reproduced with permission)

line on paternalism at the age of 18. There is no ethical reason to think that paternalism stops being justified overnight when an adolescent turns 18. However, the law has to draw a line somewhere. If, though, the reason to allow teenagers to refuse treatment is based on their best interests, that will mean that, in some cases, it would not be right to provide treatment. For example, in the case of H, doctors may have decided not to proceed with the court case because they viewed that forcing her to have a heart transplant against her will (including the need to take long-term anti-rejection drugs) would be contrary to her best interests.

How much weight should we give to the wishes of parents?

The legal framework allows parents to make decisions about medical treatment for children. One reason in support of this is that typically parents know their children well – they know how much a health condition is causing problems for the child, and can anticipate how well or poorly they would tolerate medical treatment. Another reason is that parents are usually strongly motivated to protect their children and promote their well-being. It is generally thought to be good for children to be raised by their parents, without health professionals or wider society intruding on family life and decision-making. It is also usually good for parents to allow them to make decisions about their families. Parents often have deeply held views about how they would like to raise their children. It would be bad for parents if health professionals or society infringed on parents' rights without good reason. It is also the parents, after the child, who must bear the costs (emotional, physical and financial) of medical decisions about their child.

However, parental rights have their limits. Sometimes parents make decisions that would not be best for a child. They may be mistaken, misinformed or misguided. They may make decisions that are motivated by their own interests (or the interests of other family members), and not those of the child. It is unquestionably good for children for there to be clear processes within society to intervene if parents are making decisions that would be risky or harmful for the child.

When should parents be free to make medical decisions for their children, and when should they not be permitted to do so? One answer to that question would draw on a child's 'best interests' – parents should be allowed to make decisions as long as they are making choices that would be best for a child. The legal framework appears to endorse this answer (according to the Children Act, the child's best interests are a 'paramount consideration'). However, there are several problems with this. First, in many situations it is not clear what would be best for a child. Second, this approach appears actually to give no weight to parents' views or interests. Third, it conflicts with the way that society approaches other domains of parental decision-making; parents make sub-optimal decisions for their children all the time, e.g. feeding them junk food, but the state does not intervene. Fourth, this conflicts with the way that health professionals usually work with families, allowing families to make decisions that are not always 'best' for a child.

Paediatric ethicist Lynn Gillam has described what she calls the 'Zone of Parental Discretion' (Gillam 2015). This is a term for the range of situations where parents are permitted to make decisions for their children, even if those decisions appear to be sub-optimal. The outer limits of this zone are defined primarily by harm to the child – this means that parents may choose treatment (or refuse treatment), even if that would not necessarily be best for the child (Fig. 11.3). However, if the

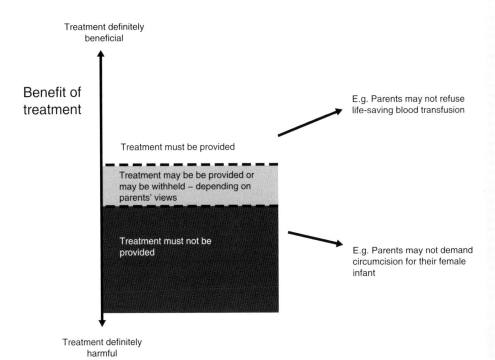

Figure 11.3 The Zone of Parental Discretion and treatment for children. The grey area on the figure indicates the range of decisions where parents' views are crucial and should be respected.

parents' choice would pose a significant risk of serious harm to the child, they should potentially be overruled. Only 'potentially' overruled, because there is a further question about what harm would come to the child from overriding the parents' decision. In some situations, parents' decision may be harmful (perhaps they are refusing medical treatment, or subjecting the child to unproven alternative therapies), but it would be *even more harmful* to the child to take the case to court or to remove the child from their parents (McDougall, Delany, and Gillam 2016).

Table 11.1 provides some examples of situations where decisions are often thought to be within the Zone of Parental Discretion (and hence treatment may be provided or not, depending on the views of parents). Male circumcision is included within this list of treatments, though there remains considerable ethical controversy about this (Earp 2015, Foddy 2013, Mazor 2013). For arguments for and against non-therapeutic male circumcision, see Up for Debate Box 11.1.

How should disputes be resolved?

Case 11.4

A critically ill infant, C, has been diagnosed with a severe genetic disorder causing paralysis, respiratory failure and seizures. All previous infants with this condition died. The doctors believe that it is not in C's best interests to keep him alive with intensive forms of medical treatment. They believe that it would be best to allow C to die. However, C's parents do not agree. They have identified an overseas specialist who is offering a treatment that has been tried in animals and in children with other health problems. They wish to take C overseas.

What should happen when parents and doctors disagree?

This is based on the case of Charlie Gard, Great Ormond Street Hospital v Yates & Ors [2017].

Table 11.1 Examples of medical treatment decisions for children and the Zone of Parental Discretion

Within the zone of parental discretion	Outside the zone of parental discretion
Routine immunization	Newborn hepatitis B immunization (where a mother is hep B–positive and there is a high risk of transmission)
Male circumcision (see text)	Female circumcision/female genital mutilation
Antibiotics for an ear infection	Antibiotics for pneumonia
Complex cardiac surgery for a newborn with a very severe congenital heart defect	Blood transfusion for severe anaemia

Up for Debate Box 11.1 Should infant male circumcision (for non-therapeutic reasons) be permitted?

In favour:
1. Male circumcision has enormous cultural significance to some communities – particularly those of Jewish or Muslim faith. Banning circumcision would contravene the freedom of those individuals to maintain a very long-standing cultural tradition. It would also be contrary to their freedom of religion.
2. Male circumcision is minimally harmful – we allow parents to make decisions for their children that are not necessarily in their child's best interests and may involve some risks. (For example, parents may drive their children in a car, or take them out in a boat, even though there are small risks of an accident that could be harmful or even lethal.)
3. Male circumcision provides some medical benefit to boys (even when it is not being done for medical reasons), including a lower risk of urinary infection and a potentially lower risk of transmission of certain sexually transmitted infections (e.g. HIV).
4. Performing male circumcision in infancy is less traumatic than performing it later in childhood or in adulthood.

Against:
1. Policies that permit male circumcision but prohibit even minimal forms of female circumcision are inconsistent. Either equivalent (minimal) forms of genital cutting should be permitted in both male and female infants, or it should be permitted in neither.
2. Religious or cultural beliefs do not provide good reason to permit parents to harm their children. For example, parents are not permitted to refuse a blood transfusion for a child, even where that is seen as a central tenet of their religion. Young children have not had any opportunity to decide whether they wish to embrace the religious values of their parents. It is unreasonable to impose harm for the sake of parents.
3. Circumcision can be performed later when a young person or adult has capacity and is able to decide whether or not to have the procedure. The claimed medical benefits of reduced HIV transmission could still be achieved. (The rates of later circumcision are low – indicating that many circumcisions are performed on individuals who would never choose to have the procedure if they had the choice.)
4. Circumcision does pose a significant harm to a child – it involves removal of an area of highly sensitive genital tissue (reducing later sexual sensation), and imposes a risk of scarring, penile amputation, haemorrhage and death.

Where parents and health professionals do not agree about what medical treatment would be best for a child, and where this is felt to be outside the Zone of Parental Discretion, there is then a question about how to resolve the disagreement. If parents have difficulty accepting the views of treating consultants, it may be helpful to seek internal or external second opinions. Hospital clinical ethics committees may provide valuable input, particularly in helping to consider whether the family's requests would pose a significant risk of serious harm. Formal mediation may be useful where the relationship between health professionals and the family has broken down. However, if those approaches have not yielded a resolution, the next step may be to apply to the court. Health professionals may apply to the court for a specific issue order – for example, asking the Family Division of the High Court for a declaration that continued intensive care would not be in a child's best interests. If a decision is reached, but the family do not accept the decision, the family may appeal – to the Court of Appeal, the Supreme Court or even the European Court of Human Rights. This was the situation in 2017 in the highly public case of Charlie Gard, a seriously ill infant, whose parents wished to take him overseas for experimental treatment.

The companion book to this textbook, *'Ethics, conflict and medical treatment for children'*, explores the Gard case in detail, considers the challenges in conflicts about medical treatment and proposes a novel framework for resolution of future cases of conflict (Wilkinson and Savulescu 2018).

CHILD SAFEGUARDING

Children and young people may experience different forms of abuse, including physical and sexual abuse, but also emotional abuse, neglect, domestic abuse, fabricated or induced illness, online abuse, bullying, sexual grooming or exploitation and female genital mutilation (FGM). Everyone has a duty to protect children from abuse and exploitation. In addition to this general responsibility, doctors have professional duties and responsibilities (Larcher 2007).

Decisions about safeguarding can be ethically complex, since they require contested concepts such as the welfare of the child, or adjudicating between competing rights (e.g. between parent and child). They are also extremely stressful for practitioners, as public responses to past cases have included intense criticism of those (including health professionals) who failed to detect or report abuse (e.g. the Victoria Climbie, the Baby P case), as well as those who were seen to have wrongfully accused parents of abuse.

The Children Act 1989 provides the main legal structure for safeguarding children. The Children (Scotland) Act 1995 contains provisions regarding child abuse that are broadly similar to those of the English Act. The Act emphasizes the paramount concern for the welfare of the child. The threshold for intervening is if the child is suffering or at risk of suffering 'significant harm'. This is defined in the Adoption and Children Act 2002 to include impairment of physical or mental health or impairment of physical, intellectual, emotional, social or behavioural development.

All NHS trusts now have a named doctor and nurse for safeguarding, to provide expert advice for fellow professionals.

Do you need to report?

Reporting of suspected child abuse is not legally mandated in the UK (as it is in some countries). However, statutory guidance is clear that those who work with children and families should report immediately to the local authorities if they have good reason to suspect that a child may have been, or is at risk of being, abused or neglected. Failure to report suspicions may lead to professional sanction.

Specific legislation introduced in 2015 in England and Wales mandates that health and social care professionals and teachers report any known cases of FGM in a girl under age 18. Where a girl under 18 reports that FGM has been performed on her, or where physical signs lead the health professional to believe that a girl under 18 has had FGM performed, they must report that to the police. (As with other reporting, health professionals should inform the young person and her parents that they intend to report, unless it would be contrary to the young person's best interests to do so.)

Uncertainty

The doctor does not need to be certain about risk of harm to report suspicions. They need, rather, to have 'good reason' to suspect harm or risk of harm. If unsure, they should seek help from more experienced professionals.

The doctor is obliged to report suspicions to the local authority, unless it is not in the child's best interests to do so. (If the doctor believes that it is not in the child's best interests to share information, this decision and the reasons behind it should be clearly documented.)

A doctor with concerns about abuse must ensure follow-on care. Children must not be discharged from hospital without a full examination. A child at risk must not be discharged from hospital without being registered at an identified GP.

Confidentiality

The doctor should usually ask for consent before sharing confidential information, unless this would result in a delay in sharing information (which would increase the risk of harm to the child or young person), or asking for consent would increase risk of harm to the child or to others.

Where a young person reports abuse, ensure that they are aware that the health professional is obliged to report this. (Ideally, explain to young people in advance that information shared is confidential, but not in situations where there is a risk to the child or to others (see Chapter 9).)

Confidential information may be shared without consent if required by law (e.g. a case of FGM), or if the benefits of sharing information for the child or young person outweigh the individual's (and public's) interest in maintaining confidentiality.

In the case of suspected child sexual abuse or fabricated/induced illness, doctors should discuss with a senior colleague (i.e. named professional) whether to discuss suspicions with carers before reporting to the local authority.

Information shared should be necessary, proportionate, relevant, adequate, accurate, timely and secure (see Chapter 9, Confidentiality).

Decisions to share information (or not) should be clearly documented, along with the reasons for reaching them.

Medical examination

Doctors may be asked by local authorities or other doctors to carry out an assessment. They should only agree to do so if they have the core competencies (skills, knowledge) necessary for this.

If medical examination is required, consent should be obtained from the young person (if aged 16 or 17, or if younger and Gillick competent), or from a parent or carer (if not Gillick competent).

If the parent refuses an examination that the doctor believes is necessary, or the young person declines consent, the professional should discuss and reach a strategy with the local authority.

Types of protection or court orders

If they have reason to suspect that a child needs urgent protection, Section 46 of the Children Act gives police the power to place a child in police protection for up to 72 hours.

The local authority may respond to reports of suspected abuse via a court application. The court has several options:

An **emergency protection order** enables a child at urgent risk of significant harm (if they are not removed from their family) to be taken to a safe place.

A **care order** enables a local authority to take over the care of a child and gives that authority PR. Courts may make such an order if they are satisfied that a child is suffering or is likely to suffer 'significant harm', attributable to care given that is not 'what it would be reasonable to expect a parent to give'.

A **supervision order** authorizes a social worker to regularly visit the family and ensure the child is safe.

A **child assessment order** is appropriate when there is suspicion of harm but lack of evidence; otherwise, it is appropriate to go directly to a care order. Medical assessment may be part of the assessment directed by the court.

Liability for reporting

In a situation where a doctor reports a suspicion of abuse or neglect, but on further assessment the child is not found to be at risk of abuse or neglect, the doctor is not likely to be found liable as long as concerns were in good faith, honestly held and reasonable; consent was obtained for information sharing (where appropriate); and only relevant information was shared.

REVISION QUESTIONS

1. A 14-year-old attends a doctor's surgery. She is pregnant, requests a termination of pregnancy and does not want anyone to know. What are the ethical considerations?
2. Doctors caring for a seriously ill newborn infant believe that continued treatment is not in the infant's best interests; however, his parents do not agree. How should this disagreement be resolved?
3. A young person who is Gillick competent can consent to medical treatment, but if they refuse treatment, this can be overridden. Is this justified?
4. Parents have a right to make medical decisions about their children. Is that correct? Do you agree?

Alex is a 13-year-old who was born biologically female. However, Alex has, over a number of years, identified as being male. He tries to avoid going to the toilet at school as he does not wish to use the female bathrooms. He has been diagnosed with gender dysphoria.

Alex wishes to have sex change surgery. His doctors have recommended puberty suppression medication that would delay the development of secondary sexual characteristics, prior to administering masculinizing hormones and later surgery (after age 18).

Are these proposed interventions in the best interests of Alex?

If he is Gillick competent, should he be permitted to consent to puberty-blocking drugs? What if his parents are opposed?

Should this intervention require court approval?

Should sex change surgery be performed prior to age 18?

This case is based on the case of Re Alex: Hormonal Treatment for Gender Identity Dysphoria [2004] (Giordano 2008, Ikuta 2016, Anon 2014).

REFERENCES

Anon. 2014. "AJOB case presentation: Andrea/Arthur was born male." *The American Journal of Bioethics* 14 (1): 42. doi: 10.1080/15265161.2014.862407.

An NHS Trust v Child B and Others [2014] EWHC 3486 (Fam).

B (A Child: Immunisation) [2018] EWFC 56.

Earp, B. D. 2015. "Do the benefits of male circumcision outweigh the risks? A critique of the proposed CDC guidelines." *Frontiers in Pediatrics* 3: 18. doi: 10.3389/fped.2015.00018.

Foddy, B. 2013. "Medical, religious and social reasons for and against an ancient rite." *Journal of Medical Ethics* 39 (7): 415. doi: 10.1136/medethics-2013-101605.

Gillam, L. 2015. "The zone of parental discretion: an ethical tool for dealing with disagreement between parents and doctors about medical treatment for a child." *Clinical Ethics* 11 (1): 1-8. doi: 10.1177/1477750915622033.

Gillick v West Norfolk & Wisbeck Area Health Authority [1986] AC 112 House of Lords.

Gilmore, S. and Herring, J. 2011. "No is the hardest word: consent and children's autonomy." *Child and Family Law Quarterly* 23 (1): 3-25.

Giordano, S. 2008. "Lives in a chiaroscuro. Should we suspend the puberty of children with gender identity disorder?" *Journal of Medical Ethics* 34: 580-4.

Great Ormond Street Hospital v Yates & Ors [2017] EWHC 972 (Fam) (11 April 2017).

Ikuta, E. 2016. "Overcoming the parental veto: how transgender adolescents can access puberty-suppressing hormone treatment in the absence of parental consent under the Mature Minor Doctrine." *Southern California Interdisciplinary Law Journal* 25 (1): 179-228.

Larcher, V. 2007. "Ethical issues in child protection." *Clinical Ethics* 2 (4): 208-12.

Larcher, V. and Hutchinson, A. 2010. "How should paediatricians assess Gillick competence?" *Archives of Disease in Childhood* 95: 307-11.

Mazor, J. 2013. "The child's interests and the case for the permissibility of male infant circumcision." *Journal of Medical Ethics* 39 (7): 421-8. doi: 10.1136/medethics-2013-101318.

McDougall, R., Delany, C. and Gillam, L. (Eds). 2016. *When doctors and parents disagree: ethics paediatrics and the zone of parental discretion.* Sydney: Federation Press.

Re Alex: Hormonal Treatment for Gender Identity Dysphoria [2004] FamCA 297.

Re J (child's religious upbringing and circumcision) [2000] 1 FCR 307.

Re P (Medical treatment: Best interests) [2003] EWHC 2327 (Fam).

Re R (a minor) (wardship: medical treatment) [1992] Fam 11.

Re S [1993] 1 FLR 377.

Re W [1992] 4 All ER 627.

Re SL (Permission to Vaccinate) [2017] EWHC 125 (Fam).

Retter, E. 2013. "Hannah Jones at 18: I turned down heart transplant aged 13 but I'm so glad I changed my mind." The Mirror, 13 Jul 2013. Accessed 15/2/2018. https://www.mirror.co.uk/news/real-life-stories/hannah-jones-18-turned-down-2049160.

Verkaik, R. 2008. "Girl, 13, wins right to refuse heart transplant." Independent, 11 November 2008. Accessed 14/2/2018. http://www.independent.co.uk/life-style/health-and-families/health-news/girl-13-wins-right-to-refuse-heart-transplant-1009569.html.

Wilkinson, D. and Savulescu, J. 2018. *Ethics, conflict and medical treatment for children: from disagreement to dissensus*. Elsevier.

Chapter **12**

Disability and disease

Case 12.1　Body integrity dysphoria (BID)

A Scottish surgeon, Mr S, amputated a healthy leg from each of two patients suffering from body integrity dysphoria (BID), a body dysmorphic disorder in which the patient feels incomplete with four limbs and wishes to have at least one limb removed. The patients had received psychiatric and psychological treatment prior to the operation, but had failed to respond to these methods. Both operations were carried out privately and not publicly funded, and the patients were satisfied with the results.

Should surgeons amputate healthy limbs from patients with BID?

(This case is based on Dyer 2000.)

What treatments or procedures should health professionals provide? One answer to that question is that doctors and surgeons should treat *disease*. They should not, however, provide treatments to people without disease just because they want that treatment.

Is body integrity dysphoria (BID) a disease? We could look to official classifications. The latest edition of the psychiatric text the Diagnostic and Statistical Manual (DSM 5) decided not to include it, but the International Classification of Diseases (ICD 11) did. But of course, that leaves open the question of which is right, and what should count as a disease.

In this chapter, we discuss some fundamental concepts in medicine such as disease, illness and disability. Our interest, however, is not in semantics but in ethics. For example, in 1973 the American Psychiatric Association asked its members to vote on whether homosexuality was a mental illness (at the time it was included in the second edition of DSM). This question, however, was not simply a semantic one, nor simply a scientific one: it also involved social and ethical values. Not far beneath the surface of this question lay issues such as whether doctors should be involved in trying to change a person's sex or sexual orientation via so-called 'conversion therapies' (Earp, Sandberg, and Savulescu 2014). These types of questions, and the closely connected, broad issue of the goals of medicine, need to be reviewed frequently in the light of both social and scientific developments (for detailed discussion see Savulescu 2007). (After its 1973 convention, the American Psychiatric Association removed homosexuality from DSM.)

In this chapter, we will investigate the question of what are disease and disability. However, we will need to go further than that. Doctors have, for some time, been involved in practices which do not involve treating or preventing disease: contraception, sterilization, abortion and euthanasia. The World Health Organization has defined health as 'a state of complete physical, mental and social well-being and not merely the absence of disease or infirmity'. The goals of medicine and the best interests of the patient have been broadening beyond disease and medical interests to include more broadly construed well-being. Furthermore, medical ethics is increasingly concerned not merely with well-being, but also the values and autonomy of the patient. Sex selection, surrogacy and enhancement are paradigm case of interventions which either promote well-being or autonomy, but do not treat disease. In the 21st century, medicine will require a new ethic of doctors' involvement in promoting people's values.

DISEASE

Is BID *really* a disease? Or is it a personal preference or fetish, more like the desire for body modification by plastic surgery for aesthetic or other reasons? If it is not a disease, is surgery warranted? Comparison can be made with gender dysphoria, and the same questions can be asked. And should the ethical question of whether it is right to amputate the healthy limb of a person with BID, or the penis of a person with gender dysphoria, depend on the answer to whether these are diseases or not?

One response to increasing requests for medical treatment has been to expand the number of diseases or lower the threshold for their diagnosis. For example, in psychiatry, there has been an epidemic of psychiatric disease. One in five US adults takes psychiatric medication (Frances 2013). By age 32, 50% of people surveyed qualified for an anxiety disorder, more than 40% for a mood disorder and more than 30% for substance dependence (Moffitt et al. 2010). Over the 15 years to 2013, cases of attention deficit/hyperactivity disorder in US children tripled, cases of autism increased 20-fold and cases of childhood bipolar disorder increased 40-fold (Frances 2013).

One highly influential definition of disease is Christopher Boorse's biostatistical theory. It is a naturalistic account that is based on the concept of *species-typical functioning* – i.e. disease is present when an organism is not able to function at a level that is typical for the species (Box 12.1).

According to Boorse, disease is intended to be a value-free scientific concept, and illness a value-laden (normative) concept. For Boorse, the fact that someone

> **Box 12.1** The Boorsian account of disease (species-typical functioning) and some criticisms
>
> For a detailed overview and response to his critics, see Boorse (1997).
>
> There are four elements to Boorse's account:
>
> 1. The *reference class* is a natural class of organisms of uniform functional design; specifically, an age group of a sex of a species.
> 2. A *normal function* of a part or a process (eg normal lung function) is the statistically typical contribution of that process to the survival or reproduction of the individual.
> 3. A *disease* is a type of internal state that is either an impairment of normal functional ability, i.e. a reduction of one or more functional abilities below typical efficiency, or a limitation on functional ability caused by environmental agents.
> 4. *Health* is the absence of disease (Boorse 1997).
>
> Boorse distinguishes disease from illness. *Illness* (or 'therapeutic abnormality') is a subclass of disease serious enough to have certain normative (that is, value-laden) features. A disease is an illness only if it is serious enough to be incapacitating, and therefore is:
>
> - undesirable for its bearer
> - a source of entitlement to special treatment
> - a valid excuse for normally criticizable behaviour.
>
> This is a biological, evolutionary account of what pathologists classify as disease. Evolution aims at survival only long enough to enable reproduction or to confer reproductive advantages. It might appear that such a definition omits those areas of medical practice devoted solely to improving quality of life. For example, rheumatoid arthritis may not kill, but causes pain. Is it a disease according to Boorse's account? It might be argued that it makes us less fit for survival, so counts as a disease on that basis. However, even if arthritis does not affect survival or reproduction, many people would still want to consider it a disease because of the chronic pain it causes.
>
> There is another important value in Boorse's naturalistic conception: it draws a line at 'statistically significant' sub-functioning. This is typically defined as functioning more than two standard deviations below the mean. Thus, intellectual disability is described as an IQ less than 70, where the mean is 100 and one standard deviation is 15 points. This means that around 2% of people are intellectually disabled. But one could draw the line differently. One could define disease as three standard deviations below the mean, in which case 0.15% of people have intellectual disability, or one standard deviation, in which 16% of people have intellectual disability. Which line one choose depends on how bad that level of function is, and that is a value judgement. It should be made with respect to the relationship between that level of function and well-being or autonomy. Today 'low-normal IQ' is used to describe those below one standard deviation because, in a technologically advanced society, even having a 'normal' IQ of 80 reduces options. For example, one needs an IQ of about 95 to complete a tax return in the US.

has a disease does not necessarily imply that she should receive treatment; the fact that someone has an *illness,* however, does have this implication. Boorse argues that many writers conflate disease with what doctors see as justifying treatment, but other goals may motivate doctors besides promoting health. He points out that doctors might legitimately prevent conception or perform abortion without classifying pregnancy or fertility as diseases. It might be helpful, therefore, to distinguish between core therapeutic medicine (involving the treatment of disease) and 'enhancement'. Enhancement aims at either promoting the well-being of people (broadly construed) or promoting their autonomy (Savulescu 2007). Enhancement could include contraception, circumcision, cosmetic surgery and even euthanasia.

There have been many objections to Boorse's account of disease. Boorse has claimed that his account is *naturalistic.* One objection is that it involves *covert normativism,* that is, the importing of value judgements about the goals of medicine (Fulford 1989). The values that are endorsed as the goals of medicine are those of survival and reproduction. Values that are rejected are those relating to reduced quality of life (such as chronic pain), where these do not affect survival and reproduction.

Even though there is disagreement over whether the concept of disease is value-free or not, values cannot be avoided in deciding when doctors should treat. Medicine is inherently and irreducibly a value-laden practice. And values are the domain of ethics.

If doctors rightly do things in addition to treating disease, it seems that we need new concepts, such as well-being and autonomy, to evaluate the impact of conditions on people's lives that are amenable to medical interventions. Aspects that decrease well-being include pain, disability, loss of freedom and loss of pleasure. Thus, pregnancy, menopause, teething and menstruation can all impact negatively on well-being for some people, and these negative impacts can, at least to some extent, be ameliorated by medical interventions. And where they do not adversely affect well-being, people may have values which can be promoted by the use of medical technologies, with family planning being an obvious example of reproductive autonomy.

Is BID a disease?

Some argue that the request for amputation of healthy limbs is a mental disorder, a form of psychosexual disorder involving sexual attraction to amputees (Elliott 2003). Bioethicists Bayne and Levy (2005) agree that it is a mental disorder, but of a different kind, representing 'a mismatch between their body and their body as they experience it', or BID. They argue that this condition is poorly studied, and treatments for it are typically ineffective. According to Boorse's definition, it is a disease because these people's psychology causes them to harm themselves, rendering them less fit for survival.

But is the question of whether this is, or is not, a disease (or disorder) relevant to the question of whether it is right for a surgeon to amputate a limb (or indeed right for the state to pay for it)? In the real case of Mr S, the National Health Service Trust responsible for the hospital banned further amputations. Bayne and

Levy argue that individuals with this condition are often driven to destructive and dangerous practices (such as self-amputation by placing the limb over a rail track). When no other more effective treatments are available, surgeons ought to be permitted, they argue, to amputate such healthy limbs.

According to this view, doctors should perform surgery, not because it is necessarily in the person's *medical* interests (i.e. treating a medical condition), but because it is in his or her overall interests or respects their autonomy.

DISABILITY

The question of when medical approaches to a problem are appropriate has been a contentious issue, over the past 40 years or so, in the context of disability (see also Chapter 18 for discussion of disability in the context of genetic testing and selection).

Case 12.2 Intentionally having a deaf child

A. Agnes and Andrew are a deaf couple. Each has a genetic cause of deafness. They request IVF and pre-implantation genetic diagnosis to see if their embryos will be deaf. However, rather than implanting a hearing embryo, they want to deliberately transfer a deaf embryo (they plan to call the child Annie). This is illegal in the UK. They object to the law, saying: 'Deafness is a difference not a disability. The disadvantages deafness causes are the result of injustice and prejudice. We are a part of the Deaf community, and we are proud of our culture which includes sign language. It is a natural expression of pride in our community that we should wish to have a child like ourselves'.

B. Beatrice and Benny are a deaf couple who are a part of the Deaf community. Their child, Boxer, is deaf. He is 6 months old. Doctors wish to insert cochlear implants so that Boxer will be able to hear and speak. Beatrice and Benny refuse to consent, saying that Boxer will be able to sign and be a part of their community. There have been numerous discussions between parents and doctors. Should doctors apply for a court order to insert cochlear implants?

Naturalistic accounts of disability

The traditional approach to defining disability has been to see it as a property of an individual. As with the Boorsian concept of disease, some have given a naturalistic account, defining disability in terms of a statistical deviation from a biological standard, appealing to the idea of species-typical functioning (see Box 12.1, and Buchanan et al. 2000). Although naturalistic accounts may account well for the concept of disease as described by pathology textbooks, they work less well as an account of disability (and indeed of mental illness; see Chapter 8).

Deviation from the biologically or statistically normal does not have intrinsic ethical significance. Loss of hearing with old age fits with the biological and statistical norm, but is hardly less disabling for that. Around 34% of all men aged 40–70 years have some erectile dysfunction, which is also a part of normal ageing. As a result, millions of men worldwide use Viagra. More recently, flibanserin has been purported to increase female sexual desire, and a new disease (hypoactive sexual desire disorder) has been invented, for which it is a treatment (Earp and Savulescu 2019). Evidently some men and women are not satisfied with the abilities that come with species-typical normal functioning.

Evolution is not directly concerned with how well our lives go. What is normal for us as a species is what has, over human history, been conducive to our survival and reproduction. But, for us as rational beings capable of forming and acting on our own conception of the good life (that is, being free and autonomous), deviation from such a statistical standard matters only when it is likely to affect the quality of a life – by making it worse or, sometimes, better. The account of disability based on species-typical functioning offers us little assistance in answering ethical questions.

Welfarist accounts of disability

As with the concept of disease, an alternative approach is to see disability as an inherently normative, or value-laden, concept. One such approach is the welfarist account of disability, which links disability to a reduction in well-being, rather than to a statistical deviation from normal functioning. Savulescu and Kahane provide such a definition as follows: a disability is a relatively stable physical or psychological condition X of person P in circumstances C if X tends to reduce the amount of well-being that P will enjoy in C. C describes the natural and social circumstances of the person (Kahane and Savulescu 2009, 2016, Savulescu and Guy 2017, Savulescu and Kahane 2009).

This definition differs from the species-typical functioning definition in two important ways. First, it relates disability to reduction in well-being rather than in terms of deviation from normal. Second, disability is relative to circumstances: it does not reside purely within an individual.

Social models of disability

The importance of circumstances is central to social models of disability (for a detailed account and critique of various models, see Shakespeare 2006). These models highlight, to various extents, the importance of social circumstances in defining disability.

The British social model of disability uses two concepts, impairment and disability, where impairment refers to a deviation from the species-typical norm with limitation of function. According to this model, however, disability combines two things: it refers to 'the disadvantage or restriction of activity' (which by implication is related to the impairment), but also includes a further causal component in that the disadvantage or restriction of activity is caused by 'contemporary social organisation which takes little or no account of people who have physical impairments and then excludes them from participation in the mainstream of social activities' (Paul Hunt, quoted in Shakespeare 2006, p. 13).

The political purpose of these definitions is to focus attention on eliminating the disadvantages to people with impairment through social changes rather than through 'curing' the impairment. For example, rather than treating (or preventing) dwarfism, the focus, according to this model, should be on changing society (both attitudes and environments) so that people with very short stature suffer no disadvantages as a result.

The mere difference view of disability

A recent development from the social model of disability is the so-called mere difference view. Many believe that disabilities such as deafness, blindness, paraplegia and severe intellectual impairment are harmful and have a significant negative impact on a person's life. Some disability theorists respond that disability itself does not make a person overall worse off; rather, it is merely a difference, like race, hair colour, gender and sexual orientation. It is thus not an impairment. This is the mere difference view, famously articulated by Elizabeth Barnes (2014). See Up for Debate Box 12.1 for arguments in favour of and against the mere difference view.

It can be difficult to clarify precisely what the points at issue are in the rather polarized area of disability studies, and where there are areas of agreement. Most agree that there are physical impairments, such as severe brain damage, that are undesirable for the person who suffers them. Most also agree that the degree to which (and even whether) a person with an impairment suffers disadvantage depends on features of society, such as social attitudes and physical environment. It is this disadvantage that is being referred to by the term 'disability', as defined in the social models. So what are the disagreements? They are of three types.

Conceptual disagreements

There are disagreements as to what should count as an impairment (using the above definition). For example, there is dispute over whether deafness or very short stature are impairments (see below).

Ethical disagreements

The main areas of disagreement are over issues that are ethical in nature, and in particular the extent to which disability should be reduced (or eliminated) through changes in society, or through treating or preventing impairment. At one end of the spectrum (the extreme social model) is the view that society should change – through adapting the environment, work practices, payments and attitudes, so that no one with an impairment is disadvantaged compared with anyone else. According to one version of this view, medical science and medical research should not be used to tackle impairments or disabilities. At the other end of the spectrum (the extreme medical model) is the view that disabilities should be reduced entirely through tackling impairments (treating or preventing the impairment), and that society should not be expected to change in order to accommodate people with impairment. Between these extremes there is a spectrum of views as to how much is it reasonable for society to change, and in what ways; and what medical interventions to reduce both impairments and disabilities should be developed and used.

Factual disagreements

Some of the disputes appear to involve factual disagreements, for example whether there is in fact a possible society in which a person with a particular impairment

✕ Up for Debate Box 12.1 Is disability a mere difference?

For

Experience and testimony from disabled people indicate that many are satisfied with their lives and report being as happy, or nearly as happy, as those without disabilities. They claim that it is wrong to appeal to or privilege the evaluation of disability by those who are not disabled (Fricker 2007). Rather, we should give greater weight to the views of disabled people about disability.

Many disabled people take pride in their disability, have a community and identify with their disability. Thus, some would not wish to be 'cured' of their disability. Even if it might bring functional advantages, it would undermine their authentic self.

In the past, people (including doctors) have regarded people as worse off if they were female, non-white, homosexual or left-handed. However, with time it has become clear that such views were the result of prejudice, and that any disadvantage was the result of the way that society was arranged. These are mere differences. With time it will become clear that disability is also a mere difference.

It would be wrong to try to prevent the existence of people with a disability, just as it would be wrong to try to prevent the existence of left-handed people.

It would also be wrong to try to 'cure' someone's disability without their consent. To use a parallel, to change someone's sex or sexual orientation without their consent would be to undermine their identity.

Against

The mere difference view has unacceptable and morally repugnant implications. It would mean, for example, that it would not be wrong to cause a non-disabled person to become disabled, or to fail to prevent or remove disability when this is possible. It would mean that, in Case 12.2, Agnes and Andrew would be right to select a deaf embryo, and Beatrice and Benny would be right to refuse a cochlear implant for their young child.

Since deafness is a difference, like hair colour, it would not be seriously wrong to deafen a newborn baby, just as it would not be seriously wrong to change its hair colour. And it would also mean that it is misguided to exert so much effort to develop ways of preventing or removing disability.

The mere difference view claims that, if the world were just, disabled people would not be disadvantaged. This requires a commitment to a view that any difference in advantage is the result of injustice. But regardless of how just social arrangements were, the deaf would not hear music or auditory warnings. For more serious physical (and especially cognitive) disabilities, it is hard to believe that, even in a perfectly egalitarian society, there would be no disadvantage. It may be possible (with a great deal of effort) to reduce or ameliorate the disadvantages of someone who is quadriplegic or profoundly cognitively impaired. But eliminate those disadvantages entirely? That seems implausible.

(Barnes 2014, Kahane and Savulescu 2016)

(blindness, for example) suffered no disadvantages (disabilities) compared with those without the impairment. There might be further disagreements about whether, even if there is theoretically such a possible society, it is achievable politically.

Is deafness an impairment?

Using the terms outlined above, there is dispute over the question of whether deafness is an impairment. Some people in the Deaf community, such as those mentioned in Case 12.2, claim that deafness does not reduce the quality of life, nor does it necessarily make it more difficult to interact with others, because signing is a unique form of communication that creates its own world of advantages. Such people often claim, further, that deafness represents a unique culture that can be fostered only by being deaf (Lane 2002). According to a naturalistic account of impairment (species-typical functioning), deafness is an impairment, and the ethical implication is that it should be treated or prevented (although it is logically possible to hold a naturalistic account of impairment whilst also believing that impairment should not be treated.) According to a welfarist account, the key issue is whether deafness is likely to increase or decrease the chances of having a good life.

It is arguable that deafness reduces welfare in two ways. First, it prevents access to the world of sound. In a world without sound, deafness would not be bad. It is the *exercise* of the capacity to hear that is valuable, not the capacity itself. But the capacity to hear is, obviously, a necessary condition for enjoying those intrinsic goods that are necessarily auditory. Second, deafness reduces the chances of realizing a good life because it makes it harder to live, to achieve one's goals and to engage with others in a world that is based on the spoken word. Being able to hear does not necessarily prevent such activities and goods. But it is nevertheless significantly harder to get a job, move through the world, respond to emergencies where the alarm is aural and so on.

The quality of life of a deaf child may depend on whether her parents are themselves deaf. Some argue that children of deaf parents would be better off deaf because they would then share with their parents the experience of being part of the Deaf community. The argument against this position is that nothing prevents the hearing children of deaf people from learning to sign and communicate with their deaf parents, just as children of English parents who are brought up in China can learn Chinese as well as English. Is it not better to have the capacity to speak two languages rather than one, and to understand two cultures rather than one? It would be disabling for a child of English parents living in China if the child spoke only English, even though it might be easier for her parents to communicate with her. Even if a condition is an advantage in the narrow context of the child's home, it may still be a significant disadvantage in the larger world.

It is no doubt true that the badness of disability has been exaggerated, and the role of prejudice and injustice ignored or underplayed. And identity and authenticity are important values for doctors to consider.

How then should we view the choices in Case 12.2?

In the case of deafness, the hearing can become deaf, but the deaf cannot become hearing (after a very early age when cochlear implants have the chance to provide some hearing). Moreover, even if the Deaf community does have a unique language, with unique forms of expression and art, a hearing child could be a member of both the hearing and Deaf communities. It is better to be bilingual rather than monolingual. From the child's perspective, it is better to have an open future with more valuable options (Davis 1997). It promotes autonomy, as well as well-being. It would be wrong, according to this view, to deny a child cochlear implants. In some cases, a court might authorize their insertion without parental consent. There are no UK cases of this. In a case in the US, a court declined to overrule a deaf mother's refusal of cochlear implants for her two deaf children (though the judge indicated that these would be in the children's best interests) (D'Silva, Daugherty, and MacDonald 2004). The children were later adopted, and received cochlear implants.

What about selecting a deaf embryo rather than a hearing embryo, like Annie (Case 12.2)? According to some views of reproductive ethics, such as procreative beneficence (Savulescu and Guy 2017), this is wrong (see Chapter 13). However, note that this is different to deafening a hearing child or failing to insert a cochlear implant (e.g. Boxer in Case 12.2). Boxer is harmed by being denied a cochlear implant because he is made worse off than he would otherwise have been: he is more disadvantaged, even in a just world. However, Annie is not harmed by being selected as a deaf embryo. She is not made worse off than she would otherwise have been. If the parents had selected a hearing embryo, a different child would have been born (perhaps 'Henry' rather than Annie). This is the so-called 'Non-Identity Problem' (Parfit 1984). Thus, even if Agnes and Andrew's choice is wrong, they should not legally be prevented from selecting a deaf embryo, as no person is harmed (Savulescu 2002). Paradoxically, though, they would potentially be under an obligation to provide a cochlear implant to Annie if one were available. Sometimes logic leads in unexpected directions (Hope and McMillan 2012).

One important point of agreement in disability ethics between those who hold the welfarist view and those who hold either the social models or the mere difference view is that social and natural circumstances can severely reduce opportunity and well-being. Much more needs to be done to reduce the disadvantage that disabled people face. Indeed, at some point of technological advance, the disabled might become the superabled with the integration of technology (Minerva and Giubilini 2018). Many disabled people would reject such technological interventions, and the debate will become more complex as the values of identity, authenticity, autonomy and well-being pull in different directions.

Is it ever right to increase a person's impairment?

Case 12.3

A 7-year old girl, Ashley, with severe physical and cognitive disability, is unable to walk, talk, eat, sit up or roll over. According to her doctors, Ashley has reached, and will remain at, the developmental level of a 3-month-old baby. She can be given the best care if she can be lifted, cuddled, and fed by her parents –in other words, treated as a young baby. However, her parents are concerned that if she grows further it will become increasingly difficult to carry her and lift her in and out of her wheelchair. Development of secondary sexual characteristics would not advantage Ashley, may cause her physical discomfort (for example, if she develops menorrhagia) and put her at risk of sexual abuse. Ashley's parents and doctors have proposed a course of treatment which includes high-dose oestrogen therapy to stunt her growth, the removal of her uterus via hyster- ectomy to prevent menstrual discomfort and the removal of her breast buds to limit the growth of her breasts. Ashley's parents argue that the treatment is intended 'to improve our daughter's quality of life and not to convenience her caregivers'.

Would it be ethical for Ashley to undergo this treatment?

This case is based on the so-called 'Ashley' case. See Gunther and Diekema (2006), Liao, Savulescu, and Sheehan (2007) and Diekema and Fost (2010).

On both the welfarist definition of disability and the species-typical functioning view, Ashley was born with a severe disability. But the implications of these views radically diverge when we turn to the effect the treatment devised by her doctors will have on Ashley. According to the species-typical functioning view, the treatment would increase Ashley's disability – driving her even further from the human norm. According to the welfarist view, in the context of Ashley's brain impairment, and assuming that the claims made for the effects of the treatment on Ashley's well-being are correct, the treatment would be not disabling, but rather enhancing. According to the social models of disability, Ashley has a significant impairment that leads to socially caused disability. An implication of the extreme social model (or of the mere difference view) is that the 'Ashley treatment' is wrong: society should adapt to ensure she suffers no disability. Even less extreme social models would focus on enabling Ashley to live as good a life as possible through social rather than physical changes.

Whenever there is a mismatch between biology, psychology and social or natural environment resulting in a bad life, or even a life that is not as good as it could be, we have a choice (Kahane and Savulescu 2009): we can alter our biology, our psychology or our environment. This is occurring in medical practice when doctors advise diets that are low in fat and high in fibre and antioxidants; that is, diets that mimic the diet which our bodies are adapted to tolerate. But another approach is not to change our environment, but to change our biology through drugs. The 'polypill' is designed to allow the body to tolerate a modern diet by chemically lowering our cholesterol levels, blood pressure, etc. We can, of course, alter both biology *and* environment, and try to make judgements in each situation as to what is, overall, the best way to reduce particular disabilities. That judgement, and the balance between making biological, psychological, environmental and social changes, will depend on the view we have on the different models of disability.

HUMAN ENHANCEMENT

Should medicine be used only for the treatment and prevention of disease and impairment, or should it also be used for human enhancement?

Medicine is already, to some extent, being used for enhancement. Cosmetic surgery is used to 'beautify' people with no abnormality in the first place. Viagra, which was originally developed as an anti-hypertensive treatment, was found to be of use in diabetics with impotence. Now, millions of healthy men worldwide use Viagra to enhance erectile function beyond age-related norms. Students, scientists and business people use nicotine, caffeine or drugs like Ritalin or modafinil in the hope of improving their wakefulness, alertness and cognitive performance. The potential over the next decades for medical technologies to be used radically to alter healthy people's lives goes far beyond current practice. Is this to be welcomed?

Definitions of enhancement

What is meant by 'enhancement'? There are three main definitions that parallel those of disease, impairment and disability (for a more detailed discussion, see Savulescu 2006b).

1. Naturalistic accounts

   Naturalistic approaches define enhancement in terms of going beyond health-restoring treatment or health. They distinguish between *treatment* (which returns an individual to species-typical functioning) and *enhancement* (which exceeds species-typical function) based on a distinction contrasting *treatment versus enhancement* (Daniels 2000, Sabin and Daniels 1994).

2. Social constructivist accounts

   Some definitions of enhancement see it as a construction of social values. For example, Wolpe claims that enhancement is a slippery 'socially constructed' concept: 'concepts such as disease, normalcy, and health are significantly culturally and historically bound, and thus the result of negotiated values' (Wolpe 2002).

3. Welfarist accounts

   Another account understands human enhancement as improvement of the person's life. On the welfarist view, human enhancement can be defined as any change in the biology or psychology of a person that increases the chances of leading a good life in circumstances C.

Future prospects for radical modification of humans

Much more radical biological modification of human beings is possible. It has been possible since about the 1980s to transfer genes from one species into another. ANDi is a rhesus monkey who has had a jellyfish gene incorporated into his DNA: he glows fluorescent green. Genes from other species could be transferred to human beings, creating transgenic humans – fluorescent humans, for example (Savulescu 2003). Gene editing offers the prospect of radical modification of human beings (Savulescu 2016).

It has been hypothesized that ageing in human beings is related to the degradation of telomeres, which are the regions on the ends of our chromosomes (Blasco 2005). We may well discover genetic sequences that reduce the rate of telomere degradation. Transfer of these sequences into the human genome might radically increase lifespan.

Other psychological characteristics besides cognitive power can perhaps also be altered. Gene therapy has been used to turn lazy monkeys into workaholics by altering the reward centre in the brain (Liu et al. 2004). Genetically modified meadow voles, a species that is normally polygamous, have become monogamous.

Physical abilities might also be altered far beyond current possibilities. 'Schwarzenegger mice' of immense strength have been produced through genetic modification that blocks the production of myostatin (Lee 2004). Genetic manipulation to stop myostatin production, or the administration of blockers, would be expected significantly to increase strength in athletes, and is likely to offer real potential for doping in the future (Savulescu, Foddy, and Clayton 2004).

The ethics of enhancement

Technologies developed for medical treatments will increasingly be able to be used for human enhancement, and research aimed purely at enhancement might be funded. But is this right? What are the arguments on each side? See Up for Debate Box 12.2. For more detailed discussion, see Savulescu (2006a), Edmonds (2019) and The Nuffield Council on Bioethics (2018).

 Up for Debate Box 12.2 Should doctors enhance human beings using medical interventions?

For

1. Choosing not to enhance is wrong.

   Imagine that a child is born with a stunning intellect but requires a simple, readily available, cheap dietary supplement to sustain his intellect. His parents neglect his diet, and, as a result, his intelligence ends up normal. This is clearly wrong. Now consider another set of parents. They have a child of a normal intellect but, if were introduce the same dietary supplement, the child's intellect would rise to a stunning level (the same as the first child initially had). These parents cannot be bothered with improving the child's diet, so the child continues to have a normal intellect. The inaction of the two sets of parents is equally wrong. It has exactly the same consequence: a child exists who could have had a stunning intellect, but is instead normal. If we substitute 'biological intervention' for 'diet', we see that, in order not to wrong our children, we should enhance them if that is possible. Unless there is something special and optimal about our children's physical, psychological or cognitive abilities, or something different about other biological interventions, it would be wrong not to enhance them.

2. Consistency

   Education, diet and training are all used to make our children better people and increase their opportunities in life. We train children to be well-behaved, cooperative and intelligent. Indeed, researchers are looking at ways to make the environment more stimulating for young children in order to maximize their intellectual development. These environmental manipulations do not act mysteriously: they alter our biology. To be consistent, if we believe that it is right to enhance people through education and diet, then it is right to do so through biological means.

Continued

Up for Debate Box 12.2 Should doctors enhance human beings using medical interventions?—cont'd

3. Enhancement is no different ethically from treating disease
   If we accept the treatment and prevention of disease, we should accept enhancement. The goodness of health is what drives a moral obligation to treat or prevent disease. But health is not what ultimately matters. Health enables us to live well. Disease prevents us from doing what we want and what is good. Health is instrumentally valuable as a resource that allows us to do what really matters: to lead a good life.
   The moral obligation to benefit people that provides the grounds for treating disease also provides grounds to enhance people, insofar as this increases their chance of having a better life.

Against
1. The precautionary principle
   We are unwise to assume we can have sufficient knowledge to meddle biologically with human nature. To attempt to enhance one characteristic may have other unknown, unforeseen and deleterious effects. Unforeseen effects are particularly likely for genetic manipulations, because genes are pleiotropic, which means they have different effects in different environments. The gene or genes that predispose to manic depression may also be responsible for heightened creativity and productivity. There is a special value in the balance and diversity that natural variation affords, and enhancement will reduce this.
2. Inequity: genetic discrimination
   Enhancement will create a two-class society of the enhanced and the unenhanced, where the inferior unenhanced are discriminated against and disadvantaged all through life.
3. Enhancements are self-defeating
   Enhancements are often self-defeating. A typical example is increase in height. If height is socially desired, then everyone will try to enhance the height of their children at some cost to themselves, but no one in the end will have benefited: 'If everyone stands on tiptoe no one sees any further'. Economists have coined the term 'positional goods'. These are goods we value principally because they are markers of our success compared with others. Many enhancements will be for positional goods and will start a 'rat race', which will end in no improvement in well-being.
4. Enhancement is playing God or against nature
   Children are a gift, of God or of nature. We should not interfere with human nature. Enhancement is tampering with our nature or an affront to human dignity.

THE FUTURE OF MEDICINE

Medicine in the 20th century made huge advances in the treatment and prevention of disease. Medicine in the 21st century will continue to make significant inroads into treating and preventing disease, but it may move beyond these traditional goals. Doctors may have to take increasing account of patients' autonomous wishes and broader conceptions of human well-being. Medicine today is about promoting people's well-being and their autonomy.

To make decisions about the use of medicine beyond the treatment and prevention of disease requires robust conceptions of disease, well-being, autonomy, disability, identity, authenticity and what actually constitutes enhancement. It will also require decisions about distributive justice.

REVISION QUESTIONS

1. Some children without an underlying genetic condition or other diagnosis are smaller than other children (by definition, 1 in 100 children will fall below the 1st centile). They do not have species-typical functioning. Does this mean that they have a disease? How should we define disease?
2. Imagine that two children have short stature, and the same height. One has a genetic condition causing low growth hormone levels. The cause of the other child's short stature is not known. Should that make a difference to whether they should receive growth hormone treatment?
3. What is the difference between the medical model and the social model of disability?
4. Some people regard their disability as part of their identity, and would not wish to be cured. Does this mean that disability should be regarded as a mere difference?
5. What is the difference between treatment and enhancement? Should doctors provide enhancements? Why/why not?

Extension case 12.4

A female athlete, C, competes in the Olympics and wins multiple gold medals. However, her physical appearance and fast performance lead to suspicion. She subsequently has tests that demonstrate that she has higher than normal testosterone levels due to a congenital genetic condition (a disorder of sex development). Should C be allowed to compete against other females? Should she be required to take drugs to lower her testosterone levels to the same as other female athletes?

A female athlete, M, competes in the Olympics and World Championships and wins multiple gold medals. She later admits to taking oxandrolone, an androgen and anabolic steroid, and is banned from competition.

Should performance-enhancing drugs in sport be banned?

(Foddy and Savulescu 2011, 2007; Savulescu 2015; Savulescu, Creaney, and Vondy 2013)

REFERENCES

Barnes, E. 2014. "Valuing disability, causing disability." *Ethics* 125 (1): 88-113. doi: 10.1086/677021.

Bayne, T. and Levy, N. 2005. "Amputees by choice: body integrity identity disorder and the ethics of amputation." *Journal of Applied Philosophy* 22 (1): 75-86.

Blasco, M. A. 2005. "Telomeres and human disease: ageing, cancer and beyond." *Nature Reviews. Genetics* 6 (8): 611-22. doi: 10.1038/nrg1656.

Boorse, C. 1997. "A rebuttal on health." In *What is disease?*, edited by J. M. Humber and R. F. Almeder. Humana Press: 3-134.

Buchanan, A. E., Brock, D. W., Daniels, N., Wikler, D. and Sober, E. 2000. *From chance to choice: genetics and justice*. Cambridge: Cambridge University Press.

D'Silva, M. U., Daugherty, M. and MacDonald, M. 2004. "Deaf is dandy: contrasting the deaf and hearing cultures." *Intercultural Communication Studies* XIII (2): 111-7.

Daniels, N. 2000. "Normal functioning and the treatment-enhancement distinction." *Cambridge Quarterly of Healthcare Ethics* 9 (03): 309-22. doi: 10.1017/s0963180100903037.

Davis, D. S. 1997. "Genetic dilemmas and the child's right to an open future." *The Hastings Center Report* 27 (2): 7-15. doi: 10.2307/3527620.

Diekema, D. S. and Fost, N. 2010. "Ashley revisited: a response to the critics." *The American Journal of Bioethics* 10 (1): 30-44.

Dyer, C. 2000. "Surgeon amputated healthy legs." *BMJ* 320 (7231): 332.

Earp, B. D., Sandberg, A. and Savulescu, J. 2014. "Brave new love: the threat of high-tech 'conversion' therapy and the bio-oppression of sexual minorities." *AJOB Neuroscience* 5: 4-12. doi: 10.1080/21507740.2013.863242.

Earp, B. and Savulescu, J. 2019. *Brave new love: science, ethics, and the future of relationships*. Redwood City: Stanford University Press.

Edmonds, D. 2019. "Human enhancement." In *Ethics and the contemporary world*, edited by D. Edmonds. Routledge.

Elliott, C. 2003. *Better than well: American medicine meets the American dream*. 1st ed. New York; London: W. W. Norton.

Foddy, B. and Savulescu, J. 2007. *Ethics of performance enhancement in sport: drugs and gene doping principles of health care ethics*. 2nd ed.

Foddy, B. and Savulescu, J. 2011. "Time to re-evaluate gender segregation in athletics?" *British Journal of Sports Medicine* 45: 1184-8. doi: 10.1136/bjsm.2010.071639.

Frances, A. 2013. *Saving normal an insider's revolt against out-of-control psychiatric diagnosis, DSM-5, Big Pharma, and the medicalization of ordinary life*. New York: Harper Collins.

Fricker, M. 2007. *Epistemic injustice: power and the ethics of knowing*. Oxford: Oxford University Press.

Fulford, K. W. M. 1989. *Moral theory and medical practice*. Cambridge: Cambridge University Press.

Gunther, D. F. and Diekema, D. S. 2006. "Attenuating growth in children with profound developmental disability: a new approach to an old dilemma." *Archives of Pediatrics & Adolescent Medicine* 160 (10): 1013-7. doi: 10.1001/archpedi.160.10.1013.

Hope, T. and McMillan, J. 2012. "Physicians' duties and the non-identity problem." *American Journal of Bioethics* 12 (8): 21-9. doi: 10.1080/15265161.2012.692432.

Kahane, G. and Savulescu, J. 2009. "The welfarist account of disability." In *Disability and disadvantage*, edited by A. Cureton and K. Brownlee. Oxford: Oxford University Press: 14-53.

Kahane, G. and Savulescu, J. 2016. "Disability and mere difference*." *Ethics* 126 (3): 774-88.

Lane, H. L. 2002. "Do deaf people have a disability?" *Sign Language Studies* 2 (4): 356-79. doi: 10.1353/sls.2002.0019.

Lee, S.-J. 2004. "Regulation of muscle mass by myostatin." *Annual Review of Cell and Developmental Biology* 20 (1): 61-86. doi: 10.1146/annurev.cellbio.20.012103.135836.

Liao, S. M., Savulescu, J. and Sheehan, M. 2007. The Ashley Treatment: best interests, convenience, and parental decision-making. *Hastings Center Report* 37 (2): 16-20.

Liu, Z., Richmond, B. J., Murray, E. A., Saunders, R. C., Steenrod, S., Stubblefield, B. K., Montague, D. M. and Ginns, E. I. 2004. "DNA targeting of rhinal cortex D2 receptor protein reversibly blocks learning of cues that predict reward." *Proceedings of the National Academy of Sciences* 101 (33): 12336-41. doi: 10.1073/pnas.0403639101.

Minerva, F. and Giubilini, A. 2018. "From assistive to enhancing technology: should the treatment-enhancement distinction apply to future assistive and augmenting technologies?" *Journal of Medical Ethics* 44: 244-7. doi: 10.1136/medethics-2016-104014.

Moffitt, T. E., Caspi, A., Taylor, A., Kokaua, J., Milne, B. J., Polanczyk, G. and Poulton, R. 2010. "How common are common mental disorders? Evidence that lifetime prevalence rates are doubled by prospective versus retrospective ascertainment." *Psychological Medicine* 40: 899-909. doi: 10.1017/S0033291709991036.

Parfit, D. 1984. *Reasons and persons*. Oxford: Oxford University Press.

Sabin, J. E. and Daniels, N. 1994. "Determining "medical necessity" in mental health practice." *The Hastings Center Report* 24 (6): 5-13. doi: 10.2307/3563458.

Savulescu, J. 2002. "Deaf lesbians, "designer disability, " and the future of medicine." *BMJ* 325: 771. doi: 10.1136/bmj.325.7367.771.

Savulescu, J. 2003. "Human–animal transgenesis and chimeras might be an expression of our humanity." *American Journal of Bioethics* 3 (3): 22-5. doi: 10.1162/15265160360706462.

Savulescu, J. 2006a. "Genetic interventions and the ethics of enhancement of human beings." In *The Oxford handbook on bioethics*, edited by B. Steinbock. Oxford: Oxford University Press: 516-36.

Savulescu, J. 2006b. "Justice, fairness, and enhancement." *Annals of the New York Academy of Sciences* 1093: 321-38. doi: 10.1196/annals.1382.021.

Savulescu, J. 2007. "Autonomy, the good life, and controversial choices." In *The Blackwell guide to medical ethics*, edited by R. Rhodes. Blackwell Publishing Ltd: 17-37.

Savulescu, J. 2015. "Healthy doping." In *The Routledge handbook of drugs and sport*, edited by V. Moller. Abingdon: Routledge: 350-62.

Savulescu, J. 2016. "Why we should fine-tune the DNA of future generations." Cosmos Magazine.

Savulescu, J., Creaney, L. and Vondy, A. 2013. "Should athletes be allowed to use performance enhancing drugs?" *BMJ* 347: f6150. doi: 10.1136/bmj.f6150.

Savulescu, J., Foddy, B. and Clayton, M. 2004. "Why we should allow performance enhancing drugs in sport." *British Journal of Sports Medicine* 38 (6): 666-70. doi: 10.1136/bjsm.2003.005249.

Savulescu, J. and Kahane, G. 2009. "The moral obligation to create children with the best chance of the best life." *Bioethics* 23 (5): 274-90. doi: 10.1111/j.1467-8519.2008.00687.x.

Savulescu, J. and Kahane, G. 2017. "Understanding procreative beneficence: the nature and extent of the moral obligation to have the best child." In *The Oxford handbook of reproductive ethics*, edited by L. Francis. Oxford: Oxford University Press.

Shakespeare, T. 2006. *Disability rights and wrongs*. London: Routledge.

The Nuffield Council on Bioethics. 2018. "Genome editing and human reproduction: social and ethical issues", accessed 19/7/18. http://nuffieldbioethics.org/project/genome-editing-human-reproduction.

Wolpe, P. R. 2002. "Treatment, enhancement, and the ethics of neurotherapeutics." *Brain and Cognition* 50 (3): 387-95.

Chapter **13**

Reproductive medicine

Case 13.1

A couple, A and A, who are both deaf, are seeking artificial fertility treatment. The woman is not able to conceive naturally. They would like any embryo successfully created through the fertility treatment to be tested for the genetic form of deafness that affects them. However, if they are able to identify such an embryo, they would choose to implant it rather than one without the gene.

Should parents be permitted to select an embryo with a disability?

(This case is based on the case of Tom Lichy and Paula Garfield (Hinsliff and McKie 2008).)

In the last chapter, we considered a version of the above case when thinking about disability (Case 12.2). Here, we are interested in a different question – about the ethics and regulation of reproduction.

Most parents have their children without interference from the state. The main role of medicine in the process of reproduction is to ensure that mother and baby are healthy. Medical technology, however, can promote reproductive or procreative liberty or autonomy: the freedom to decide whether to have children, when to have children, how many children to have and what kind of children to have. This is achieved by:

1. contraception, sterilization or termination of pregnancy (abortion)
2. assisted reproduction, such as in-vitro fertilization (IVF)
3. genomic or other testing of the embryo or fetus, for disease or non-disease states.

To what extent should health professionals support or limit procreative freedom?

ETHICAL APPROACHES TO THE ISSUE OF REPRODUCTIVE CHOICE

Procreative autonomy – the interests of parents

This approach emphasizes the value, or perhaps the right, of adults to make their own reproductive choices. According to this approach, state or professional interference should be kept to a minimum and exercised only in rather extreme situations. This position has been taken by a number of liberal philosophers (e.g. Agar 2004, Dworkin 1993, Harris 1997, 1998). It would support allowing A and A to choose to implant a deaf embryo in Case 13.1.

Procreative beneficence

A different approach (the principle of procreative beneficence (Savulescu 2001, Savulescu and Kahane 2017)) claims that couples have a moral obligation to make reproductive choices that will maximize the welfare of the children they conceive. They should select the best child of the possible children they could have. Procreative beneficence articulates one moral reason which must be balanced against other reasons such as the health of the mother, the implications for society in terms of equality and solidarity, etc. However, when these reasons are not significant, it implies that couples should select not only the healthiest embryo, but the embryo with the genes associated with the best chance of the best life, such as genes for general intelligence or impulse control. According to this principle, parents A and A should not select a deaf embryo (Savulescu 2002b).

The interests of the future child

An alternative viewpoint (perhaps in between procreative autonomy and beneficence) is the idea that reproductive decisions should be made with the interests of the future child in mind. Some might feel that this would argue against A and A's choice. We should limit access to reproduction where preventing access is in the interests of the potential or future child. However, as noted in the last chapter, A and A's decision would not harm their future child (if born with congenital deafness) – he or she would not otherwise exist. Indeed, it would be in the interests of that child to be born.

However, the interests of the child might affect other decisions more. Future children can be negatively affected by some actions that are taken before their birth (such as drinking alcohol or taking drugs in pregnancy) or even before their conception (such as exposing gametes to radiation). We would not allow someone to harm a child who has already been born. When a harm occurs is morally irrelevant, so that may mean that certain risky choices should be avoided or limited.

The interests of the state

Reproductive choices affect the composition of the future population. The state therefore has an interest in what choices are made. Such interests may be relevant where the future child will require significant resources for its care, or where allowing couples choice (for example, in selecting the sex of their children; see Chapter 18) could have undesirable consequences for the population as a whole. Someone might argue that A and A's choice should not be allowed, as that would generate additional costs for the state (for example, in special educational needs, assistive technology or even cochlear implantation (see previous chapter)). However, limiting reproductive freedom on that basis may raise concerns about eugenics (see Chapter 18).

Preserving life

Central to many questions in reproduction is the morality of killing a fetus or embryo. Even if considerable weight is given to procreative liberty, many would take the view that reproductive choice should not be enabled through killing an already existing fetus or embryo.

ABORTION

Case 13.2

A mother in Northern Ireland bought medicine online for her teenage daughter that would induce a medical termination of pregnancy. (Her daughter had been in an abusive relationship and did not wish to continue the pregnancy.) This medicine is legally available within the health system in other parts of the UK. The daughter terminated her pregnancy. Several years later, the mother was criminally prosecuted for supplying the pills, with a potential jail sentence of five years.

Should abortion be legal? Should laws be consistent across a country?

(This case is based on one in Belfast court in late 2018 (Carroll 2018).)

At the heart of much of the debate around abortion, embryo experimentation and IVF are questions of the moral status of the embryo and fetus. Is it wrong to kill human embryos and fetuses, and, if it is, is that wrong significant enough to outweigh other goods?

Many different positions are taken on this issue. What all agree on is that there are very few justifications for killing a child or adult. Such killing is a serious wrong. (One major exception is self-defence, and that is a major strand of argument in the legal literature as to why abortion should be legal.) The child (normally) develops from the fertilized egg. At what stage in the development of the human

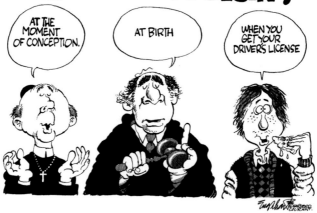

Figure 13.1 When does life begin? (© Bob Engleheart, reproduced with permission)

organism from egg to child does it become a significant wrong to kill the organism (Figure 13.1)? Some answer this question by identifying a point in the developmental process when such killing passes from being morally unimportant (or almost so) to being morally extremely serious – on a par with the killing of a child. Others deny that there is a point at which there is a sudden large change in moral status. Instead, through the developmental period, the wrong of killing increases so that there has to be increasing justification for allowing an abortion. Whichever of these two positions is taken, grounds have to be given for why it is that the moral status is different at different times in development.

Four views on what is important in determining the moral status of the embryo

Identity as a human organism

According to this view, there are no good grounds for according a different moral status to the human being at different stages in its development. If it is wrong to kill the child, then it would have been just as wrong to kill that child at any stage in its existence. The fundamental reason, according to this view, is that the embryo is the same entity – it has the same identity – as the child into which it develops. Because it is the same being, it should have the same moral standing.

Most supporters of this position put the moment at when the embryo attains full moral status as conception. Some have argued that an individual cannot be said to exist until the potential for twinning is lost and the neural streak begins to develop. (This is on the grounds that, until this point, the embryo could become two different people, as well as this being the earliest point of nervous system development. If a single embryo develops into two different people, it can't be the case that either is 'identical' to that early embryo.)

According to this view, Case 13.2 would be just as bad as another case where a grandmother supplied medication used to kill her 10-year-old grandchild.

The potential to be a person

This argument is that, if you kill an embryo or fetus, at any stage, you are carrying out an act that will mean that a potential future child will not exist. You are in effect killing a potential child. This argument differs from the preceding argument in that it does not accord fetuses and embryos moral status for what they are, but because of what they have the potential to become.

A related argument is the 'future of value' argument. Don Marquis argues that it is wrong to kill an embryo because it has a future like ours (Marquis 1989, Savulescu 2002a). What is wrong with killing persons is cutting short a valuable future. An embryo, Marquis argues, has the same future of value.

Again, according to this view, the mother in Case 13.2 was an accessory to the killing of a potential person.

Identity as a person

The view that an embryo, from the point of conception, has the same moral status as a child is sometimes called the right-to-life, or the pro-life position. The main alternative is the view that the moral status of an embryo depends on its properties, and not on its identity or potential. This view is often expressed as follows: it is very wrong to kill a *person* (in most situations), but a human embryo is not a person. A 'person' is a human being that has certain characteristics. The important moral issue is: what determines the stage during development when a human organism becomes a person?

Many different answers have been given to this question. Most proponents of this approach hold that being a person must involve some degree of *consciousness*. We, as persons, are conscious minds as well as physical bodies. Conscious life, or at least the perception of pain, is thought to start at about 24 weeks' gestation (Anand and Hickey 1987). According to most forms of this view, therefore, fetuses aged less than 24 weeks do not have moral status.

However, consciousness in the sense of feeling pain seems a rather minimal condition for being a person. Even quite primitive animals feel pain, and yet we do not accord them anything like the status of human persons in terms of the morality of killing. What is it that distinguishes a human being from a non-human animal, such that the one has a strong right to life and the other does not? Features such as the number of chromosomes seem irrelevant.

Some philosophers have focused on *self-consciousness* as the hallmark of being a person (Singer 1993, Tooley 1972). These philosophers argue that what is wrong with killing a self-conscious being is the frustration of the desires that the being has for its own future: its future-directed plans and goals. Other candidates for the mental capacities that are important to being a person include rationality (the ability to reason) and the ability to form relationships.

A different basis for the start of personhood is given by some religious traditions that confer moral status at the point when the soul enters the body (ensoulment).

Various times, from conception to birth, have been proposed as the moment of ensoulment.

The value given to the human organism by others is crucial (conferred moral status)

Some have argued that moral status need not be based only on intrinsic properties of the entity, but that it can be conferred by others (Strong 1997). Benn and Feinberg have argued that conferring moral status at birth can be justified in terms of the consequences for others and in terms of fostering concern, warmth and sympathy for others (Benn 1984, Feinberg 1984). Feinberg argues that it is because infants are so similar to persons that we should confer status on them in a symbolic way. Engelhardt argues that, at birth, the infant takes on an important social role, and that this justifies conferring moral status (Engelhardt 1973).

According to all these closely related views, a strong prohibition on killing infants is justified, both because those close to the infant care strongly for it, and because without such strong prohibition there is a danger that we will relax the strong prohibition on killing older babies and children.

However, because the fetus has not yet been recognized as a member of society, nor granted social standing, it would be acceptable to terminate the pregnancy in Case 13.2.

Problems with these four views

Each of the four views outlined above faces problems, which is why the issue of abortion remains so difficult. The first position confers moral status on what is just one cell or a few cells. It implies that killing that cell (or that early embryo) is, from a moral point of view, the same as killing a 10-year-old child. Such a position faces particular difficulties when the reasons a woman has for wanting an abortion are very powerful – for example, that she has become pregnant as a result of rape. This view also implies that taking post-coital contraception (such as the 'morning-after pill') or using an intrauterine contraceptive device amounts, morally, to murdering an adult.

The second position faces the same difficulties as the first, and other problems as well. The argument is likely to prove too much. A single sperm about to be injected into an egg constitutes a potential person, but it seems absurd to object to the disposal of either the egg or the sperm on the grounds that they constitute a potential person. Furthermore, each couple could give birth to many potential people. Contraception and sexual abstinence both prevent some of these potential persons from coming into existence. Are they therefore morally wrong (Singer and Kuhse 1986)? Cloning raises further problems for this position, as all somatic human cells are potential people. It seems absurd to suggest that destroying somatic cells would be (a serious) wrong.

If the first two positions appear to give too much moral protection to very early embryos, the third may give too little protection to infants and people with severe learning difficulties. Infants may not be self-conscious; does that mean infanticide should be permitted on the same basis as abortion (Giubilini and Minerva 2013)?

It also faces problems in justifying the particular feature, or group of features, that is taken to characterize a person.

The fourth position helps justify some of our intuitions about the moral importance of infants. However, to many it seems to justify these intuitions for the wrong reasons. It seems to suggest that we should not kill an infant on grounds such as that the infant's parents (and a few others) would be terribly upset. For many this is not the fundamental reason why we should not kill newborn children. Would it be ethical to end the life of an infant if they were orphaned, or if their parents did not wish them to live?

One view that is intuitively attractive to many people is that the moral status of the fetus develops as the fetus itself develops. According to this view, it may be wrong to kill even an early fetus, but the degree of wrong would be very much less than killing a late fetus. Furthermore, the grounds that would justify killing a fetus need to become stronger and stronger as the fetus develops. According to that view, the permissibility of termination in Case 13.2 depends on how advanced the pregnancy was at the time.

The morality of abortion

When is it wrong for a woman to have an abortion? When should the state prevent a woman from having an abortion? Although these questions are related, they are not the same. We may consider that it is morally wrong to lie to our friends, in many circumstances, without believing that it should be made illegal.

The answer to the first of the above questions is often taken to be: once the embryo or fetus acquires moral status. However, for many people this is only part of the picture, because the reasons why the woman wants the abortion are also crucial (Box 13.1). Those who believe that the grounds that justify abortion must be increasingly powerful as the fetus develops must take the view that the moral status of the embryo increases (either in stepwise or continuous fashion) during development.

Box 13.1 Some circumstances and reasons for an abortion that might affect its ethical status

1. The pregnancy is the result of rape.
2. The woman is only 16 years old.
3. Having a child would interfere with the woman's education or career.
4. The expected time of birth coincides with a planned holiday.
5. The woman would be a single mother and very poor.
6. The couple already have three children. This pregnancy was the result of carelessness, by the couple, over contraception.
7. As for 6, but the pregnancy resulted from a failure of contraception.
8. The woman is depressed and feels unable to cope with motherhood.
9. Pre-natal testing has revealed that the child will have a severe physical disability/illness and is highly likely to die in childhood or early infancy.
10. Pre-natal testing has revealed that the child will have severe learning disabilities.

The rights and interests of women

Despite the wide range of quite different views on abortion considered above, they all share one assumption. This is that, if the fetus had the same moral status as a normal adult, then it would be (almost always) wrong for a woman to have an abortion, and (almost always) right for the state to prevent the woman from having an abortion. Some philosophers, for example Judith Jarvis Thomson, have denied this assumption (Thomson 1971). Consider Case 13.3.

Case 13.3 (Fig. 13.2)

Imagine that you wake up one day with your circulatory system connected to another person, V. It transpires that he is a famous violinist. His fans have kidnapped you and connected you in order to save his life. V has a fatal kidney condition. However, if V remains connected to your circulatory system, he will eventually be cured. You are the only person who can save his life. 'But,' they say, 'good news. It is only for 9 months and then V will be fully recovered and you can be disconnected.'

Are you ethically obliged to remain connected to life support for 9 months in order to save the violinist?

(This is based on a famous thought experiment proposed by Judith Jarvis Thomson (Thomson 1971).)

Thomson argues that it would be highly laudable if you were to choose to remain connected to the violinist and thus save his life, but you are not morally required to remain connected. The key point of this analogy is to suggest that, even if we grant the fetus full moral status as a human person (the violinist has full moral status), it does not necessarily follow that a woman has an obligation to continue with a pregnancy. You have a right to control what happens to your

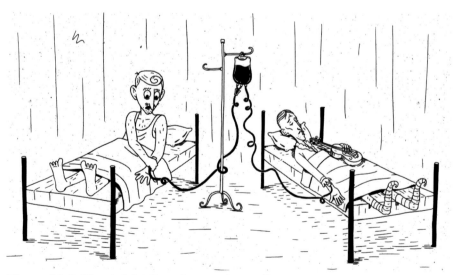

Figure 13.2 The violinist thought experiment (Reproduced with permission from SRF/Nino Christen (www.srf.ch/filosofix))

body. Thus, the abortion debate should not depend exclusively on the issue of the moral status of the embryo.

Many feminists argue that a woman has a right to choose abortion on more general principles. Benschof claims that a right to abortion is grounded in a right to 'privacy, autonomy and bodily integrity' (Benshoof 1985). Warren argues that making abortion illegal fails to respect women's right to liberty, self-determination and freedom from bodily harm, because pregnancy is arduous and risky (Warren 1991). See also Holmes and Purdy (1992).

Abortion law

There are different approaches to the law on abortion in different parts of the world. A small number of countries ban abortion completely (e.g. Nicaragua, Vatican City). Approximately 25% of countries have highly restrictive laws (for example, permitting abortion only to save the woman's life). Other countries (about 40%) may permit abortion for a wide range of reasons, including most or all of the reasons in Box 13.1. Nevertheless, in most of those countries, there are limits to the gestations at which abortion is permitted.

There are three key statutes relevant to abortion in England and Wales: the Offences Against the Person Act, the Infant Life (Preservation) Act and the Abortion Act. The first two statutes create criminal offences in relation to abortion, while the Abortion Act sets out exceptions when an abortion will be legal. The Abortion Act also covers abortion in Scotland. In Northern Ireland (at the time of writing) abortion remains a criminal offence, except in cases where it has been performed to preserve the life of the mother (or avoid serious long-term harm to her).

The Abortion Act 1967, amended 1990

The Abortion Act was designed to tackle the problem of 'back-street abortions', which were occurring despite their being illegal. These were often medically quite unsafe, and an increasing number of women were being admitted to hospital with complications resulting from such abortions. It was also aimed to address the lack of clarity over when a doctor could carry out an abortion for the sake of the mother's health. Doctors, acting in good faith in the interests of their patients, faced the possibility of criminal charges.

The Act gives immunity from prosecution to a doctor ('medical practitioner') who carries out an abortion within the terms of the Act. It does not decriminalize abortion in general. Nor does it provide protection for anyone other than the doctor (and nurses as well, following the House of Lords ruling in Royal College of Nursing of UK v DHSS [1981]).

Box 13.2 lists some of the important sections of the amended Act as set out in professional guidance. There are several points worth noting. Before 24 weeks' gestation, a doctor may carry out an abortion, with the woman's consent, on very wide grounds (Ground C). (That is because pregnancy almost always poses some risks to a woman's health.) In 2017, 98% of abortions in England and Wales were performed on this basis (Department of Health and Social Care 2018). After 24 weeks, abortion is lawful only to prevent risk of considerable harm to the mother, or for the sake of the fetus/child (see Box 13.2 for exact wording). In practice,

---

> **Box 13.2** Statutory grounds for termination of pregnancy (Royal College of Obstetricians and Gynecologists 2011)
>
> Abortion is legal in the UK if two doctors decide in good faith that, in relation to a particular pregnancy, one or more of the grounds specified in the Abortion Act are met, as follows:
>
> A. The continuance of the pregnancy would involve risk to the life of the pregnant woman greater than if the pregnancy were terminated: Abortion Act 1967 as amended, Section 1(1)(c).
> B. The termination is necessary to prevent grave permanent injury to the physical or mental health of the pregnant woman: Section 1(1)(b).
> C. The pregnancy has not exceeded its 24th week, and the continuance of the pregnancy would involve risk, greater than if the pregnancy were terminated, of injury to the physical or mental health of the pregnant woman: Section 1(1)(a).
> D. The pregnancy has not exceeded its 24th week, and the continuance of the pregnancy would involve risk, greater than if the pregnancy were terminated, of injury to the physical or mental health of any existing child(ren) of the family of the pregnant woman: Section 1(1)(a).
> E. There is a substantial risk that, if the child were born, it would suffer from such physical or mental abnormalities as to be seriously handicapped: Section 1(1)(d).
>
> The Act also permits abortion to be performed in an emergency if a doctor is of the opinion formed in good faith that termination is immediately necessary:
>
> F. to save the life of the pregnant woman: Section 1(4).
> G. to prevent grave permanent injury to the physical or mental health of the pregnant woman: Section 1(4).

most abortions after 24 weeks are done on grounds of fetal impairment (Ground E) – these comprised nearly 2% of abortions in 2017. Except in an emergency, two doctors are required to agree that abortion is justified on one of the grounds stated in the Act. Box 13.3 provides some additional points on abortion and the law.

MATERNAL–FETAL RELATIONS

> **Case 13.4**
>
> A pregnant woman, AP, with a history of mental illness, developed psychosis in the late stages of pregnancy. She was detained under the Mental Health Act (see Chapter 8). AP had previously had two caesarean sections. Delivery of the baby was imminent, but AP was judged to lack capacity because of her mental illness. The hospital believed that a caesarean section would be in AP's best interests because there was a risk of uterine rupture (estimated at 1%) if she had a vaginal delivery. Her treating psychiatrist also judged that it would be a potential risk to AP's mental health if her baby were to die as a result of this complication.
>
> Should a court authorize a caesarean section against AP's wishes (including restraint if necessary)?
>
> (This is based on the case of Re AA [2012]. See also the closely related Case 8.2 in Chapter 8.)

Box 13.3 Additional points in the law on abortion

1. Doctors may refuse to carry out an abortion on grounds of conscientious objection (Section 4 of the Abortion Act). The burden of proof lies with the doctor to show that he or she did have a conscientious objection. Conscientious objection is not a defence, however, if the abortion 'is necessary to save the life or to prevent grave permanent injury to the physical or mental health of a pregnant woman'.
2. The Abortion Act does not give a woman the right to demand an abortion. However, a doctor might be found negligent either for not advising a woman (in appropriate circumstances) of the possibility of an abortion, or for not carrying out an abortion, where appropriate, under Section 1 (1b, 1c) (unless due to conscientious objection; see above).
3. The fetus has no right to life. Thus, its status in law is dramatically affected by birth. A fetus cannot be the subject of child protection under the Children Act (see Chapter 10).
4. A fetus probably has no legal right to be aborted. In other words, damages could not be claimed on the grounds that, had doctors acted differently (e.g. advised abortion), the child would not have been born, and that it would have been better for the child not to have been born.
5. A woman has a legal right to refuse an abortion.
6. The father of a fetus has no legal right to prevent a woman from having an abortion – and no right to be consulted about it. Under Article 8 of the Human Rights Act (see Chapter 4) it may be possible for a father to claim some rights with regard to abortion. Such a claim, made in 1980 to the European Commission, was, however, rejected.

Intrauterine contraceptive devices and 'morning-after' pills

The combined effect of R (on the application of Smeaton) v The Secretary of State for Health [2002] and the Prescription Only Medicines (Human Use) Amendment Order 2000 is that:
1. It is legal for a pharmacist to dispense emergency contraception without a doctor's prescription.
2. Methods of contraception, such as the intrauterine contraceptive device and the morning-after pill, which are designed to prevent implantation, are classified as contraceptive techniques. As such they are not governed by the Abortion Act 1967.

A number of cases have been heard in the courts about the legality of enforcing a caesarean section on an unwilling woman. The Royal College of Obstetricians and Gynaecologists produced guidelines that state:

In caring for the pregnant woman, an obstetrician must respect the woman's autonomy and her legal right to refuse any recommended course of action … The use of judicial authority to implement treatment regimens in order to protect the fetus violates the pregnant woman's autonomy and should be avoided unless stringent criteria are met (Royal College of Obstetricians and Gynecologists 2006).

In an earlier case, the Court of Appeal Judges stated:

A competent woman, who has the capacity to decide, may, for religious reasons, other reasons, for rational or irrational reasons or for no reason at all, choose not to have medical intervention, even though the consequence may be the death or serious handicap of the child she bears, or her own death. In that event, the courts do not have the jurisdiction to declare medical intervention lawful and the question of her own best interests, objectively considered, does not arise... (in Re MB (An Adult: Medical Treatment) [1997]).

The courts have indicated that a woman with capacity has the right to refuse treatment even where the life of the fetus is at grave risk. The interests of the fetus are not taken into consideration by the court.

However, judges have often (in cases that reached the court) judged the woman to lack capacity to make a decision – perhaps, to justify saving the fetus, and perhaps with the view that the woman will be glad afterwards that that was the decision taken. For example, in the case of MB, severe needle phobia was judged to impair her decision to refuse caesarean section. In AP's case (13.4), the judge authorized elective caesarean section, with restraint if necessary.

What about other actions that pregnant women take that might affect the fetus?

Case 13.5

A woman with a history of alcohol and substance abuse drank heavily while she was pregnant (half a bottle of vodka and eight cans of strong lager per day). Her child, CP, was subsequently diagnosed with developmental disabilities from fetal alcohol syndrome.

The local authority, who were caring for CP, sought compensation from the Criminal Injuries Compensation Authority for what they claimed was effectively a form of attempted manslaughter.

This is based on CP (A Child) [2014].

Under the Congenital Disabilities (Civil Liability) Act 1976, a damaged child can make a claim and recover damages from a negligent defendant (for example, a doctor) who has caused or contributed to the child's disability. This Act specifically *excludes* the case where the damage is a result of actions by the mother (except in the case of negligent driving). In the case of CP, the court ruled that the child should not be eligible for compensation, either from his mother or from the compensation authority.

But is that ethically correct? Should pregnant women who make choices that will lead to significant harm to the future child be liable for the consequences, or constrained to prevent the harm? Up for Debate Box 13.1 summarizes some of the ethical arguments for and against such interventions.

ASSISTED REPRODUCTION

Assisted reproduction has come of age. Louise Brown, the first 'test-tube' baby, was 40 years old in 2018. Since Louise Brown's conception, which was made possible through IVF, even more sophisticated techniques have been developed. There was initially intense ethical debate about whether assisted reproduction should be provided (largely on the basis of concerns about the moral status of

Up for Debate Box 13.1 Should a pregnant woman's behaviour be constrained for the sake of the fetus (or future child)?

Against

1. *Autonomy* – such constraints infringe on the woman's autonomy. This argument could be supplemented using a similar argument to that of Thomson (see Case 13.3) in the context of abortion.
2. *Privacy* – the woman has a right not to have her body invaded or even touched without consent. Many constraints on her behaviour would involve such battery (for example, forced caesarean section).
3. *Fetal status* – in English law the fetus has no status as a person until birth. The rights of a person (the woman) should not be subjugated to the rights, if any, of an entity that is not a person.
4. *Public policy* – the likely consequences of allowing fetal interests to affect the legal provisions for restraining people's behaviour are undesirable. A liberal society rightly draws back from the spectre of either imprisoning or impoverishing pregnant women for behaviour that would be tolerated in men, or in women who are not pregnant.
5. *Impact on abortion law* – recognition of the interests of unborn children might have the consequence of leading to restrictions in abortion law.
6. *Morality versus law* – Even if it is morally wrong for a pregnant woman to behave in ways that might harm the fetus or future child, it does not follow that such behaviour should be the subject of legal restraint.

For

1. *Consistency* – a classic example of justified state restraint is the banning of the sedative thalidomide. This sedative had no significant adverse effects on mothers. However, if taken during fetal gestation, it interfered with limb development. Rather than informing women of these possible effects and allowing them to choose whether to take this sedative, the state rightly banned it in the interests of future people.
2. According to the *principle of temporal neutrality,* the timing of a harm, or when a harm occurs, is morally irrelevant. It would be wrong to administer large amounts of alcohol to a young child or to cause brain damage to them by administering a poison. It would be equally wrong to cause the same degree of brain damage prior to the child's birth. Just as we have reasons to prevent child abuse, we have reasons to restrain people from taking actions whose harmful effects will be manifest in the future (Wilkinson et al. 2016).
3. *Abortion is different from causing harm to a future child* – while abortion does not lead to any future child who is harmed, non-lethal but damaging behaviour can result in a child existing in the future who has been harmed. The principle of preventing harm to others articulated by John Stuart Mill licences the use of state power to prevent such harm.

embryos that might be destroyed). However, there is now wide acceptance of the ethical acceptability of IVF. Debate now more often focuses on questions such as the funding of IVF (should it receive public funding), who should be eligible for treatment and (as highlighted in Case 13.1) whether different forms of embryo selection should be permitted.

Who should be helped to conceive?

Case 13.6

A 57-year-old retired teacher, ST, wished to become pregnant, but had age-related infertility. She was not eligible for publicly funded IVF (NICE guidelines offer treatment up to age 42), and most UK private fertility clinics do not offer treatment after age 50. She eventually sought treatment overseas and successfully conceived using a donor egg and sperm from her husband.

Should there be an age limit on IVF?

(This is based on the case of Sue Tollefsen (Anon 2010).)

There are different reasons that women or couples might seek fertility treatment. In deciding whether, or when, it is right to veto a request for help, or in deciding priorities for treatment, there are three main interests that are potentially important: those of the (potential) child, those of the couple and those of society more generally.

The interests of the (potential) child

Most discussions, and the law, consider the interests of the child that may result from the assisted reproduction to be of paramount importance. However, it is not as clear as might at first be thought what these interests are.

One approach sees the issue as broadly analogous to that of adoption. The central question is: which couple, out of all the available couples wishing to adopt, is likely to provide the best parents for this baby? Some might feel that an older mother (as in Case 13.6) is not the best prospective parent. There are two major problems with the analogy with adoption. The first is the nature of the judgements and the evidence on which they are based. What is the evidence that children brought up by a single mother or an older mother are less happy (or whatever) than a child brought up by a couple or a younger mother? Is the fertility clinic in a position to decide which of the couples or individuals will make the best parents? The second problem is more profound. This is to deny that the adoption model is the appropriate model in the first place. There is a crucial difference between adoption and fertility treatment. For adoption, we have the same baby whichever couple we choose as parents; in the case of fertility treatment it is a different baby in each case. This is the non-identity problem mentioned in the previous chapter.

In the case of ST, what are the interests of the potential child? If we refuse help, the child will not come into existence. If we help, the child will be born to a mother aged 57. Which represents the best interests of the potential child? Although it might be preferable, if there were a choice, for the child to have a younger mother, that choice does not exist. According to this analysis, the criterion of the best interests of the potential child, which is given such a central place in most discussions about fertility treatment, is of little value. It would rule out assisting reproduction only in some rather extreme situations, for example when the potential child is likely to suffer either from a very serious genetic disorder or from very bad parenting, when it might be worse for the child to exist than never to exist.

The interests of the potential parent(s)

Fertility clinics are often faced with couples who want IVF, although there are reasons for thinking that this would not be in their best interests – for example, if pregnancy would pose an increased medical risk, or if the chance of success is very low (e.g. because of the woman's age). From the professionals' point of view, it does not seem worth the risks or costs of the treatment, given the very low chance of success.

What should the professionals do? This situation, if we are considering only the interests of the couple, is similar to a situation frequently met with in medicine: a patient making a decision that the professionals believe is not in his or her best interests (see Chapter 5). One response to such situations is to provide the couple with relevant information and to explain the reasons for the professional opinion. However, if the couple, after due deliberation, still want to go ahead with fertility treatment, and will pay the costs, it would be providing paternalistic to deny them treatment.

The interests of the state

The state has interests in the people who are born, even if the couple are paying for the entire costs of the fertility treatment. This may be significant, for example, if the child has profound impairments requiring considerable welfare provision. But the state's interests go further than this. When is it in the interests of society that a particular couple or individual should not be helped to conceive? Should a single mother, or a same-sex couple or a woman aged 60 be allowed access to fertility treatment if the total costs are met by the couple or the individual?

The starting point in a liberal society is that the state needs a good reason to interfere in individual liberty. It might be claimed that, in allowing fertility treatment to single women, same-sex couples or older women, there would be harm to wider society. Reasons would need to be given not only as to why it is thought that such family life is wrong, but also why it is the kind of wrong that justifies state interference.

Assisted reproduction and the law

The Human Fertilisation and Embryology Act 1990

The Human Fertilisation and Embryology Act (HFEA) 1990, in addition to providing most of the key aspects of legislation in this area, set up the *Human Fertilisation and Embryology Authority*. This Authority regulates much of the provision for assisting reproduction, some of which is summarized in Box 13.4.

Case 13.7

A woman, S, enters into an informal arrangement with a gay couple who wish to have a child. She agrees to gestate the child (conceived with sperm from one of the men and a donor egg), with the plan for the child to be cared for by the couple. However, later, S changed her mind and did not wish to hand over the child.

Should surrogacy be permitted? (Should surrogacy arrangements be enforced? What about commercial surrogacy? Should payments to surrogates be permitted?)

> **Box 13.4** The Human Fertilisation and Embryology Act 1990 (HFEA)
>
> **Areas covered by the act**
>
> 1. Treatment that involves the use of donated genetic material (eggs, sperm or embryos), stored genetic material or embryos created outside the body (e.g. by IVF). Such treatments have to be *licensed*.
> 2. The storage of human eggs, sperm and embryos.
> 3. Research on human embryos.
>
> **The Human Fertilisation and Embryology Authority**
>
> This was set up by Parliament under the Act. It is funded partly by centres licensed to provide fertility treatment, and partly from taxation. The Authority has 19 members appointed by the Secretary of State for Health. The functions of the Authority include the following:
>
> 1. Inspecting and licensing centres involved in the areas covered by the Act (see above).
> 2. Keeping a confidential register of information about donors, patients and treatments.
> 3. Publishing a code of practice.
> 4. Giving information and advice to those seeking fertility treatment.
> 5. Keeping the whole field under review.
>
> **Research on embryos**
>
> 1. Research on human embryos more than 14 days old (i.e. from the appearance of the primitive streak) is illegal.
> 2. Research leading to the production of identical individuals by genetic replacement is illegal.
> 3. It is illegal to attempt to produce embryos by combining the gametes of humans with animals.
>
> **HFEA guidance**
>
> The HFEA Code of practice provides detailed guidance for IVF clinics based on the Act.
>
> For example, Section 13(5) of the HFEA states that: 'a woman shall not be provided with treatment services unless account has been taken of the welfare of any child who may be born as a result of the treatment (including the need of that child for a father) and of any other child who may be affected by the birth'.
>
> The Code of Practice gives more detailed guidance as to when treatment should be refused, i.e. if the child who may be born or any existing child in the family is likely to be at risk of significant harm or neglect. The guidance explicitly states that patients should not be discriminated against on grounds of gender, race, disability, sexual orientation, religious belief or age.

The Surrogacy Arrangements Act 1985

Surrogacy is covered by the Surrogacy Arrangements Act (SAA) 1985. This makes any commercial basis for surrogacy a criminal offence. Thus, facilitators of commercial surrogacy would be committing an illegal act, and advertising for such arrangements is illegal. However, the Act specifically gives immunity to the actual parties themselves. The HFEA made amendments to the SAA, stating: 'No surrogacy arrangement is enforceable by or against any of the persons making it …'. Thus, the surrogate mother (whatever the genetic relationships) will remain the child's mother if she wishes to do so.

Reform of the SAA is long overdue. Three areas in particular are problematic. First, the prohibition against commercialization has failed to prevent payments being made (of up to £50,000). Second, the HFEA's definition of motherhood and fatherhood does not adequately cover surrogacy arrangements. Third, the rules governing the transfer of legal parenthood are complex and costly. Whilst the government has accepted the need to reform the Act, it has so far failed to propose new legislation.

REVISION QUESTIONS

1. In England, abortion is permitted, with little restriction, until 24 weeks' gestation. Why has this point been chosen? Is it ethically justified?
2. Ethical arguments around abortion often centre on the question of the 'moral status' of the fetus. What does this mean? Could abortion be permitted even if the fetus had full moral status?
3. Is a father's consent required prior to an abortion? Do you agree with existing law on that?
4. A trans-sexual man wishes to have IVF. Should it be provided to him?
5. Are age cut-offs for fertility treatment justified?
6. How should the 'welfare of the child' be considered when making decisions about fertility treatment?

Extension case 13.8

A. A young woman presents to a fertility clinic requesting tubal ligation. She is clear that she does not wish to have children, has never wished for children and does not believe that she will change her mind. She has capacity and is fully informed that reversal of the tubal ligation may be difficult, complicated and not necessarily possible.

The surgeon refuses to perform the tubal ligation. Is this justified?

B. A young woman presents to a fertility clinic requesting egg freezing. She does not currently have a long-term partner. She believes that she may like to have children one day, but intends to focus on her career for the next decade. She would like to maximize her future options and minimize the chance that she would need fertility treatment in the future.

The fertility clinic tells her that she may pay privately to have her eggs frozen, but that they would only be stored for 10 years and then destroyed.

Should public health systems or insurers subsidize or pay for egg freezing? Is the time limit on egg storage justified?

Read Benn and Lupton (2005), Ehman and Costescu (2018), Savulescu (2002a) and Jackson (2016).

REFERENCES

Agar, N. 2004. *Liberal eugenics: in defence of human enhancement*. Maldon, MA; Oxford: Blackwell.

Anand, K. J. and Hickey, P. R. 1987. "Pain and its effects in the human neonate and fetus." *The New England Journal of Medicine* 317 (21): 1321-9. doi: 10.1056/NEJM19871119 3172105.

Anon. 2010. "Risks are too great to have another IVF child, says mother, 59." Evening Standard, 17 May 2010. https://www.standard.co.uk/news/risks-are-too-great-to-have-another-ivf-child-says-mother-59-6470249.html.

Benn, P. and Lupton, M. 2005. "Sterilisation of young, competent, and childless adults." *BMJ (Clinical Research Ed.)* 330 (7503): 1323-5. doi: 10.1136/bmj.330.7503.1323.

Benn, S. 1984. "Abortion, infanticide, and respect for persons." In *The problem of abortion*, edited by J. Feinberg. Belmont: Wadsworth: 135-44.

Benshoof, J. 1985. "Reasserting women's rights." *Family Planning Perspectives* 17 (4): 160-4. doi: 10.2307/2135239.

Carroll, R. 2018. "Northern Irish woman to challenge abortion prosecution." The Guardian, 5 Nov 2018. Accessed 12/8/18. https://www.theguardian.com/uk-news/2018/nov/05/northern-irish-woman-abortion-pills-fights-prosecution.

CP (A Child) [2014] EWCA Civ 1554.

Department of Health and Social Care. 2018. "Abortion statistics, England and Wales: 2017," accessed 12/11/18. https://assets.publishing.service.gov.uk/government/uploads/system/uploads/attachment_data/file/714183/2017_Abortion_Statistics_Commentary.pdf.

Dworkin, R. 1993. *Life's dominion: an argument about abortion and euthanasia*. London: HarperCollins.

Ehman, D. and Costescu, D. 2018. "Tubal sterilization in women under 30: case series and ethical implications." *Journal of Obstetrics and Gynaecology Canada* 40 (1): 36-40. doi: 10.1016/j.jogc.2017.05.034.

Engelhardt, H. T., Jr. 1973. "Viability, abortion, and the difference between a fetus and an infant." *American Journal of Obstetrics and Gynecology* 116 (3): 429-34.

Feinberg, J. 1984. "Potentiality, development and rights." In *The problem of abortion*, edited by J. Feinberg. Belmont: Wadsworth: 145-50.

Giubilini, A. and Minerva, F. 2013. "After-birth abortion: why should the baby live?" *Journal of Medical Ethics* 39 (5): 261-3. doi: 10.1136/medethics-2011-100411.

Harris, J. 1997. "'Goodbye Dolly?' The ethics of human cloning." *Journal of Medical Ethics* 23 (6): 353-60.

Harris, J. 1998. "Rights and reproductive choice." In *The future of human reproduction: ethics, choice and regulation*, edited by J. Harris and S. Holm. Oxford: Clarendon Press.

Hinsliff, G. and McKie, R. 2008. "This couple want a deaf child. Should we try to stop them?" The Observer, 9 March 2008. Accessed 12/8/18. https://www.theguardian.com/science/2008/mar/09/genetics.medicalresearch.

Holmes, H. B. and Purdy, L. M. 1992. *Feminist perspectives in medical ethics*. Bloomington: Indiana University Press.

Jackson, E. 2016. "'Social' egg freezing and the UK's statutory storage time limits." *Journal of Medical Ethics* 42: 738-41.

Marquis, D. 1989. "Why abortion is immoral." *The Journal of Philosophy* 86: 183-202.

R (on the application of Smeaton) v Secretary of State for Health [2002] All ER (D) 115 (Apr).

Re AA [2012] EWHC 4378 (COP).

Re MB (Caesarean Section) [1997] EWCA Civ 1361.

Royal College of Nursing of UK v DHSS [1981] AC 800.

Royal College of Obstetricians and Gynecologists. 2006. "Law and ethics in relation to court-authorised obstetric intervention. Ethics Committee Guideline No. 1." Accessed 12/8/18. http://www.aogm.org.mo/assets/Uploads/aogm/Guidelines/RCOG—UK/No-1-RCOG-Law-and-Ethics-in-Relation-to-Court-Authorised-Obsetric-Intervention.pdf.

Royal College of Obstetricians and Gynecologists. 2011. "The care of women requesting induced abortion (Evidence-based Clinical Guideline No. 7)." Accessed 12/8/18. https://www.rcog.org.uk/en/guidelines-research-services/guidelines/the-care-of-women-requesting-induced-abortion/.

Savulescu, J. 2001. "Procreative beneficence: why we should select the best children." *Bioethics* 15 (5–6): 413-26.

Savulescu, J. 2002a. "Abortion, embryo destruction and the future of value argument." *Journal of Medical Ethics* 28: 133-5.

Savulescu, J. 2002b. "Deaf lesbians, 'designer disability,' and the future of medicine." *BMJ* 325: 771. doi: 10.1136/bmj.325.7367.771.

Savulescu, J. and Kahane, G. 2017. "Understanding procreative beneficence: the nature and extent of the moral obligatiiono have the best child." In *The Oxford handbook of reproductive ethics*, edited by L. Francis. Oxford: Oxford University Press.

Singer, P. 1993. *Practical ethics*. Cambridge: Cambridge University Press.

Singer, P. and Kuhse, H. 1986. "The ethics of embryo research." *Law, Medicine and Health Care* 14 (3–4): 133-8.

Strong, C. 1997. *Ethics in reproductive and perinatal medicine : a new framework*. New Haven; London: Yale University Press.

Thomson, J. J. 1971. "A defense of abortion." *Philosophy and Public Affairs* 1 (1): 47-66.

Tooley, M. 1972. "Abortion and infanticide." *Philosophy and Public Affairs* 2 (1): 37-65.

Warren, M. A. 1991. "Abortion." In *A companion to ethics*, edited by P. Singer. Oxford: Blackwell: 303-14.

Wilkinson, D., Skene, L., De Crespigny, L. and Savulescu, J. 2016. "Protecting future childrenrom in-utero harm." *Bioethics* 30 (6): 425-32. doi: 10.1111/bioe.12238.

REPRODUCTIVE MEDICINE

Chapter **14**

End of life

Case 14.1

An elderly woman, LB, is admitted to hospital with severe rheumatoid arthritis. She is emaciated, unwell and believed to have only a short time to live. LB also has severe pain, despite very high doses of pain-relieving medication. She has recently refused all life-prolonging treatment and asks Dr C (who has treated her arthritis for many years) to end her life. Her family support her request.

Would it be either ethical or legal for Dr C to end LB's life?

(The above case is based on the case of Lillian Boyes and Dr Nigel Cox (R v Cox [1992]).)

ENDING LIFE AND THE LAW

The UK legal position relevant to end-of-life decisions in a clinical context is summarized in Box 14.1. We will discuss some of the basis for these conclusions in more detail in this section.

Active euthanasia (mercy killing) is illegal

To take an active step with the *intention* of shortening the patient's life is murder. This is the case even if the patient requests to be killed. Active euthanasia, whether voluntary or not, is illegal.

Passive euthanasia is not necessarily illegal

It is not normally illegal for a doctor to withhold or withdraw treatment (such as ventilation) if the treatment is not in the patient's best interests, or if a patient with capacity does not consent to it.

Intending relief of distress, but foreseeing death, is normally legal

To take an active step with the *intention* of relieving the patient's distress, but with the *foreseen result* that it is likely to shorten life, is normally legal.

Assisting suicide is a criminal offence

Suicide and attempting suicide are not criminal offences. It is a criminal offence, however, for anyone (not just a doctor) to 'assist or encourage' the suicide of someone else. Thus, if a patient committed suicide by taking an overdose of tablets that the doctor had left by the bedside for that purpose, the doctor could be found guilty of assisting suicide.

Some patients travel overseas to access assisted suicide. Family members who help a patient travel to access assisted dying will not necessarily be prosecuted, if it is not deemed to be in the public interest. The director of Public Prosecutions has provided guidance indicating when prosecution is more likely. This guidance suggests that health professionals who provide advice or other assistance to a patient in their care (including travel support for assisted suicide) could be prosecuted (Director of Public Prosecutions 2014).

A patient with capacity who refuses life-saving treatment is not committing suicide

A patient with capacity can refuse any, even life-saving, treatment. The doctor would be committing a battery to give the treatment in the light of the patient's refusal.

The impact of the Human Rights Act 1998

The law on euthanasia and assisted suicide has been challenged in several high-profile cases involving the Human Rights Act 1998 and the European Convention on Human Rights (ECHR). In summary, these establish that:

a. Under Article 2 ECHR, people have a right to life, and the state must take reasonable steps to prevent people being killed without their consent.

b. The European Court of Human Rights (ECtHR) has held that, under Article 8, the state must balance the right under paragraph (1) of protecting the right of a person to decide the manner and time of their death as part of the respect for their right to private life, with, under paragraph (2), the interests of vulnerable people who may be killed or commit suicide without their full consent. The ECtHR has held that the current law (permitting suicide and not always prosecuting assisted suicide) strikes a fair balance.

> **Box 14.1** Summary of the UK law relating to medical decisions at the end of life—cont'd
>
> c. In R (Nicklinson) v Ministry of Justice, the Supreme Court confirmed that, although the European Court has held that the current law strikes a *permissible* balance, that does not prevent the English courts considering whether the law strikes the *correct* balance. The Supreme Court decided to delay issuing a final decision on that question as the issue was being debated in Parliament. Those debates did not lead to a change in the law, and so litigation is currently ongoing to determine whether, under English law, the correct balance is struck. The issue is bound to return to the Supreme Court, but it is clear from Nicklinson that the Supreme Court is divided on the question.
>
> d. General Medical Council guidelines that set out good practice for doctors in withdrawing and withholding treatment (e.g. artificial hydration and nutrition) do not conflict with Article 3 (prohibition of inhuman or degrading treatment) (Burke v UK [2006]). For example, withholding or withdrawing treatment in the patient's best interests (e.g. to enable a comfortable death) can be lawful and not contrary to Article 3.

Active euthanasia (mercy killing) is illegal (murder)

It would be illegal for Dr C to take an action with the aim of ending LB's life. In the UK, in the only case of its kind, Dr Nigel Cox was convicted and found guilty of attempted murder for performing voluntary active euthanasia of his patient Lillian Boyes. He administered a dose of potassium chloride to stop her heart. The judge, in directing the jury, said: 'Even the prosecution case acknowledged that he [Dr Cox] … was prompted by deep distress at Lillian Boyes' condition; by a belief that she was totally beyond recall and by an intense compassion for her fearful suffering. Nonetheless … if he injected her with potassium chloride for the primary purpose of killing her, or hastening her death, he is guilty of [*attempted murder*] … neither the express wishes of the patient nor of her loving and devoted family can affect the position'. (Dr Cox eventually received a suspended sentence and later returned to clinical work under supervision.)

Intending relief of distress in the patient's best interests, but foreseeing death, is normally legal

What if Dr Cox had used higher doses of pain relief instead of potassium chloride? In the Cox case, the judge drew a clear distinction between intending death and foreseeing death. The former is potentially murder, the second may be good practice. Lord Neuberger in R (Nicklinson) v Ministry of Justice [2014] confirmed that 'a doctor commits no offence when treating a patient in a way which hastens death, if the purpose of the treatment is to relieve pain and suffering'.

This is based on the so-called doctrine of double effect (see below for more discussion of this).

Withholding and withdrawing treatment are not necessarily illegal

If LB's life could be extended with medical treatment, it would be legal for Dr C to stop (withdraw) treatment that is prolonging LB's life (e.g. antibiotics), or to not start (withhold) potentially life-prolonging treatment (e.g. cardiopulmonary resuscitation).

In the Bland case (Case 14.3 below), Lord Goff said: '... the law draws a crucial distinction between cases in which a doctor decides not to provide, or to continue to provide, for his patient treatment or care which could or might prolong his life, and those in which he decides, for example by administering a lethal drug, actively to bring his patient's life to an end ... the former may be lawful ...' (but not the latter). In the case of withholding or withdrawing treatment, the question is whether the treatment is in the best interests of the patient, and the intent of doctor is of no legal relevance.

(For more on withholding and withdrawing treatment, see below.)

The patient with mental capacity has a right to refuse treatment

A patient with capacity may refuse any treatment, whatever the likely consequences. They may do so if they have capacity at the time of needing treatment, or via a (valid) advance directive (see Chapter 7). In Chapter 7, we mentioned the case of a patient with capacity who had attempted suicide but did not wish medical treatment to save her life. Her doctors believed that they were obliged to respect her wishes, and a coronial inquiry supported their decision.

In another case, a paralyzed patient did not wish to be kept alive any longer. She wished to have her breathing support withdrawn, but her doctors were unwilling to carry out her wishes. The court, having determined that she had capacity to make the decision, confirmed that she had the right to demand withdrawal of treatment. The doctors had either to comply with her wishes or transfer her care to doctors who would comply with her wishes (Re B [2002]).

The patient lacking mental capacity should be treated in his/her best interests

What if LB no longer had capacity to express her wishes? In the case of a patient lacking capacity, a doctor's duty of care is to treat in that patient's best interests. How does the law tackle the situation?

There is a presumption in favour of prolonging life – sometimes called the 'sanctity of life principle'. However, the courts have accepted that there is no obligation to prolong life in all circumstances; it is not always in a patient's best interest to keep them alive.

In relation to those aged 16 years and over, the interpretation of best interests is now governed by s.4 of the Mental Capacity Act 2005 (MCA) (unless a valid advance decision applies; see Chapter 7). The patient's best interests are understood to include 'medical, emotional and all other welfare issues' (Portsmouth NHS Trust v Wyatt [2004]). This includes consideration of the patient's wishes, lifestyle and values, which will be given 'great weight' (Briggs v Briggs [2016]) (and the views of family members may be relevant to this). For example, one case noted that the patient, who during her life had attached considerable weight to her personal appearance and being 'glamorous', would have found invasive life-sustaining treatment undignified. That was a factor in deciding its provision was not in her best interests (Kings College NHS Foundation Trust v C [2015]). By contrast, a court might be persuaded that a patient with strong religious views in support of the sanctity of life would want to be kept alive unless the treatment was clearly futile. Particularly relevant in this context is s.4(5) MCA, which states that 'where the determination [*of best interests*] relates to life-sustaining treatment [*the decision-maker*] must not, in considering whether the treatment is in the best interests of the person concerned, be motivated by a desire to bring about his death'. Essentially this section enshrines the double effect doctrine (see below).

For those aged under 16 years, who are not covered by the MCA, a series of cases about disputes between parents and doctors over medical treatment make it clear that end-of-life decisions hinge on the best interests test, which is applied by comparing the reasons or considerations in favour of treatment (and prolonging life) with those reasons against treatment. Courts have often referred to a 'balance sheet' and sometimes ask doctors to provide a written list of the pros and cons of treatment. Where there is a dispute between parents and doctors about life-prolonging treatment, the court will aim to determine an 'objective' view of the child's best interests. The views of the parents will be taken into account, but ultimately the court will reach its own view on what is in the child's best interests. In a recent case (and in a number other cases of disagreement), the courts have authorized withdrawal of treatment for a child against the objections of the parents (Great Ormond St Hospital v Yates [2017]) (see also Chapter 11).

DNACPR decisions should be discussed with patients/family

Case 14.2

A 28-year-old man, Carl, with long-standing severe cerebral palsy, epilepsy and kypho-scoliosis was admitted to hospital with pneumonia. He did not have capacity to make decisions about his health. In the middle of the night, Carl was reviewed by a registrar, who concluded that if Carl deteriorated further it would not be in his interests to perform cardiopulmonary resuscitation. He believed that this would be distressing, painful and futile. The doctor documented in the patient's medical record that he should not receive resuscitation, and that this should be discussed with Carl's mother in the morning.

Can doctors make unilateral decisions to withhold life-sustaining treatment (e.g. resuscitation in the event of a cardiac arrest)?

(This case is based on Winspear v City Hospitals [2015].)

In the past, doctors were inclined to view DNACPR ('do not attempt cardiopulmonary resuscitation') orders as 'medical' decisions that did not necessarily require discussion or the agreement of families or patients. Two recent cases have clarified the legal position (Butler-Coles 2018).

1. Doctors *can* make decisions about cardiopulmonary resuscitation (CPR). They are not obliged to provide treatment that they believe would be futile (R (*Burke*) v *General Medical Council* [2005]), nor to provide treatment that they believe would be contrary to the patient's best interests.

2. However, DNACPR decisions must (ordinarily) be disclosed and discussed. Such decisions must be discussed with the patient (if he or she has capacity and if it would not cause physical or psychological harm to do so) or with carers (if the patient does not have capacity and it is practical and appropriate) (R (Tracey) v Cambridgeshire [2014]; Winspear [2015]). In the case of Carl Winspear, the court found that it would have been practicable for the registrar to contact his mother in the middle of the night, and that failure to do so was a breach of the doctor's duties under the MCA as well as of Article 8 of the European Convention on Human Rights. Why do doctors need to discuss DNACPR if they have already decided that they are not going to resuscitate? First, the courts have found that a patient is entitled to know that such a decision has been made. Second, if CPR is being withheld on the basis of the best interests of the patient, it would be important to incorporate the patient's wishes into this assessment. Third, it gives the patient (or family) the option of seeking a second opinion. If family members disagree with a decision, doctors must explain the reasons for their decision and options available to them (e.g. a second opinion or court involvement) (Re M [2017]). See also discussion of futility below.

Even if a DNACPR order is not in place, there is no obligation to provide resuscitation if a doctor believes that doing so is not in a patient's best interests.

(In the actual case of Carl Winspear, the DNACPR decision was revoked after his mother spoke with a consultant the next morning. He was moved to intensive care later in the day, but died that evening.)

Treatment may be withdrawn in prolonged disorders of unconsciousness

Case 14.3

A 21-year-old man, AB, was seriously hurt when crushed by overcrowding at a football stadium. While AB was able to be resuscitated, he was left unconscious and with no prospect of ever regaining consciousness (persistent vegetative state). He required artificial feeding and hydration, as he was unable to swallow. This medical treatment was keeping AB alive (he was not dependent on other, more intensive, forms of life-prolonging treatment). After AB had been in this state for about 3 years without any sign of improvement, the hospital Trust applied to the court for a ruling as to whether it would be lawful to discontinue AB's life support (artificial hydration and nutrition), which would inevitably lead to his death.

Would it be ethical or lawful to stop artificial feeding in a patient with severe brain injury?

This is based on the Case of Anthony Bland (Airedale NHS Trust v Bland [1993]).

Following severe illness or injury to the brain, patients may be left in a state of reduced or absent consciousness. There is a spectrum of severity, including coma (absent wakefulness and awareness), persistent vegetative state (PVS; wakefulness, but absent awareness) and minimally conscious state (MCS; wakefulness, minimal awareness) (Royal College of Physicians 2015). Patients in such states usually require assistance in order to remain alive. Such assistance will include, at a minimum, artificial nutrition and hydration. It may also include mechanical ventilation and other life support measures.

The question arises as to whether it is lawful to withdraw life support measures, allowing the patient to die. The patient may not be suffering as a consequence of continued life, but nor may they gain any positive benefit. This was the situation in the case of Tony Bland (Case 12.3). The Bland case went to the House of Lords, where the Lords judged that life support could be stopped, allowing Bland to die on the basis that treatment was not 'in' his interests (as he did not have any interests).

The judgement in the Bland case is important in medical law in at least four respects:

1. Three of the five judges indicated that the doctors' intention if they withdrew treatment would be to end Tony Bland's life.
2. However, the judges found that withdrawal of treatment would be an 'omission' rather than a positive act. An omission would not give rise to a conviction for murder (even if death was intended), unless the doctor had a duty to act.
3. As Tony Bland was permanently unconscious, he did not have any interest in continued treatment – the doctors did not have a duty to provide such treatment.
4. Nutrition and hydration, i.e. what might be called basic care, were judged to be part of 'medical treatment'. They could be withdrawn.

The Scottish case of Law Hospital NHS Trust v Lord Advocate [1996] followed the precedent set in the Bland case.

Until recently, it was thought to be necessary for doctors to obtain permission from the Court of Protection prior to withdrawing treatment from patients with PVS. It was also thought that life-prolonging treatment would be deemed to be *in* the best interests of a patient with a MCS. Recent cases in the Court of Protection support the view that life-prolonging treatment is not necessarily in the best interests of a patient with MCS (where the patient would not have wanted such treatment) and may be withdrawn (Re M; Briggs). There is also no longer an obligation to obtain a court order authorizing the withdrawal of treatment from such patients, where both the clinical team and the patient's family agree that this would be in the patient's best interests (in cases of uncertainty or dispute, an application to the court would be wise) (Royal College of Physicians 2017) (An NHS trust and others v Y [2018]). This means that decisions about continuing or withdrawing nutrition and hydration can be made on the same basis as decisions about stopping other life-prolonging treatment (e.g. mechanical ventilation).

The ethical principles embedded in English law

English law looks at end-of-life issues mainly from the perspective of a doctor's duty of care to her patients. That duty of care is primarily to act in the patient's best interests. However, there are three ethical principles that are adopted to some extent by the law which are contentious and subject to considerable ethical debate: a qualified principle of sanctity of life; the doctrine of double effect; and the moral difference between acts and omissions.

THREE MORAL PRINCIPLES RELEVANT TO END-OF-LIFE DECISIONS

The principle of the sanctity of life

There are differing versions of the principle (or doctrine) of the sanctity of life. While the term is often associated with religious views, it is not a traditional religious concept (Jones 2016). The most extreme version is sometimes called *vitalism*. According to vitalism, human life is of absolute or even infinite value. It is always wrong to take human life, and whenever possible, human life should be maintained (Gormally 1985). This view would seem to commit us to maintaining a person's life no matter what burden it is to that person. It would also imply putting enormous resources into even trivial extensions of human life.

A less extreme form of the sanctity-of-life principle is one that sees life as intrinsically valuable but not an absolute good. By denying that life is an absolute good, it is meant that preserving life does not necessarily outweigh all other considerations. By asserting that life is intrinsically valuable, it is meant that the value of life cannot be accounted for completely in terms of a person's experiences and beliefs (i.e. instrumentally). There is therefore value to a person's simply being alive, no matter what state that person is in, even, for example, if he or she is in a state of permanent unconsciousness.

Other expressions of the sanctity of life principle endorse an attitude of respect or reverence towards life (rather than an expression of value). These views often express the idea that certain actions (particularly intentional ending of innocent life) are always wrong, as they represent a lack of respect for life (Jones 2016).

Case 14.4

A pair of 2-month-old conjoined twins, Jodie and Mary, share a circulation. One of the twins, Jodie, is relatively healthy, whereas the other, Mary, has a number of abnormalities, including a very poorly functioning heart and lungs. If the twins remain joined, it is likely that Jodie will develop heart failure and both will die. If the twins are separated electively, it is expected that Jodie will survive; however, it seems inevitable that Mary will die. Can it be morally right to carry out an operation that will, inevitably, kill Mary?
(This case is based on Re A [2000].)

The moral distinction between foresight and intention: the doctrine of double effect

The doctrine of double effect was developed in mediaeval Catholic theology. The core of the doctrine can be summarized as two moral claims (Glover 1990). The first is that performing a bad act in order to bring about good consequences is always wrong: the end does not justify the means. The second is that performing a good act that is predicted to lead to bad consequences may sometimes be right. In order for both of these claims to be held consistently, a moral distinction must be made between intending an outcome and foreseeing an outcome.

Those who hold a broadly consequentialist morality (see Chapter 2) are likely to argue in favour of separation of the conjoined twins on the grounds that this has the better consequences (one twin surviving rather than both dying). Many non-consequentialist ethical theories (see Chapter 2) require the evaluation of acts independently of outcomes. According to many such theories, some acts are morally wrong even if, overall, they bring about the better outcome. One act that is widely held as wrong, in this sense, is the act of killing. Can a moral theory that considers killing a child wrong nevertheless defend separation of the twins in the example given above? The doctrine of double effect might be used to provide such a defence.

According to this doctrine, it may be right to separate the twins, despite the inevitable result that the Mary will die, if and only if four conditions hold:

1. The action is good in itself or at least permitted. (Separating conjoined twins is generally permitted.)
2. The intention is solely to produce the good effect (i.e. the intention is to save Jodie, and not to kill Mary).
3. The good effect is not achieved through the bad effect (i.e. the saving of Jodie is not achieved directly through killing Mary; Mary's death is a 'side-effect' of the action taken to save the twins. After all, the doctors would wish to separate the twins even if Mary would survive.)
4. There is sufficient reason to permit the bad effect (i.e. the good of saving Jodie provides sufficient grounds to justify the bad result – the death of Mary). The doctrine does not justify an intended good action if the unintended foreseeable result is worse than the good achieved.

At the core of the doctrine of double effect is the claim that there is a moral distinction between *foreseeing* a result and *intending* a result. Thus, it may be forbidden on moral grounds to bring about a bad result if that result is intended (even if as a means to a better overall outcome), but not forbidden to bring about the same result if the result is foreseen but not intended.

There are two main ethical criticisms of the doctrine of double effect. The first is that it is confused or ambiguous; the second is that, although clear, it is morally wrong. A third, empirically based criticism is that, in many situations in palliative care, it is unnecessary.

The argument that the doctrine of double effect is confused or ambiguous

In the case of Lillian Boyce (14.1), Dr Cox's intentions were clear. However, in many situations, individuals' intentions may be ambiguous. If a doctor separates the twins, do they *intend* the death of Mary, or merely foresee it? Similarly, if a doctor provides terminal sedation (sedation to unconsciousness until death in a dying patient), do they intend to kill the patient, or merely relieve their suffering (Jansen 2010)? The focus on intentions may lead health professionals to redirect their intentions (describing or documenting their actions in a socially sanctioned way, though their actual intentions are otherwise). Some may worry that, in this way, the doctrine of double effect permits actions that are actually morally impermissible. It certainly raises the question of whether the doctrine is helpful in law, which requires clear guiding rules that are susceptible to proof in a court room (Foster et al. 2011). It should be clear that, at the present time, the law does permit the lethal separation of conjoined twins and terminal sedation.

The argument that the doctrine of double effect is morally wrong

The doctrine of double effect is part of a moral theory that considers some acts as always wrong, if carried out intentionally, whatever the consequences. Killing is the key example of such an act. However, such theories seem problematic to many in the face of severe suffering at the end of life, as in cases like Lillian Boyes' or counter-examples such as the 'trapped lorry driver'. (A driver is trapped in a blazing lorry. There is no way in which he can be saved. He will soon burn to death. A friend of the driver is standing by the lorry. This friend has a gun and is a good shot. The driver asks this friend to shoot him dead. It will be less painful for him to be shot than to burn to death. *Should the friend shoot the driver dead?*)

The worry is that the doctrine of double effect rules out actions that seem to be morally permissible. In these cases, the doctrine seems to give priority to the purity of the intention of the bystander at the expense of the suffering of the lorry driver, or to the doctor at the expense of the dying woman. Many people may be drawn to the view that, even if killing is usually wrong, and there is good reason for a strong moral rule against killing, there may be exceptions to that rule.

The argument that the doctrine of double effect is (often) unnecessary

A commonly cited example of the doctrine of double effect is the use of opiates (e.g. morphine or diamorphine) in dying patients. That was cited in the Dr Cox case (though it was not relevant, as he used potassium rather than morphine!). Doctors sometimes worry that opiates will hasten death, and are reassured that this could be defended on the basis of the doctrine of double effect. However, studies in palliative care suggest that patients who receive opiates (or higher doses of opiates) do not necessarily die sooner than others who do not receive opiates. In fact, there is some evidence that good pain control may prolong life in patients with terminal illness (Fohr 1998). Although opiates can depress breathing, patients rapidly develop tolerance to this, while pain itself stimulates breathing. On the other hand, in a small number of patients with severe pain or breathlessness in the dying phase, respiratory depression may be a genuine possibility; this risk needs to be balanced against the benefits of symptom control (Quill 1998, Quill, Dresser, and Brock 1997). (For some patients, perhaps many, the risk of inadequate symptom control is the much more serious harm in the face of inevitable death.)

In the actual legal case of the conjoined twins, most of the judges did not find the doctrine of double effect helpful. They did, however, ultimately allow separation of the twins (arguing that Mary's death would not be intended by the surgeons, and hence that this would not be murder). Jodie survived, while Mary died 3 months later.

The moral distinction between acts and omissions

According to the acts–omissions distinction, 'in certain contexts, failure to perform an act, with certain foreseen bad consequences of that failure, is morally less bad than to perform a different act which has the identical foreseen bad consequences. It is worse to kill someone than to let them die' (Glover 1990).

The distinction is relevant in English law (see above). It accords with common intuitions. Acting to kill a patient, even for good reasons, may seem wrong, whereas omitting to act, for example by withholding life-saving treatment, may seem the right thing to do. The moral distinction between active and passive euthanasia rests principally on the distinction between acts and omissions.

Below are two pairs of cases, one of which (Robinson and Davies) provides intuitive support in favour of the moral distinction between acts and omissions. The other pair (Smith and Jones) provides support against such a distinction.

Case 14.5

The cases of Robinson and Davies

This pair of cases is based on an article by Foot (1967) and discussed in Glover (1977, p. 93).

Robinson does not give £100 to a charity that is helping to combat starvation in a poor country. As a result, one person dies from starvation who would have lived had Robinson sent the money.

Davies does send £100, but also sends a poisoned food parcel for use by a charity distributing food donations. The overall and intended result is that one person is killed from the poisoned food parcel, and another person's life is saved by the £100 donation.

Is there a moral difference between what Robinson and Davies do? If there is, is this because Davies acts to kill, whereas Robinson only omits to act?

The cases of Smith and Jones (Rachels 1975)

Smith stands to gain a large inheritance from the death of his 6-year-old cousin. He sneaks into the bathroom of his cousin and drowns him, arranging things so that it will look like an accident.

Jones stands to gain a similar large inheritance from the death of his cousin. Like Smith, Jones sneaks into the bathroom with the intention of drowning his cousin. The cousin, however, is startled by the arrival of Jones, accidentally slips, knocks his head and falls under the water. Jones could easily save his cousin, but instead stands by and waits for his cousin to drown before calling an ambulance.

Is there a moral difference between what Smith and Jones do? If there is, is this because Smith acts to kill, whereas Robinson only omits to act?

The cases of Smith and Jones provide a 'controlled experiment': everything is kept the same, except that Smith *acts*, whereas Jones *omits to act*. The distinction between an act and an omission seems morally irrelevant in this pair of cases. Many consequentialists would hold that we are just as responsible for omissions as we are for acts. Essentially, when faced with a problematic situation we could pursue two or more paths. If we choose one path, whether this is to act or to omit to act, both are 'active' choices, and both carry equal moral weight. Sometimes it is less certain what will happen if we omit to act. However, where the outcome is certain (and the same), omitting to act is just as bad (or just as good) as acting.

In practice, it is not always conceptually clear when something is an act or an omission. Is switching off a ventilator or removing a breathing tube an act or an omission? At first sight it appears to be an act, but suppose the ventilator needs to be switched off for a few seconds to correct some electrical fault. If the responsible person intentionally fails to switch it back on (an omission), is it meaningful to consider this different from switching it off (an act)?

However, if we reject the acts–omissions distinction, that may leave us morally to blame for a great deal. All of us are guilty of failing to do as much good as we could. For example, there are many lives that we could save by donating regularly to charity. If there is no moral difference between acts and omissions, it seems from the Robinson–Davies pair of cases that we should either be incredibly guilty for all the good we fail to do, or else we must be less censorious about people who carry out evil acts and harm others. (See (Glover 1990) for a detailed analysis and criticism of the acts–omissions distinction.)

Some (particularly non-consequentialists) find a difference between the Smith and Jones cases. A conceptually clear – if complex – account can be given of the distinction between acts and omissions (Stauch 2000). The law operates the distinction, and in practice there is no difficulty in classifying a doctor who gives a lethal injection (see Case 14.1) as having actively killed a patient, whereas doctors who withdraw life support (for good reasons) are classified as acting legally in omitting to provide burdensome treatment.

The act–omission distinction might be one reason why doctors, patients and families are more averse to stopping (withdrawing) life-sustaining medical treatment than they are to withholding the same treatment. In fact, as noted above, the law regards both withdrawing and withholding as 'omissions'. (We will return to withdrawing/withholding shortly.)

THE ETHICS OF EUTHANASIA

Arguments concerning euthanasia are often muddled by insufficient clarity over terms (Box 14.2). Voluntary active euthanasia remains illegal in the UK, despite multiple debates in parliament. In other countries, it can be carried out legally under certain conditions (Box 14.3). The debate over whether or not it should be legalized in the UK is unlikely to go away. Doctors will play an important part in such debate. As mentioned in Box 14.1 the issue is likely to be considered by the Supreme Court in the near future. Up for Debate Box 14.1 summarizes some of the principle arguments for and against voluntary active euthanasia.

MEDICAL FUTILITY, 'DO NOT RESUSCITATE' ORDERS AND OTHER LIMITATIONS TO TREATMENT

A DNACPR order is a specific example of a limitation of treatment. It a written instruction designed to communicate that a patient should not be resuscitated in the event of an arrest. Above, we noted the law around such orders.

> **Box 14.2** Euthanasia and suicide: terminology
>
> **Killing:** To intentionally cause the death of someone.
> **Euthanasia:** To intentionally cause or permit the death of someone, for their sake.
> *Passive euthanasia:* To withhold or stop medical treatment that could prolong someone's life. (Other terms: letting die, allowing to die.) For example, stopping life support.
> *Active euthanasia:* To take active steps with the intention of causing someone to die. (Other terms: deliberate ending of life, mercy killing.) For example, giving a lethal injection.
> *Voluntary euthanasia:* Euthanasia at the request of a conscious patient with capacity (subtypes: voluntary active euthanasia, voluntary passive euthanasia).
> *Non-voluntary euthanasia:* Euthanasia performed for a patient who is not conscious or who lacks capacity.
> *Involuntary euthanasia:* Euthanasia performed for a conscious patient with capacity, despite their request to continue to live. (Many people would not classify this as 'euthanasia' – rather as a form of wrongful killing.)
> **Suicide:** To intentionally cause your own death.
> *Assisted suicide:* To help someone to end their own life.
> *Physician-assisted suicide:* A doctor provides medical assistance to a patient to take their own life (for example, by prescribing a drug that the patient administers to themselves). (Other terms: medically assisted dying.)
> **Voluntary stopping eating and drinking:** A conscious patient decides to stop drinking liquids and eating food in order to hasten their death.
> **Palliative (or terminal) sedation:** A patient has a terminal illness and severe and refractory symptoms. A doctor provides the patient with sedation until they are unconscious, with the intention of relieving symptoms until the patient dies. This may be accompanied by withdrawal of artificial nutrition and hydration.

DNACPR orders are sometimes considered in isolation. Such orders in themselves do not mean that other interventions should be withheld. However, there is a strong argument to consider decisions about CPR within a wider discussion and end-of-life care plan (Fritz, Slowther, and Perkins 2017). There is evidence that patients with DNACPR orders are less likely to receive other interventions (e.g. blood cultures, monitoring, intensive care admission), even though these are not specified in the DNACPR document. Broader advance care plans (e.g. Recommended Summary Plan for Emergency Care and Treatment, ReSPECT (Fritz, Slowther, and Perkins 2017)) can allow documentation of patient values and priorities and indicate clearly which interventions should be provided, as well as those that should be withheld.

Potentially life-prolonging treatments may be withheld for four separate ethical reasons:

1. Autonomy. Where treatment is not in accord with the wishes of a patient with capacity (or for a patient without capacity, in accord with a valid advance directive (see Chapter 7)).
2. Futility. Where treatment will not be successful in prolonging life.

Box 14.3 End-of-life law in other jurisdictions

Netherlands: Law in the Netherlands since 2002 permits voluntary active euthanasia and assisted suicide, though doctors are obliged to report all cases to regional review committees. If physicians follow due care criteria, they are exempt from criminal prosecution. Patients must have unbearable suffering with no prospect of improvement. They must be at least 12 years old. Patients can request euthanasia via an advance directive. Non-voluntary euthanasia is not legal (though guidelines support euthanasia in newborns in restricted circumstances (Verhagen and Sauer 2005)).

Switzerland: Active euthanasia is prohibited in Switzerland, though assisted suicide is permitted (including for foreigners). The patient must have capacity, but there are no limitations relating to incurable or terminal illness. Non-profit organizations check that the patient has capacity, is not depressed and is not being coerced.

Canada: Following a challenge by two women with severe incurable illness, a Supreme Court decision in 2015 found that Canada's law against assisted suicide breached section 7 of the Canadian charter of rights (to 'life, liberty and security'). A subsequent law was passed by the Canadian parliament in 2016, permitting assisted suicide for patients with 'grievous and irremediable medical conditions'. Death must be 'reasonably foreseeable'. This law permits assisted suicide, as well as active euthanasia, in situations where patients are physically unable to kill themselves.

Israel: Law in Israel prohibits active euthanasia and assisted suicide. Some forms of passive euthanasia are accepted (withholding of treatment). Withdrawal of continuous life-prolonging treatment (e.g. mechanical ventilation) is not generally permitted (Doron et al. 2014). This is sometimes avoided by attaching timers to ventilators that would allow doctors to withhold resetting the ventilator (Ravitsky 2005).

3. Best interests. Where treatment may be successful in prolonging life, but the quantity or quality of that life means that it would not be in the patient's interests to provide it.
4. Distributive justice. Where treatment cannot be provided because of scarce resources (see Chapter 10).

Is there any ethical difference between withholding and withdrawing treatment? Doctors sometimes find decisions to stop treatment more difficult than decisions not to start treatment (Wilkinson and Savulescu 2012). However, there are serious consequences for patients if doctors are more reluctant to stop treatment than not start it (e.g. trials of treatment may not be provided because doctors are worried that they will not be able to stop them). It is possible that doctors' reluctance to stop treatment may be a form of cognitive bias (Wilkinson, Butcherine, and Savulescu 2019). Professional guidelines (e.g. British Medical Association 2007) state that there is no ethical distinction between withdrawing and withholding treatment. Box 14.4 provides a set of practical strategies for doctors to use to assess and address reluctance to withdraw treatment.

Doctors often find it difficult to talk to patients and families about resuscitation and end-of-life care. However, the importance of patient autonomy is one reason

Up for Debate Box 14.1 Should voluntary active euthanasia be legal?

14

END OF LIFE

For

Consistency

Suicide is accepted and no longer illegal. Some suicidal acts are rational. However, those who are most disabled are often unable to take their own life without assistance. The more disabled a person is by disease and illness, the more she requires the assistance of others to die. It is discriminatory to deny these individuals the right to end their lives.

Suicide tourism is permitted. Patients with terminal illnesses are legally able to access assisted suicide overseas, e.g. in Switzerland, and many travel each year to do this (Gauthier et al. 2015). It is unreasonable for the UK to export its assisted dying to other countries. It is unfair for patients who are unable to travel to be denied the option of choosing to end their lives.

From passive to active euthanasia. Withdrawing and withholding life-prolonging treatment (passive euthanasia) are widely accepted and practiced. Doctors already make decisions that will lead inevitably to the death of the patient (on the basis of the patient's request, or their best interests). However, a slow death after treatment is withdrawn may cause more suffering for the patient than a more rapid death would. Therefore, active euthanasia would often be preferable.

From sedatives to lethal injections. It is widely accepted that actions may be taken even if it is foreseen that life may thereby be shortened. For example, it is ethical to provide terminal sedation to dying patients with severe suffering despite palliative care. If we reject the doctrine of double effect (see text), then this practice provides grounds for allowing the use of purely life-shortening drugs in those circumstances.

Appeal to principles

Euthanasia can be justified by appeal to two principles:

Mercy/beneficence. Euthanasia is often described as 'mercy killing'. The suffering associated with some diseases is so great that it outweighs the benefits of continuing to live. If active euthanasia will result in less suffering, it is preferable to perform passive euthanasia in these cases. Even with modern pain control and other palliative care measures, patients can still suffer near the end of life (for example from persistent breathlessness or psychological pain). Palliative care may take some time to relieve symptoms, or may only do so at the cost of leaving the patient confused, delirious or semi-conscious. If patients are determined to die, but doctors refuse to help them, they will often attempt to end their own life using means that cause them pain/suffering or lead to considerable suffering for family members.

Autonomy. Doctors are obliged to respect patient autonomy, because individual freedom is fundamentally important. A decision about whether to continue living is arguably the most important decision that an individual could make. Doctors must respect the wish to refuse treatment of a patient with capacity, even if the treatment would be simple and free from side-effects and certainly save the patient's life. Why, then, would a doctor refuse a suffering patient's request to end their life? Respect for patient autonomy should include respecting their wish for active euthanasia, at least when the patient's grounds for preferring death to continuing illness are reasonable.

Continued

Up for Debate Box 14.1 Should voluntary active euthanasia be legal?—cont'd

Against

Palliative care makes euthanasia unnecessary

One of the main arguments for euthanasia is relief of suffering. Great advances have been made in palliative care, and many argue that this obviates the need for euthanasia (House of Lords Select Committee on Medical Ethics 1994). Patients who request assistance in dying are often afraid of being in pain, but palliative care is able to relieve the suffering of almost all patients with severe or terminal illness (Quill 1998). Where patients have persistent pain despite palliative care, there is always the option of deep sedation to unconsciousness (terminal sedation). Countries that pass assisted dying laws may not be motivated to provide good quality palliative care because it is easier or cheaper to help patients to die.

Manipulation or exploitation by others, impact on disabled

Those who are severely disabled and ill are vulnerable to exploitation. There may be coercion or pressure on an ill (especially an elderly or disabled) person to ask for euthanasia. Even if no-one is putting direct pressure on patients to choose euthanasia, they may decide that they want to die to spare family members the burden of looking after them. Views differ as to whether euthanasia in such circumstances is highly undesirable, or a laudable respecting of autonomy.

Moreover, where assisted dying is permitted for patients with severe illness or disability, that reinforces a view within society that it is better to die than to be severely disabled. Many disabled individuals already feel devalued by society. They fear that disabled people who do not wish to die will find their choices criticized, or their lives will be stigmatized as not worth living.

Slippery slope objections

If active voluntary euthanasia were legalized, this might be the first step on a slippery slope which would take us to non-voluntary mercy killing of people with severe disability. From the perspective of public policy, we need laws prohibiting euthanasia to protect vulnerable innocents. This argument has a *logical* version and an *empirical* version (see Chapter 2). The logical version is that there is no clear boundary between permissible and impermissible forms of euthanasia; it is not possible to safely or consistently distinguish between them. The empirical version holds that, as a matter of psychological fact, when we loosen the constraints on killing, doctors will be inclined to end the lives of patients in other situations. Once some forms of assisted dying are allowed, society will be more inclined to allow euthanasia in other situations.

Contrary to the aims of medicine

The aims of medicine include the promotion of health and life. These aims are central to the practice of medicine, and to society's attitude towards health professionals. Allowing active euthanasia would be opposed to the key values of medicine, and, as a consequence, patients would lose their trust in doctors.

> **Box 14.4** Practical strategies to address physician reluctance to withdraw treatment (Wilkinson, Butcherine, and Savulescu 2019)
>
> 1. **The Equivalence Test.** If patient A is currently receiving treatment, imagine that another patient (B) were to present tomorrow with identical features to A (identical preferences, illness, prognosis, etc.). Would you be prepared to withhold treatment from B? If so, on the basis of ethical consistency you should be prepared to withdraw treatment today from A.
> 2. **The 'if I'd only known' test.** If Patient A is currently receiving treatment, think back to before they started. Imagine that you knew then what you know now about the patient (in terms of response to treatment, prognosis, etc.). Would you have been prepared to withhold treatment then? If so, you should be prepared to withdraw treatment from A now.
> 3. **The peer review test.** In a situation where you are not prepared to withdraw treatment (but would withhold), consider whether any of your professional peers (for example, other specialists) would withdraw treatment in a patient with features similar to the current patient. If so, you should consider whether your own personal values are influencing your ethical evaluation. You should potentially offer withdrawal of treatment as an option, or referral to another physician (Wilkinson and Truog 2013).
> 4. **Conditional offer of treatment.** At the time of commencing therapy, identify the goals of treatment, along with potential reasons (triggers) to discontinue treatment. Offer treatment on the condition that measurable progress towards those goals is able to be discerned within a set period. After the set period, if the conditions are not met, withdraw treatment.
> 5. **Defined treatment period.** Provide treatment for a set period. At the end of that period, the default would be for treatment to be withdrawn. There would need to be an active decision to reinstitute therapy or to embark on a further period of treatment.

why such conversations are vital – they prevent patients receiving treatments that they would not want at the end of their life.

Patient autonomy does not mean, however, that patients can demand treatment. It is generally accepted that, where doctors believe that treatment would have no chance of working, they are not obliged to provide it (even if strongly desired). 'Futility' is, in practice, a common reason cited by doctors for limiting treatment. However, there are several problems with the concept of futility (Wilkinson 2017). One problem is that it can be very difficult to determine if a treatment (for example, CPR) has no chance of working. Studies of past cases may not be relevant to the patient in front of you (because the patient has different features, or because medical treatment has advanced). They can also be influenced by self-fulfilling prophecies; for example, treatment may have been stopped or withheld in those past cases because it was regarded as futile – but then you cannot tell what would have happened if treatment had been provided (Wilkinson 2009).

The other problem with 'futility' is that the term often contains value judgements. For example, what counts as a successful outcome of CPR? Is it return of spontaneous circulation, short-term survival (e.g. for a matter of hours or days), survival to hospital discharge or survival with a particular quality of life? What probability of success is so low as to make resuscitation futile – 5%, 1%, 0.1%? Some patients might want to take the chance of the resuscitation being successful, no matter how small. Although doctors might use the label 'futile', more commonly there is some chance of treatment succeeding, but the probability of benefit or the magnitude of that benefit is so low that the medical team believe that it would be 'potentially inappropriate' to provide it.

Life-prolonging treatment might not be in the best interests of a patient for two broad groups of reasons (Table 14.1). CPR might merely delay inevitable death. Or, it may lead to restoration of circulation, but to prolongation or worsening of a quality of life that is deemed to be unacceptably poor. However, as any evaluation of the patient's interests is going to involve value judgements, that determination should include consideration of the priorities and wishes of the patient, and discussion with the patient and/or family.

Finally, in some situations, treatment that is desired by the patient and potentially in their best interests may need to be limited because of scarcity of medical resources. CPR might, in some situations, take specialist medical teams away from other patients in need of urgent attention. Of perhaps more concern, a patient who has had successful resuscitation is likely to need admission to the intensive care unit (ICU). However, it may not be deemed a reasonable use of limited ICU beds to admit a patient who is predicted to die regardless within a short time, or who has a very poor quality of life. See also Chapter 10 and Wilkinson and Savulescu (2018).

Table 14.1 Situations where it could be in a patient's best interests to limit life-prolonging treatment (Larcher et al. 2015).

Limited quantity of life

Brain death	A patient has irreversibly lost their capacity for consciousness and their capacity to breathe, and fulfils neurological criteria for death
Imminent death	A patient is physiologically deteriorating and expected to die within minutes or hours (e.g. multi-organ failure despite maximal treatment)
Inevitable death	A patient is expected to die despite treatment (e.g. within a period of days or weeks)

Limited quality of life

Burdens of treatment	Life can only be sustained at the cost of significant pain or distress (e.g. with unpleasant chemotherapy or invasive forms of life support)
Burdens of illness or underlying condition	The severity or impact of an underlying condition causes pain and distress that would outweigh the benefits of sustaining life
Lack of ability to derive benefit	The nature or severity of a patient's underlying condition makes it difficult or impossible for them to enjoy the benefits of continued life (e.g. severe dementia, minimally conscious state)

REVISION QUESTIONS

1. A terminally ill patient has severe pain and is requesting pain relief. Her doctor is concerned that, if she prescribes opiates, this might hasten death, and that this would be unlawful. Is the doctor's concern justified?
2. A patient with end-stage emphysema has an indwelling cardiac pacemaker for severe heart block. He asks for the pacemaker to be deactivated. Would it be lawful to do this?
3. A frail, elderly patient with multiple morbidities and dementia has been admitted to the medical ward with renal failure. Nursing staff have asked you to complete a DNACPR order. No family members have been able to be contacted. Should you complete a DNACPR form?
4. A young adult presents to hospital unconscious following a car accident. He is severely anaemic and needs an urgent transfusion; however, he has a bracelet on indicating that he is a Jehovah's Witness. Should he be transfused?

Extension case 14.6

A patient, T, with long-standing motor neurone disease no longer wishes to live, but is physically unable to end his own life. He wishes to die in his own home and decides not to travel overseas to access assisted suicide.

T decides to stop eating and drinking, with the expectation that this will lead to his death. However, he does not wish to experience distress (for example from hunger/thirst). He asks his doctor to provide him with palliative care, including sedation to the point of unconsciousness if his suffering becomes unbearable.

Is this a form of suicide?

Should T be admitted to hospital and force-fed, if necessary?

Would it be ethical or legal for T's doctor to agree to his wishes?

For further discussion of this issue, see White, Willmott, and Savulescu (2014) and Quill, Ganzini, and Truog (2018).

REFERENCES

Airedale NHS Trust v Bland [1993] AC 789.

An NHS trust and others (respondents) v Y (by his litigation friend, the official solicitor) and another (appellants) [2018] UKSC 46.

Briggs v Briggs [2016] EWCOP 53.

British Medical Association. 2007. *Withholding and withdrawing life-prolonging medical treatment: guidance for decision making*. 3rd ed., Malden, Mass. Oxford: Blackwell.

Butler-Coles, V. 2018. "DNACPR and the law." Medium.

Director of Public Prosecutions. 2014. "Policy for prosecutors in respect of encouraging or assisting suicide." accessed 26/01/2018. https://www.cps.gov.uk/legal-guidance/policy-prosecutors-respect-cases-encouraging-or-assisting-suicide.

Doron, D., Wexler, I. D., Shabtai, E. and Corn, B. W. 2014. "Israeli dying patient act: physician knowledge and attitudes." *American Journal of Clinical Oncology* 37 (6): 597-602.

Fohr, S. A. 1998. "The double effect of pain medication: separating myth from reality." *Journal of Palliative Medicine* 1 (4): 315-28. doi: 10.1089/jpm.1998.1.315.

Foster, C., Herring, J., Melham, K. and Hope, T. 2011. "The double effect effect." *Cambridge Quarterly of Healthcare Ethics* 20 (1): 56-72.

Fritz, Z., Slowther, A. M. and Perkins, G. D. 2017. "Resuscitation policy should focus on the patient, not the decision." *BMJ* 356: j813.

Gauthier, S., Mausbach, J., Reisch, T. and Bartsch, C. 2015. "Suicide tourism: a pilot study on the Swiss phenomenon." *Journal of Medical Ethics* 41 (8): 611-7. doi: 10.1136/medethics-2014-102091.

Glover, J. 1990. *Causing death and saving lives.* Harmondsworth: Penguin.

Gormally, L. 1985. "Against voluntary euthanasia." In *The principles of health care ethics*, edited by R. Gillon and A. Lloyd. Chichester: John Wiley: 761-74.

Great Ormond Street Hospital v Yates & Ors [2017] EWHC 972 (Fam) (11 April 2017).

House of Lords Select Committee on Medical Ethics. 1994. "Report of the Select Committee on Medical Ethics." https://api.parliament.uk/historic-hansard/lords/1994/may/09/medical-ethics-select-committee-report.

Jansen, L. A. 2010. "Disambiguating clinical intentions: the ethics of palliative sedation." *Journal of Medicine and Philosophy* 35 (1): 19-31. doi: 10.1093/jmp/jhp056.

Jones, D. A. 2016. "An unholy mess: why 'the sanctity of life principle'should be jettisoned." *The New Bioethics* 22 (3): 185-201.

Kings College Hospital NHS Foundation Trust v C and Another [2015] EWCOP 80.

Larcher, V., Craig, F., Bhogal, K., Wilkinson, D. and Brierley, J. 2015. "Making decisions to limit treatment in life-limiting and life-threatening conditions in children: a framework for practice." *Archives of Disease in Childhood* 100 (Suppl. 2): s1-23. doi: 10.1136/archdischild-2014-306666.

Law Hospital NHS Trust v Lord Advocate [1996] 2 FLR 407.

Quill, T. E. 1998. "Principle of double effect and end-of-life pain management: additional myths and a limited role." *Journal of Palliative Medicine* 1 (4): 333-6. doi: 10.1089/jpm.1998.1.333.

Quill, T. E., Dresser, R. and Brock, D. W. 1997. "The rule of double effect – a critique of its role in end-of-life decision making." *The New England Journal of Medicine* 337 (24): 1768-71. doi: 10.1056/NEJM199712113372413.

Quill, T., Ganzini, L. and Truog, R. D. 2018. "Voluntarily stopping eating and drinking among patients with serious advanced illness – clinical, ethical, and legal aspects." *JAMA: The Journal of the American Medical Association* 178 (1): 123-7. doi: 10.1001/jamainternmed.2017.6307.

R v Cox [1992] 12 BMLR 38.

R (Burke) v General Medical Council [2005] EWCA Civ 1003.

R (Nicklinson) v Ministry of Justice [2014] UKSC 48.

R (Tracey) v Cambridgeshire Hospital [2014] EWCA 822.

Ravitsky, V. 2005. "Timers on ventilators." *BMJ* 330 (7488): 415-7.

Re A (conjoined twins) [2000] EWCA Civ 254.

Re B [2002] EWHC 429 (Adult: refusal of medical treatment).

Re M [2017] EWCOP 17.

Royal College of Physicians. 2015. "Prolonged disorders of consciousness: national clinical guidelines." https://www.rcplondon.ac.uk/guidelines-policy/prolonged-disorders-consciousness-national-clinical-guidelines.

Royal College of Physicians. 2017. "Interim guidance on clinically assisted nutrition and hydration," accessed 13/8/18. https://www.rcplondon.ac.uk/guidelines-policy/prolonged-disorders-consciousness-national-clinical-guidelines-interimguidance.

Stauch, M. 2000. "Causal authorship and the equality principle: a defence of the acts/omissions distinction in euthanasia." *Journal of Medical Ethics* 26 (4): 237-41.

Verhagen, E. and Sauer, P. J. 2005. "The Groningen protocol – euthanasia in severely ill newborns." *The New England Journal of Medicine* 352 (10): 959-62. doi: 10.1056/NEJMp058026.

White, B., Willmott, L. and Savulescu, J. 2014. "Voluntary palliated starvation: a lawful and ethical way to die?" *Journal of Law and Medicine* 22 (2): 376-86.

Wilkinson, D. 2009. "The self-fulfilling prophecy in intensive care." *Theoretical Medicine and Bioethics* 30 (6): 401-10. doi: 10.1007/s11017-009-9120-6.

Wilkinson, D. J. C. 2017. "Medical futility." In The international encyclopedia of ethics.

Wilkinson, D., Butcherine, E. and Savulescu, J. 2019. "Withdrawal aversion and the equivalence test." *American Journal of Bioethics* forthcoming.

Wilkinson, D. and Savulescu, J. 2018. *Ethics, conflict and medical treatment for children: from disagreement to dissensus.* Elsevier.

Wilkinson, D. J. and Truog, R. D. 2013. "The luck of the draw: physician-related variability in end-of-life decision-making in intensive care." *Intensive Care Medicine* 39 (6): 1128-32. doi: 10.1007/s00134-013-2871-6.

Wilkinson, D. and Savulescu, J. 2012. "A costly separation between withdrawing and withholding treatment in intensive care." *Bioethics* 26 (1): 32-48. doi: 10.1111/j.1467-8519.2010.01811.x.

Winspear v City Hospitals Sunderland NHS Foundation Trust [2015] EWHC 3250 (QB).

END OF LIFE

Chapter **15**

Organ transplantation and definitions of death

Case 15.1

Mrs M is a 71-year-old woman who collapses at home after complaining of a severe headache. On arrival of the ambulance, she is obtunded, and is intubated and transferred urgently to hospital. In the ED, a CT scan shows extensive sub-arachnoid haemorrhage. She is comatose, with fixed dilated pupils, but has intermittent respiratory effort. Neurosurgeons have assessed and discussed Mrs M's prognosis with her family. Surgery is possible, but her outcome is thought to be very poor. In accordance with Mrs M's wishes, the family and neurosurgeons have decided that she should not have surgery, and should have treatment withdrawn.

Mrs M has an organ donation card in her purse, but her family do not agree to organ donation.

Should organ donation proceed for Mrs M, despite family objections?

DONATION STATISTICS

As of March 2017, 6388 people in the UK were on organ transplant waiting lists. In the preceding year, 2456 people donated organs (NHS Blood and Transplant 2017a). Overall, 4025 organs were transplanted; kidneys were the commonest organ (3348 transplants), and there were 985 liver transplants, 376 heart or lung transplants and 224 pancreas transplants.

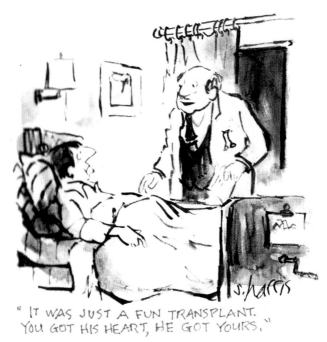

" IT WAS JUST A FUN TRANSPLANT. YOU GOT HIS HEART, HE GOT YOURS."

Figure 15.1 Fun transplant (© Sidney Harris, reproduced with permission from ScienceCartoonsPlus.com)

However, organ supply continues to fall short of demand. The average (median) wait for a kidney transplant was 864 days. Over 450 patients died in 2016 while on the transplant waiting list, and 875 were taken off the waiting list before receiving a transplant – usually because of deteriorating health. Other patients who might benefit from a transplant are not offered the option because of the length of the waiting list.

There are also many patients who could donate, but do not do so. In 2016–2017, of 5681 patients dying in UK hospitals who were deemed to be potentially eligible donors, only 1413 actually donated organs (NHS Blood and Transplant 2017a). There are 23.6 million people in the UK who have indicated a desire to donate (opt-in or 'consent-in') by registering with the NHS organ donor register. Two hundred thousand people have registered a desire *not* to donate (opt-out), including approximately 6% of the population in Wales and 1% in other areas of the UK (the higher rate in Wales may reflect the different law around consent – see below).

Types of donation

There are different types of solid organ donation (Box 15.1). Approximately half of the people who donated in the UK in 2016 had died (deceased donors), while half were living donors. Living donors may donate kidneys or part of their liver. Deceased donors may donate heart, lungs, liver, kidneys, pancreas, intestine or combinations of organs. Donation after Brain Death (DBD) donors (see Box 15.1) typically donate more organs per donor than Donation after Circulatory Death

> **Box 15.1** Types of solid organ donation
>
> **Living donation:** living patient consents to donate a single non-critical organ (or part of an organ)
> *Living related* – donation to a family member
> *Living unrelated* – donation to a non-family member; sometimes undertaken as part of a paired exchange or donation chain (Reese, Boudville, and Garg 2015)
> **Deceased organ donation:** donation after death (often multiple organs)
> - *Donation after brain death* (DBD, also called heart-beating donation) – death diagnosed on the basis of neurological criteria
> - *Donation after circulatory death* (DCD, also called non-heart-beating donation) – death diagnosed on the basis of circulatory criteria, most commonly after withdrawal of mechanical ventilation

(DCD) donors (average: 3.8 versus 2.8) (NHS Blood and Transplant 2017a). Other types of non-solid organ donation include blood, bone marrow or tissue donation (e.g. cornea, heart valve). We will mostly focus on solid organ donation in this chapter, though some of the same issues apply.

If Mrs M were diagnosed with brain death (see below), and organ donation were proceeding, life support would usually be continued until she could be transferred to an operating theatre for organ retrieval. (Note that at the time of Case 15.1, Mrs M would not meet brain death criteria because of her intermittent respiratory effort.)

If Mrs M were to proceed with donation after circulatory death, intensive care would first be withdrawn. After she had been asystolic for several minutes, death would be declared, and organ retrieval would need to proceed immediately. For this reason, for potential DCD donors, life support is sometimes withdrawn adjacent to operating theatres.

THE LEGAL FRAMEWORK

Organ donation in the UK is governed by the Human Tissue Act 2004 and the Organ Donation (Deemed Consent) Act 2019 (for England and Northern Ireland), the Human Tissue (Scotland) Act 2006 and the Human Transplantation (Wales) Act 2013.

Deceased donation

England/Northern Ireland/Scotland

The Human Tissue Acts were passed in the wake of controversial cases in the late 1990s and early 2000s involving the retention of body parts and organs from dead children without their parents' knowledge or permission. The Acts set out a legal framework for the storage and use of tissue from the living, and for the removal, storage and use of tissue and organs from the dead. They also set up a body, the Human Tissue Authority (HTA), to advise and oversee compliance with the Act.

The Acts make consent a fundamental principle both for donation and research. For deceased donors, consent is required, however, after the Organ Donation

(Deemed Consent) Act 2019 consent will be assumed, unless a person in a 'qualifying relationship' (e.g. a close relative) 'provides information that would lead a reasonable person to conclude that the person concerned would not have consented'. Relatives are ranked in a hierarchy headed by the spouse or partner; then parent or child (of any age); brother or sister; grandparent or grandchild; niece or nephew; stepfather or stepmother; half-brother or half-sister; or friend of long standing (s.27(4)). Minors can consent to organ donation after death (if Gillick competent, see Chapter 11), otherwise parents may consent for a deceased child.

Where the deceased would not have consented, donation cannot occur. On the other hand, if the deceased is deemed to consent to donate organs, there is no obligation to proceed to organ retrieval. Families do not have a legal right to veto donation, so in the case of Mrs M, it would be legal to proceed with donation. However, in practice, family members are still usually asked, and if they oppose donation, their wishes are usually respected (Shaw et al. 2017).

Wales

The Welsh Assembly introduced legislation in 2013 that endorses an opt-out approach to organ donation consent. Patients are assumed to support organ donation if they have not opted out during life. However, families are still asked for their agreement to donate, so if Mrs M were in Wales, donation might still not proceed. (See below for discussion of organ donation consent.)

There is no statutory definition of death in the UK. Professional guidelines have set forth criteria for diagnosis of death by neurological criteria ('brain death'). The concept of brain death was accepted as the legal definition of death in Re A [1992]. Family members cannot insist on continued treatment for a patient diagnosed with brain death in the UK (though that is different elsewhere – see Case 15.3). In 2015, the High Court heard a case of a family who disagreed on religious grounds with a diagnosis of brain death in a 19-month-old infant (Re A, A child [2015]). The court accepted the doctors' diagnosis and authorized withdrawal of mechanical ventilation. See also 'Definitions of death' below.

Living donors

Case 15.2

Miss Y was 25 years old, but had hydrocephalus and a severe learning disability and was living in a care home. She could speak and sign a few words. Her older sister, aged 36, suffered from a myelodysplastic syndrome and needed an urgent bone marrow transplant (there was a high chance that she would progress to acute myeloid leukaemia within 3 months). Miss Y was the only family member who was a potentially compatible donor. (Search of the bone marrow registry had also not identified any potential donors.) The sister sought a court declaration that it would be lawful for Miss Y to have blood tests with a view to possible bone marrow extraction for donation, in order to treat the disorder, despite the fact that Miss Y did not have the capacity to give consent.

Is living donation by a patient lacking capacity ethical or legal?

This is based on the case of Re Y [1996].

Live donations are governed mainly by s.33 of the Human Tissue Act 2004, but also by the common law.

Two important legal principles apply. The first is that it is not lawful to consent to a procedure that causes death or serious injury. Thus, for example, it would be unlawful for a parent to donate his or her heart to a child, or for a surgeon to carry out such a procedure. It would probably be unlawful for a surgeon to remove both kidneys for transplant (even if the patient consented to it), even though the parent could remain alive on dialysis. Lesser injuries or risks, however, can be lawful, such as donating one kidney. The second is that valid legal consent must be obtained (see Chapter 6). In this context, that means that the donor must fully understand the processes involved.

Whether live donations are lawful for an adult lacking capacity or for a child ultimately turns on whether they are in the best interests of the donor (as defined by the Mental Capacity Act 2005; see Chapter 7). The Human Tissue Act indicates that they also require approval of at least three members of the HTA. Donation from an adult lacking capacity would require a court's approval, except in the most unusual circumstances.

In the case of Miss Y, the judge said that such tests (and subsequent transplantation) would be illegal unless in the best interests of Miss Y; the interests of Miss Y's sister had no weight. In fact, the judge allowed that Miss Y's best interests were served by the tests going ahead, because there were reasons to suppose that Miss Y would get better care if her sister lived (e.g. her mother would visit regularly).

There is no case law on the specific issue of live donations by children and young people aged less than 18 years. The lawfulness of using children as living donors is therefore uncertain. However, it seems that, before the removal of a solid organ from a child, whether competent or not, it is good practice for court approval to be obtained. In theory, a Gillick competent young person could consent to organ donation, although in practice such procedures are very rare (unlike skin or blood donations, which are more common).

Payment

Section 32 of the Human Tissue Act explicitly prohibits commercial exchanges of human material for transplantation. It would be illegal in the UK to offer (or to receive) payment in exchange for donation of an organ or other human tissue. The definition of 'controlled material' in the Act potentially would include donation of blood or blood products.

THE ETHICAL FRAMEWORK

The definition of death

Until the 1960s, doctors diagnosed people as dead in essentially only one way: by confirming that the patient was pulseless and apnoeic, with fixed pupils and no heart sounds. This is the traditional diagnosis of death by cardio-respiratory criteria.

However, the advent of modern forms of intensive life support led to two concerns with the traditional cardio-respiratory definition of death. First, high-tech

A Californian teenage girl, JM, has a cardiac arrest after suffering complications of a tonsillectomy. She suffers severe hypoxic brain injury and is subsequently diagnosed with brain death. However, her parents do not accept that she is dead. Her heart is still beating, and they regard this as evidence that she is alive. They wish JM to have a tracheostomy, and for respiratory support to continue.

Is the patient really dead? Should patients or families be permitted to apply different criteria for death?

This is based on the case of Jahi McMath (Luce 2015, du Toit and Miller 2016).

forms of organ support mean that it is possible to sustain patients' heart and lungs for long periods of time, despite such profound brain damage that they will never recover consciousness or be able to survive without life support. Second, patients who are anticipated to die in intensive care might have a desire to donate their organs. However, waiting until a patient's heart beat has stopped may lead to organ damage from lack of perfusion and mean that transplantation is not possible (or is less successful).

These concerns led to the medical profession adopting a new and separate way of diagnosing death. In 1968, an ad hoc committee of the Harvard medical school proposed a set of criteria for a condition that they initially labelled 'irreversible coma', and subsequently called 'brain death' (1968, Wijdicks 2003). Similar criteria were adopted by medical professional groups in many countries around the world, including the UK. The latest code of practice from the Academy of Medical Royal Colleges (2008) equates death with irreversible loss of consciousness combined with irreversible loss of the capacity to breathe. It sets out a set of criteria for diagnosing death based on signs of irreversible loss of brain-stem function (Box 15.2).

There are some international differences in the definition of brain death (Smith 2012, Wijdicks 2002). For example, most countries (e.g. USA) use a 'whole brain' definition, whereby brain death is seen to be synonymous with loss of function of the entire brain (including brain-stem). Patients with some electrical activity of the brain or some intracranial blood flow would not be considered brain dead in such countries (though they could in countries with 'brain-stem' criteria such as the UK). The clinical testing for brain death is, however, very similar in countries with whole brain or brain-stem definitions (Smith 2012).

While brain death has wide professional acceptance, there are some ethical criticisms (Up for Debate Box 15.1). This includes some who feel that patients who meet neurological criteria are not 'dead', but that organ donation is still permissible (e.g. Truog and Robinson 2003). (They therefore reject the so-called 'dead donor rule' – that patients must be dead before organ donation may occur.) Other critics claim that patients who meet neurological criteria are alive but profoundly disabled, and that much currently practiced organ donation is not ethical (Symons and Chua 2018, Verheijde and Rady 2011).

> **Box 15.2** Diagnosis of death by neurological criteria (Academy of Medical Royal Colleges 2008)
>
> - The patient has a known cause of irreversible brain damage.
> - Potentially reversible causes have been excluded (e.g. CNS-depressant drugs, muscle relaxant, hypothermia, metabolic derangement).
> - Clinical testing must reveal absent brain-stem reflexes:
>   - Pupillary light reflex (pupils are fixed and dilated)
>   - Corneal reflex (absent blink in response to touching cornea)
>   - Oculovestibular reflex (no eye movement in response to injection of ice-cold water into auditory canal)
>   - Motor responses in cranial nerve distribution in response to painful stimulus e.g. supraorbital pressure
>   - Gag reflex (absent response to stimulation of posterior pharynx with spatula)
>   - Cough reflex (absent response to tracheal suctioning)
>   - Apnoea test (absent respiratory response to hypercarbia).
> - Testing must be performed twice by two medical practitioners with relevant experience (one must be a consultant).
> - Irreversible loss of brain-stem function does not always coincide with complete loss of other brain functions. Additional tests (e.g. EEG, angiography or brain blood flow scans) are not required, though may sometimes be helpful if the clinical testing of brain-stem reflexes is difficult.
> - Diagnosis of death may occur on the same basis in children and infants.

Most religions support the diagnosis of death by neurological criteria. However, some (e.g. some orthodox Jewish authorities, some Roman Catholics, some evangelical Protestants, some Islamic scholars and some Native Americans) prefer the traditional cardio-respiratory definition of death (Olick, Braun, and Potash 2009). This raises the question of whether societies should accommodate families who disagree with a diagnosis of brain death. In the case of Jahi McMath, her family arranged transfer to New Jersey (where a legal clause allows families with a religious objection to brain death to ask for cardio-respiratory criteria to be applied instead). Somatic support continued for more than 4 years while legal disputes were ongoing. This was finally ceased (and a second death certificate applied) after she developed internal bleeding secondary to liver failure.

Definitions of death by circulatory criteria have also led to ethical debate. For example, there are questions about how long doctors should wait after the development of asystole before declaring death. Shorter durations (e.g. 1–2 minutes) may increase the viability of organs for transplantation, but raise questions about whether circulation has irreversibly ceased. Cardiac transplantation after circulatory death has been performed, and this leads to similar questions; if the heart has been restarted in another patient, the donor could not have had 'irreversible' cessation of circulation. Interventions have been suggested to improve donation success – these include insertion of catheters prior to withdrawal of life support, or administration of heparin. These raise questions about whether such interventions are in the best interests of the donor.

Up for Debate Box 15.1 Are patients who meet neurological criteria for death actually dead?

For

Patients who fulfil neurological criteria for death have permanently lost the capacity for consciousness and independent respiration. There are no credible cases of recovery of consciousness in patients who have had brain death diagnosed rigorously according to official professional guidelines. Without intensive forms of medical treatment and life support, brain dead patients all inevitably deteriorate and meet cardio-respiratory criteria for death. Brain function (unlike the function of other organs) is necessary for the vital work of a living human organism. If a human has lost the capacity to receive signals from the world, to respond to them and to engage in self-preservation (e.g. by breathing), the organism can no longer be viewed as alive.

Against

Patients who meet criteria for brain death can be sustained with forms of organ support, including artificial ventilation, for months or years. Although many functions of the brain may be lost, some brain activity can remain in patients who meet neurological criteria, e.g. hypothalamic function. Patients diagnosed with brain death can show physical growth, menstruate and even gestate a fetus over a period of several months. This suggests that the 'vital work' of the organism can continue after brain death. While it is true that such patients will inevitably deteriorate without intensive medical support, that is also true of many other patients with severe chronic health conditions who are not regarded as deceased. It may be ethical to withdraw organ support from patients who meet neurological criteria, and it may also be ethical for them to donate their organs; however, this is because of their loss of consciousness and personhood, not because they are dead.

Consent for deceased organ donation

Recent ethical debates about organ donation in the UK have focused on whether there should be an opt-in or opt-out approach to consent. In an opt-in system, patients become organ donors through an active decision during life (or by their family after death). In an opt-out system, patients become organ donors if they are eligible to do so *unless* they have made an active decision that they do not wish to donate organs. The ethical arguments around opt-in/opt-out donation are summarized in Up for Debate Box 15.2.

Even in opt-in systems, consent for organ donation is typically much less stringent than consent for surgery during life (see Chapter 6). For example, a person can become an organ donor by signing up on a website or by ticking a form on a driving license application. Neither of these would usually be regarded as representing sufficient evidence of informed consent for a medical procedure to take place.

There might be three different justifications for relaxing consent requirements around organ donation. The first is that, unlike procedures performed during life, donation of organs after death does not have any side-effects and cannot harm the donor. The second is that more stringent consent rules would likely reduce the number of donors and harm those in need of organs. The third is that, in

Up for Debate Box 15.2 Should consent for organ donation be presumed (opt-out)?

For

In countries like the UK, the majority of the population are supportive of organ donation. For example, in a 2017 survey, 81% of people supported organ donation in principle. However, only 36% of the population had opted in to the register. When families are approached, they agree to organ donation in only 63% of cases (NHS Blood and Transplant 2017a). This means that some people who would have wanted to donate do not end up donating. Countries with opt-out donation systems have higher donation rates on average (Shepherd, O'Carroll, and Ferguson 2014). Approaching families to agree to organ donation places an extra burden on them to make a decision at an extremely stressful time. There are different forms of opt-out system – for example, in a 'soft' opt-out system (e.g. Wales), families are still asked about organ donation.

Against

Some patients do not wish to donate their organs. However, they may not get around to opting out during life. This means that some people who would not have wanted to donate end up donating organs in an opt-out system. This may be more common in patients from ethnic minorities, or for whom English is not their first language.

There is not clear evidence that an opt-out system in itself increases donation rates. Countries with opt-out systems often have pursued other measures to increase donation, so it is not clear which factor causes higher donation (Rithalia et al. 2009). Some countries with opt-out consent have low donation rates (e.g. Sweden). Change to an opt-out system might lead to a backlash, with paradoxical reduced rates of consent to donation. If families are asked about donation anyway, there may not be any advantage of an opt-out process. If families are not asked about organ donation, that could cause considerable additional distress when they are already having to cope with the death of a loved one.

the majority of cases, patients have to make a decision about organ donation a long time in advance, while the actual chance of donation is very small. At the time of potential donation, the patient will almost invariably lack capacity (and potentially be deceased), so consent from surrogates (e.g. family) will be required. This may mean that consent during life simply indicates the general preference of the deceased, while informed consent will need to be taken from the family.

The allocation of organs for donation

There are insufficient organs for all those who could benefit from receiving them. Decisions therefore have to be made as to who should have priority for the organs that are available. NHS Blood and Transplant (NHSBT) has developed guidelines to help guide patient selection (for entry onto the transplant waiting list) and allocation of organs (amongst those on the waiting list) (Transplant Policy Review Committee 2015). If entry onto waiting lists is unrestricted, there will be a greater demand for organs, and many patients listed will not receive an organ. On the other hand, more restrictive selection for transplantation leads to a greater challenge in defining which patients are eligible. These are ethical, not purely medical, decisions. The UK has elected to have more restricted waiting lists for organs, on the grounds that this approach is preferred by patients.

Patient selection for transplant waiting lists is typically made by multi-disciplinary teams in transplant centres. Selection criteria are different for different organs. They include conditions associated with positive outcome from transplantation. Clinical criteria are also used to establish urgency (e.g. 'urgent' or 'super-urgent' categories). Co-morbidities that are associated with poor outcome after transplantation are considered, including medical conditions (e.g. malignancy, other organ failure) but also (more controversially) other factors (including social factors, non-adherence to treatment, mental illness or mental capacity) that are predicted to result in poor outcomes (NHS Blood and Transplant 2017b). Alcohol-associated liver disease is not in itself a contraindication to listing, since the policy notes that outcomes may be as good in selected patients (e.g. without ongoing alcohol abuse) as in patients with other illnesses.

Factors that are taken into account in allocating the organs include: urgency (patients with a high chance of death within a short period without transplantation may be prioritized); the chance of success of the transplant (for example, as predicted from the degree of compatibility between donor and recipient); the age of the donor (those under 18 years are given priority, however, patients are not excluded solely on the basis of age); the difference in age/size between the donor and the recipient (partly on the grounds of most effective use of the organ) and the proximity of the centre that is the source of the donor and the centre undertaking the transplant.

Other ethical questions and future developments

Box 15.3 lists several such issues.

Box 15.3 Other ethical questions that arise in organ donation and future developments

Donors lacking capacity

The legal standard allows organ donation only where the donor can give consent or where donation is in the donor's best interests. Is it right to give no weight to the recipient's interests?

Markets in organs

The Human Tissue Act 2004 prohibits (as did previous legislation) the commercial dealing in human organs, of any kind, except for 'expenses and loss of earnings incurred by the donor'. However, people are free to engage in a range of risky activities in exchange for compensation or payment. Are markets in organs necessarily unethical? See (Richards 2012) for a compelling case in favour of allowing organ sales. [This is also one of the best books written on method in medical ethics.]

How should scarce organs be allocated?

In the UK there is an elaborate process of allocation. Is the method of allocation right? Should those under 18 years old, for example, be given priority over those aged more

---

Box 15.3 Other ethical questions that arise in organ donation and future developments—cont'd

than 18 years? And if they should, would it not be consistent to give higher priority to, say, a 22-year-old than to a 40-year-old?

Should a person be allowed to refuse consent for their organs to be used after their death?

An organ may save someone's life. Removing an organ from someone after their death does them no harm. Even if a person does not want their organs to be used after their death, it could be argued that this should not preclude the use of the organ. According to this view, saving someone's life should take precedence over whatever interest a person can have over how their body is used after their death.

What power of veto should relatives have?

Under the Human Tissue Act, relatives do not have the legal right to veto a deceased's wishes. Should they have such power?

Should donors be allowed to donate conditionally?

Suppose a donor said: you may use one of my kidneys (in the case of a live donor), or you may use both my kidneys after my death, but only if the recipient is Jewish, a woman, white, etc. Should such conditional donations be accepted?

Should registered organ donors receive priority?

Patients can be eligible to receive organs even if, in different circumstances, they would not be prepared to donate organs. This seems hypocritical. Should people who have been on the organ donor register get higher priority for organs?

Elective ventilation

In some patients (e.g. Mrs M, discussed at the start of this chapter), provision of life-sustaining treatment (e.g. ICU admission) might facilitate organ donation; for example, additional time might help to discover the wishes of the patient, help families consider the option of donation or allow a patient with raised intracranial pressure to progress to brain death. Is it ethical to start or continue treatment that is not for the medical benefit of the patient, but rather to allow organ donation (Coggon 2012)?

Xenotransplantation

Organ transplants from other animals (e.g. pigs) have been performed in the past. Recent developments may overcome come of the medical challenges of xenotransplantation. For example, gene editing of pigs using CRISPR may reduce the possibility of transmitting retroviruses. They could also be engineered to reduce problems of immune rejection. That could include chimeric animals designed to grow human organs. Is it ethical to genetically modify animals for the purpose of organ transplantation?

Artificial organs

Alternatives to organ transplantation may become available. This could include advances on current mechanical devices (e.g. ventricular assist devices, which can replace the function of failing hearts), or novel bio-synthetic organs (e.g. 3-D printed organs or synthetic organs grown on artificial scaffolds). However, such organs are likely, in the short term at least, to be highly expensive. Is it an acceptable use of limited public health resources to spend large amounts of money on artificial organs? If artificial organs are available privately, is it acceptable for wealthy patients to be able to circumvent organ transplant waiting lists?

REVISION QUESTIONS

1. Can children donate organs after death?
2. In a Welsh intensive care unit, a patient is diagnosed as brain dead. He is not on the organ donation register. Can his organs be donated?
3. An adult has been diagnosed as brain dead, but his family have a religious objection to brain death. Can they object to organ donation? What if they wish intensive care to continue?
4. An adult with capacity wishes to donate a kidney to a stranger. Should that be allowed? (What if he wanted to donate two kidneys, and understood that this would leave him requiring dialysis?)

Extension case 15.4

In some countries that permit voluntary active euthanasia, patients are able to request voluntary euthanasia with subsequent organ donation. As part of this process, euthanasia is performed first, with organ donation occurring after criteria for circulatory death are met (Bollen et al. 2016).

Should this be permitted? Is it ethical to combine organ donation and voluntary euthanasia?

Imagine the following case:

Professor D is a philosophy professor living in a country that permits voluntary euthanasia, as well as allowing patients to use advance directives to request assisted dying in future situations where they have lost capacity. Professor D has a strong desire to be able to donate his organs if he were ever in a position to do so. He completes an advance directive requesting active euthanasia combined with organ donation in the event that he is ever unconscious in intensive care and withdrawal of active treatment is planned. He has made a specific request that organ donation occur under general anaesthesia *prior to* euthanasia, with donation of any viable organs (including heart, lungs, liver, kidneys). Euthanasia would occur via the organ donation procedure when cross-clamping of the aorta occurs.

Should organ donation euthanasia advance directives be permitted?

For further discussion of this issue, see Wilkinson and Savulescu (2012).

REFERENCES

Academy of Medical Royal Colleges. 2008. "A code of practice for the diagnosis and confirmation of death", accessed 18/11/2008. http://www.aomrc.org.uk/publications/reports -guidance/doc_download/42-a-code-of-practice -for-the-diagnosis-and-confirmation-of-death .html.

Anon. 1968. "A definition of irreversible coma. Report of the Ad Hoc Committee of the Harvard Medical School to Examine the Definition of Brain Death." *JAMA: The Journal of the American Medical Association* 205 (6): 337-40.

Bollen, J., de Jongh, W., Hagenaars, J., van Dijk, G., Ten Hoopen, R., Ysebaert, D., Ijzermans, J., van Heurn, E. and van Mook, W. 2016. "Organ donation after euthanasia: a Dutch practical manual." *American Journal of Transplantation* 16 (7): 1967-72. doi: 10.1111/ ajt.13746.

Coggon, J. 2012. "Elective ventilation for organ donation: law, policy and public ethics." *Journal of Medical Ethics* 39: 130-4. doi: 10.1136/medethics-2012-100992.

du Toit, J. and Miller, F. 2016. "The ethics of continued life-sustaining treatment for those diagnosed as brain-dead." *Bioethics* 30 (3): 151-8. doi: 10.1111/bioe.12178.

Luce, J. M. 2015. "The uncommon case of Jahi McMath." *Chest* 147 (4): 1144-51. doi: 10.1378/chest.14-2227.

NHS Blood and Transplant. 2017a. "Organ donation and transplantation: activity report." NHSBT, accessed 6/2/2018. https://nhsbtdbe.blob.core.windows.net/umbraco-assets-corp/4657/activity_report_2016_17.pdf.

NHS Blood and Transplant. 2017b. "Policy POL229/5.1 Heart transplantation: selection criteria and recipient registration", accessed 7/2/2018. https://nhsbtdbe.blob.core.windows.net/umbraco-assets-corp/6536/pol229-heart-selection.pdf.

Olick, R. S., Braun, E. A. and Potash, J. 2009. "Accommodating religious and moral objections to neurological death." *The Journal of Clinical Ethics* 20 (2): 183-91.

Re, A. [1992] 3 Med LR 303.

Re, Y. (mental incapacity) [1996] 2 FLR 787.

Re, A. (A Child) [2015] EWHC 443 (Fam).

Reese, P. P., Boudville, N. and Garg, A. X. 2015. "Living kidney donation: outcomes, ethics, and uncertainty." *Lancet* 385 (9981): 2003-13. doi: 10.1016/S0140-6736(14)62484-3.

Richards, J. R. 2012. *The ethics of transplants: why careless thought costs lives*. Oxford: Oxford University Press.

Rithalia, A., McDaid, C., Suekarran, S., Myers, L. and Sowden, A. 2009. "Impact of presumed consent for organ donation on donation rates: a systematic review." *BMJ* 338: a3162.

Shaw, D., Georgieva, D., Haase, B., Gardiner, D., Lewis, P., Jansen, N., Wind, T., Samuel, U., McDonald, M., Ploeg, R. and Elpat Working Group on Deceased Donation. 2017. "Family over rules? An ethical analysis of allowing families to overrule donation intentions." *Transplantation* 101 (3): 482-7. doi: 10.1097/TP.0000000000001536.

Shepherd, L., O'Carroll, R. E. and Ferguson, E. 2014. "An international comparison of deceased and living organ donation/transplant rates in opt-in and opt-out systems: a panel study." *BMC Medicine* 12: 131. doi: 10.1186/s12916-014-0131-4.

Smith, M. 2012. "Brain death: time for an international consensus." *British Journal of Anaesthesia* 108 (Suppl. 1): i6-9. doi: 10.1093/bja/aer355.

Symons, X. and Chua, R. M. 2018. "Organismal death, the dead-donor rule and the ethics of vital organ procurement." *Journal of Medical Ethics* 44: 868-71.

Transplant Policy Review Committee. 2015. "Policy POL200/3 Introduction to patient selection and organ allocation policies", accessed 8/2/2018. http://odt.nhs.uk/pdf/introduction_to_selection_and_allocation_policies.pdf.

Truog, R. and Robinson, W. 2003. "Role of brain death and the dead-donor rule in the ethics of organ transplantation." *Critical Care Medicine* 31 (9): 2391-6. doi: 10.1097/01.CCM.0000090869.19410.3C.

Verheijde, J. L. and Rady, M. Y. 2011. "Justifying physician-assisted death in organ donation." *The American Journal of Bioethics* 11 (8): 52-4. doi: 10.1080/15265161.2011.585275.

Wijdicks, E. F. 2002. "Brain death worldwide: accepted fact but no global consensus in diagnostic criteria." *Neurology* 58 (1): 20-5.

Wijdicks, E. F. 2003. "The neurologist and Harvard criteria for brain death." *Neurology* 61 (7): 970-6.

Wilkinson, D. and Savulescu, J. 2012. "Should we allow organ donation euthanasia? Alternatives for maximizing the number and quality of organs for transplantation." *Bioethics* 26 (1): 32-48. doi: 10.1111/j.1467-8519.2010.01811.x.

Chapter 16

Research

Case 16.1

A trial is planned of a novel strategy that attempts to cure patients of human immuno-deficiency virus (HIV). As part of the trial, participants who have been previously diagnosed with HIV and who are stable on maintenance anti-HIV therapy would stop their medication during the trial. There is a risk that, as a consequence of the study, participants would develop a relapse of their HIV. There may be an increased risk that they would pass on HIV to any sexual partners. The treatment is experimental and is not expected to benefit participants.

Is it ethical to conduct a trial like this that would put patients at some personal risk? Would patients be acting irrationally if they took part? Should ethics committees prevent the trial from going ahead, even if participants consent?

(For more discussion of the ethics of HIV cure trials, see Eyal 2017.)

LEGAL AND REGULATORY FRAMEWORK

Medical research is subject to more complex and detailed regulation and guidelines than almost any other area of ethics or medicine. Regulation focuses on safeguarding individuals who take part in research. The central concern is to ensure that the interests of society, or the enthusiasm of the researcher, do not override the interests of the individual.

For the most part, the ethical regulation of research is set out in professional standards or guidelines, rather than in legislation. There are prominent and highly influential international guidelines. General principles in common across these guidelines are summarized in Box 16.1.

The first internationally agreed guidelines on research involving people (the Nuremberg Code (1949)) were a direct response to the appalling experiments carried out by some Nazi doctors. This code consisted of ten principles, which were incorporated by the medical profession into the Declaration of Helsinki, first published by the World Medical Association in 1964 and last updated in 2013 (World Medical Association 2013). For example, Article 23 of the Declaration mandates that research protocols are submitted to a transparent, independent and

---

Box 16.1 Summary of international and national guidelines on research ethics

1. Research participants should not be put at more than minimal risk of harm as a result of taking part in research. Guidelines suggest that it is appropriate to balance some risk of harm with other considerations, such as the potential value of the research and whether it can be carried out without exposure to harm. However, even if the research is likely to lead to enormous benefit to others, the risk to participants should be small. The only possible exception is in some therapeutic research.

2. Potential research participants should be fully informed about both the purpose of the study and what will be involved in taking part, including an honest account of risks and benefits.

3. It is difficult or even impossible to obtain individual consent to carry out some research, for example some research using data from case notes or clinical databases. Ethics committees need to be satisfied that the research is of sufficient value to justify the breach of autonomy (confidentiality), and that it cannot be carried out satisfactorily in any other way.

4. No coercion must be brought to bear on people to take part in research. Care must be taken to ensure that the potential participant does not feel an obligation to take part. It must be made clear to patients that their clinical care (outside the research study) will not be affected if they refuse to take part in research.

5. Payments may be made to patients only to offset reasonable costs, and must not be large enough to act as an inducement for the person to take part in the research.

6. Patients who are not competent to give consent for research may still be eligible to take part in research. Ethics committees will need to be satisfied that:
   - the risk of harm is very low, probably lower than the risk that would be acceptable in the case of competent participants
   - the research aims cannot be achieved by other means
   - the research is of considerable value, and
   - a relevant person (usually a close relative) gives valid consent.

qualified research ethics committee, which will approve the study only if it meets national and international standards.

In the UK, principles of good practice relating to research are set out in the following documents:

UK Policy Framework for Health and Social Care Research – sets out the high-level principles and responsibilities that apply to medical research across the UK (Health Research Authority 2018).

Governance Arrangements for Research Ethics Committees – describes the role, make-up, function and management of Research Ethics Committees (RECs), as well as when review by a REC is necessary (Health Research Authority 2012).

Guidance for Good Clinical Practice (GCP) – international standard that sets out the ethical principles for conducting clinical trials (particularly drug trials) (European Medicines Agency 2017). This incorporates the Declaration of Helsinki and is designed to ensure consistent international ethical guidelines relating to research. Health professionals who participate in clinical research in the UK are expected to undertake GCP training. The Medicines and Healthcare products Regulatory Agency (MHRA) has a responsibility to ensure that research sites comply with GCP standards.

There are additional guidelines from the Royal College of Physicians (2007) and Medical Research Council (2018).

There are some regulations that apply to medical research. These include:

The **Medicines for Use (Clinical Trials) Regulations** 2004. If research involves a 'clinical trial of an investigational medicinal product' (a so-called 'CTIMP') involving human participants, researchers must follow the requirements of these regulations. The regulations are lengthy and detailed, and aim to standardize the regulation of medical research throughout the European Union (EU), including the ethical review of research protocols. There are several key regulations covering the factors that RECs must consider before approving a clinical trial. These include, for example, the anticipated risks and benefits of the trial and its design, the procedure for obtaining consent and the suitability of the protocol. Most significantly, the regulations introduce new criminal sanctions. Sixteen principles of good practice are also identified (which largely repeat those contained in various international codes and guidance).

European Clinical Trials Regulation (Clinical Trial Regulation EU No. 536/2014). This will officially come into force from 2019, and replaces a previous European directive (which was implemented in the UK by the Medicines for Use (Clinical Trials) regulations). It applies to CTIMPs and is designed to achieve a common approach to regulation of clinical trials across Europe. (It is not clear how this regulation will apply to the UK after it leaves the EU.)

Statutes such as the Human Rights Act 1998, the Human Tissue Act 2004 and the Mental Capacity Act 2005 also apply to medical research. As we shall see below, the general principles that apply to the law of consent to treatment apply to research. Thus, for consent to be legally valid, it must be voluntary, i.e. obtained without duress or undue influence, and informed, i.e. following full and detailed disclosure.

The UK Framework (HRA 2018) makes it quite clear that neither RECs nor reviewers are responsible for giving legal advice. The responsibility for breaches of the law rests with researchers and health and social care institutions.

ETHICAL VALUES RELEVANT TO MEDICAL RESEARCH

There are three main ethical values that can be applied to research. They are compared in Table 16.1, though all three are given some weight in existing guidelines.

The autonomy of the research participant

One important value in research, as in the rest of medicine, is to respect participants' freedom to decide whether or not to participate. An approach to the ethics of research that gave exclusive weight to respecting participant autonomy is the 'libertarian position' (Table 16.1). According to this view, research would be ethical as long as a potential research participant is fully informed, competent and not coerced. This would allow participants to take part even in very dangerous research – as long as they know and accept the risks. It would, for example, allow patients to take part in HIV cure trials. In defence of this position, libertarians might point out that we allow people to take considerable risks, for example, in the pursuit of dangerous sports. It would be a patient's right to stop taking regular medication for HIV if they choose, so it would appear strange to prevent them from doing so in the context of research (where there would likely be much greater safeguards and monitoring).

The risk of harm to the research participant

A different ethical value emphasizes the duty of the researcher to ensure that the potential participant is not put at risk of harm through taking part in the

Table 16.1 A comparison of three different ethical approaches to research.

	Important research where participants knowingly expose themselves to high risk	Low-risk research, performed without consent; participants do not know they are taking risks	Low-risk research where participants are fully informed	Poor-quality research that is of little value, but where participants are fully informed
Libertarian (rights-based)	Yes	No	Yes	Yes
Paternalistic (duty-based)	No	Yes	Yes	No
Utilitarian (consequentialist)	Yes	Yes	Yes	No

research. Almost exclusive concern for such risk gives rise to what might be called the paternalistic position. The paternalist would potentially regard HIV cure trials as unethical, even if the potential participant gave fully informed consent. On the other hand, the paternalist may not be concerned with research that poses no risk of harm but took place without the consent of the participants, for example, research that involved collecting anonymized information from patients' medical notes.

The consequences for society

An important aspect of a consequentialist approach (see Chapter 2) to research is that the benefits and harms both to participants *and* to those in the future are to be considered. According to the consequentialist view, the risk of harm to research participants (who may develop a relapse of HIV) may be justified by the benefits for the large number of people in the future who could benefit from an HIV cure. Some consequentialist perspectives would give equal weight to the interests of research participants and those in the future who might benefit from the research. The Declaration of Helsinki and national guidelines reject this position. The interests of research participants are given much greater weight than the interests of people in the future.

A more complex consequentialist picture would acknowledge the impact of harmful research on societal trust and on the ability of researchers to recruit patients into trials, for example, if participants develop serious complications that could lead to scandal and intense media attention. This may lead to restrictive research policies or may simply mean that future patients are loathe to consent to trials.

The general presumption of research ethics guidelines is that participating in research is potentially harmful, or at least burdensome. However, at least for some therapeutic research, participants may benefit simply from participating in the research, because, for example, the standard of clinical care is often better within a funded research project (Chalmers and Lindley 2001).

KEY ETHICAL QUESTIONS

Is this research?

Case 16.2

A surgeon wishes to know whether a particular technique is associated with improved outcomes for patients. She collects information on her use of this technique in a series of patients. She also collects information on patients where she used a different surgical technique. She compares the two groups of patients and presents the results at a surgical conference.

Does the surgeon need ethics committee approval?

If this counts as research, the surgeon would need to apply to the local REC. That would often require completing a long, detailed and complicated form. Approval may sometimes take a long time to obtain. The surgeon may need to obtain specific consent from her patients for involvement in the study (see below). However, if this does not count as research (for example, if it is regarded as an 'audit'), the surgeon may not need to obtain approval at all, or may need only complete a much simpler and quicker outline of the proposed project for sign-off. The surgeon may not need to obtain specific consent (though, of course, she would require standard informed consent for the procedure, see Chapter 6).

Gathering information about practice, reviewing outcomes and modifying care to benefit patients are ethically essential components of medicine. However, there is a worry that, where these are construed as research, the time and effort required to obtain approval may discourage health professionals from taking part in rigorous assessment and appraisal of care. Alternatively, there is a risk that some projects that really warrant ethical review are rebadged as 'audit' to avoid the hassle of obtaining approval.

The rules that determine whether or not a study is classified as research, or requires ethics approval, are complex, and may be specific to an institution. The Health Research Authority provides a decision tool that may be helpful (http://www.hra-decisiontools.org.uk/ethics/) (though it would often be wise to discuss with colleagues and/or local REC coordinators before embarking on a study). Some of the features of different types of enquiry are summarized in Table 16.2. Three key elements that typically distinguish research are discussed next.

Intention

For the surgeon, one important question may be whether she intends to generate knowledge that would be useful for others. For example, if she aims to publish the results of her enquiry so others can decide whether or not to use this intervention, that would potentially mean this is research. (Since publication in a medical journal often requires evidence of REC approval, that also may mean that she needs to go to the REC if she proposes to do this.)

Intervention

If the technique that the surgeon wishes to analyze is different from usual care, or if she wishes to perform extra investigations to evaluate it (e.g. extra scans or blood tests in addition to the normal tests), that would likely mean this is classified as research.

Allocation

If the surgeon wishes to compare those who received the technique with those who did not (for example, because they were treated before it was introduced, or because their surgeon decided to use a different technique) that would not necessarily count as research. However, if she wishes to randomize which patients receive the technique, that would almost certainly be classified as research.

If an enquiry is classified as research, other key ethical questions are likely to be raised (Box 16.2).

Table 16.2 Different types of enquiry.

	Aim	Technique
Research	To generate generalizable or transferable knowledge	Usually collects data additional to routine
		May involve interventions (e.g. tests, procedures, medicines) in addition to usual care
	To generate or test hypotheses or to describe	May involve randomization
Service evaluation	To assess the standard of delivered care	Sometimes involves additional data (e.g. questionnaire)
		Only involves interventions provided in standard care
		No randomization
Clinical audit	To compare care against a set standard	Usually only collects existing data
		Only involves interventions provided in standard care
		No randomization
Usual practice/ surveillance (public health)	To identify health problems and their cause	Collects population data
		Existing interventions
		Statistical methods may be used

Is the research scientifically valid?

The Declaration of Helsinki (Principle 21) states:

Medical research involving human subjects must conform to generally accepted scientific principles, be based on a thorough knowledge of the scientific literature, other relevant sources of information, and adequate laboratory and, as appropriate, animal experimentation. (World Medical Association 2013)

RECs will often arrange separate scientific appraisal of research studies by those with some expertise in the area. At first glance, that might seem to be outside the scope of 'ethics' committees. However, research that is scientifically poor may be unethical on paternalistic or consequentialist grounds because it will not benefit people in the future, and so any risk of harm to participants cannot be justified, or because it may harm people in the future because the results are misleading (Table 16.1). Failing to systematically review existing evidence before conducting research potentially wastes the limited time of researchers, ethics committees, research funders and patients (Glasziou and Chalmers 2015). It can also be lethal to participants (Savulescu and Spriggs 2002).

NB: RECs do not normally insist on (or check) publication of results. However, perhaps they should. It is important that all evidence is publicly available. The failure to publish negative findings results in publication bias and is unethical. There is a moral imperative to make the results of all research publicly accessible (Savulescu, Chalmers, and Blunt 1996).

Box 16.2 Some key issues in assessing the ethical aspects of a research protocol

Scientific validity
- Are the aims worthwhile?
- Is the method appropriate to the aims?

Safety
- Are the procedures safe, and are all reasonable precautions being taken?
- Is the degree of risk for participants acceptable?
- Consent procedure

Informed
- Is the information clearly written, honest, sufficient and balanced?

Voluntary (absence of coercion)
- Is it clear to the participant that refusal to take part will not affect clinical care?
- Is the relationship between researcher and participant free from potential coercion?
- Is the payment such as to encourage participation 'against the person's better judgement'?
- Is the researcher under undue pressure to recruit participants?
- Is there sufficient time after being given information for the person to decide whether to participate?

Competent
- Are the potential participants competent to decide whether or not to take part?
- Is such competence being assessed, when relevant?
- If potential participants are not competent, are they excluded, or is the recruitment procedure adequate?

Confidentiality
- Have participants given consent for confidential data to be accessed in the research?
- Are there adequate safeguards to prevent those not involved in the research from having access to confidential information?

Is the research risky?

The Declaration of Helsinki states:

> *Medical research involving human subjects may only be conducted if the importance of the objective outweighs the risks and burdens to the research subjects. (World Medical Association 2013)*

A central ethical position taken by international and national guidelines is that research participants must be protected from being at much risk of harm, even if the benefit of the research to people in the future is considerable.

The level of risk that is deemed to be acceptable depends on whether the research is 'therapeutic', and on whether the participant is able to consent. If the research intervention (for example an experimental drug) has the potential to benefit the participant, the research would be regarded as therapeutic. Then the question is how risky the experimental intervention is compared with standard care (see 'Is there equipoise' below), and also how *much* the patient stands to benefit from treatment. If there is no direct benefit to the participant from involvement in the study, or if the patient cannot consent, it is usually felt that only 'minimal risk' research is acceptable.

The term 'minimal risk' is not always defined. The Royal College of Physicians (2007) endorsed a definition of minimal risk as research that 'would result, at the most, in a very slight and temporary negative impact on the health of the person concerned' (Royal College of Physicians 2007). For children, this has been interpreted as permitting collection of urine, or the use of blood collected as part of treatment, but not venipuncture or injections (which are seen as imposing a 'low' rather than 'minimal' risk (Paediatrics and Committee 2000)). Other accounts of minimal risk refer to the level of risk that is encountered in daily life. This needs to be interpreted with care, as children and adults may sometimes face a high degree of risk in their daily life because of their social circumstances, and this does not necessarily justify imposing a higher burden of research on those participants (Binik 2014).

In determining whether the risks of participation in research are reasonable, the following factors are relevant (Savulescu and Hope 2010):

1. Is there a known risk to participants prior to commencing the study, and what is its magnitude?
2. Should any non-human research, epidemiological research, systematic overview or computer modelling have been performed prior to the study to better estimate the risk to participants or avoid the need for human participants?
3. Could the risk have been reduced in any other way? Is it as small as possible?
4. Are the potential benefits of this study worth the risks?
5. Could this research generate knowledge that is likely to significantly harm either participants or others outside the research, now or in the future?

Is there equipoise (uncertainty)?

For therapeutic research, in particular, randomized clinical trials, questions about risk are often replaced with questions about *equipoise*. This is the idea that the investigator is in a state of balance between the two arms of a trial – they do not know whether one arm or the other is superior. By contrast, if the researcher knows that a particular study intervention is better, it would be unethical for them to randomize a participant to receive a suboptimal intervention. In practice, though, it is common for there to be some evidence to suggest that one arm of a trial would be preferable. Investigators or clinicians often have (sometimes strongly held) beliefs about the merits of one treatment or the other. That does not mean that randomization is unethical. Instead, it may be helpful to ask whether there is genuine *uncertainty* about the benefits of the different treatments. An ethics committee could look at whether there is reasonable disagreement between professionals about the treatments. (For further discussion about the role of reasonable disagreement in deliberation, see the accompanying book (Wilkinson and Savulescu 2018).)

For studies that compare two different therapies for an illness, the *absolute* risk involved in the therapy may be greater than minimal; however, the *relative* risk of receiving one therapy or the other should be small (Royal College of Physicians 2007). Imagine, for example, two different chemotherapy regimes for cancer. There are likely to be more than minimal risks involved in undergoing chemotherapy (compared to not having chemotherapy). That does not mean that a research study would be ruled out. However, guidelines suggest that the relative risks of the different regimes should be small.

Has an adult with capacity given informed consent?

Informed consent is rightly regarded as crucial for medical research. For consent to be valid, the person must have legal capacity to give the consent, must be properly informed and must be free from coercion.

The assessment of capacity in the setting of research should presumably be approached in the same way as in consent to treatment (see Chapter 7).

The Medicines for Human Use (Clinical Trials) Regulations 2004 set out information that should be provided as part of informed consent for drug trials, including 'the nature, significance, implications and risks of the trial'. This appears to be similar to the type of information required normally in consent for treatment (see Chapter 6). However, it is common for RECs to require far more detailed written information than would usually be provided in clinical care (see below for discussion of Double Standards). Importantly, failure to provide sufficient information may give rise to criminal liability. Furthermore, the participant must have an interview with the researcher, during which he must have been given the opportunity to understand the objectives, risks and inconveniences of the trial and the conditions under which it is to be conducted. Normally consent must be formally recorded on a signed, written consent form (Fig. 16.1). Consent once given can also, of course, be withdrawn at any time.

A signed consent form does not guarantee that a patient has understood information about a study, nor that consent has been freely given. There are multiple challenges in practice. Patients do not always understand the difference between research and clinical care; they may believe, mistakenly, that an experimental treatment is likely to benefit them (this is the so-called 'therapeutic misconception'). Paradoxically, long and detailed written information may mean that the participant understands and retains little.

To avoid coercion, it should be clear to participants that their medical treatment (outside the trial) will not be affected if they decide to participate. RECs often pay particular attention to the relationship between the researcher and the participant. One key question is whether the potential participant is in a special relationship with the researcher, so that it might be hard to refuse participation in the study. Examples of such special relationships are those between patient and doctor, and between student and teacher.

Are there double standards?

Several researchers have argued that different standards are being applied without good reason to therapeutic research on the one hand, and clinical practice on the other:

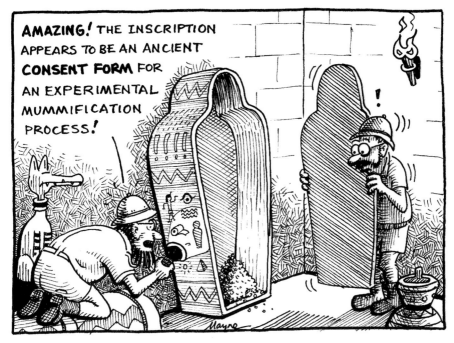

Figure 16.1 Consent form (© Don Mayne. Used with permission)

*If I give all my patients the same treatment, no one is around to stop
me, but should I decide to give only half of my patients the very same
treatment, the world seems full of people who will tell me why I should not
do this. (Chalmers and Lindley 2001)*

Double standards appear to be particularly evident with regard to the amount
of information provided to patients or participants. If the surgeon in Case 16.2
is conducting a trial of the different techniques, she is likely to be required to
provide very detailed information about both methods, the current scientific state
of understanding about each and the risks and benefits of involvement in the trial.
However, if she decides to use a new technique in all her patients, she will certainly
describe the planned intervention, but may give relatively little information about
alternatives.

Is this difference justified? Up for Debate Box 16.1 summarizes some arguments
for and against such 'double standards'.

When is research ethical in adults without capacity?

The legal position of research involving adults who lack capacity is now a complex
combination of the Clinical Trial Regulations 2004 (for CTIMPs – i.e. drug trials)
and the Mental Capacity Act 2005 (for most other research) (Fig. 16.2).

In some trials, like the one described in Case 16.3, prior consent is impossible
because the patient lacks capacity and there is no time to consult a surrogate
decision-maker. In emergency situations, the choice is between performing a trial
without consent or performing no trial at all.

Up for Debate Box 16.1 Should patients receive more detailed information about treatment that is part of a research trial than they would for treatment provided in clinical care?

For

1. Research trials and clinical practice are critically different, because, in the case of a trial, the central purpose is to benefit people in the future (the research intention). There is a pressure on the doctors and those running the trial to make decisions that are good for the trial, in addition to considering the best interests of the patient. In the case of ordinary clinical practice, the doctor has no double master. Her duty is simply to the best interests of the patient. The requirement for a more careful consent procedure arises from this difference.
2. It is likely that, if patients were not informed that they had been entered into a trial and that their treatment had been chosen using a random process, they would be extremely angry. On the other hand, it seems much less likely that patients would be concerned if the doctor, within normal clinical practice, had selected 'in good faith' what she saw as the most appropriate treatment.
3. If people were to realize that trials were being conducted without having received full information, then there would likely to be a loss of trust in doctors. This seems less likely in the case of patients realizing that doctors vary in their decisions about treatment – as long as the decisions are reasonable.

Against

The three reasons given above can each be criticized:

1. It is naive to think that the fact that a doctor acting in the best interests of her patient is sufficiently different from the doctor in the case of the clinical trial. In practice, the doctor is influenced in her prescribing by many factors. In fact, in the case of a randomized controlled trial, there will have been much more careful scrutiny of the objective data regarding efficacy than would be normal in clinical practice. There have to be safeguards to ensure that patients are no longer entered into the trial when there is good reason to suppose that one drug is better than the other. But, if these safeguards are in place, there is no good reason to demand a high standard of consent in the case of research.
2. Points (2) and (3) above are both empirical claims that may or may not be true. If it is true that patients would like a different standard of consent in the case of a trial than for normal clinical practice, then this could be seen as irrational.

Case 16.3

Researchers want to know whether adrenaline improves or worsens outcome for patients who suffer a cardiac arrest. They propose a randomized controlled trial, whereby paramedics will give adrenaline to half of patients with an out-of-hospital cardiac arrest and will give the other half placebo. They will not obtain consent prior to recruitment to the study. Families of patients who survive will be informed about the study, and given the option of consenting to follow-up. Families of patients who have died, however, will not be informed that their family member took part in the study.

Is it ever ethical to perform a study without consent?

(This case is based on the PARAMEDIC 2 trial (Perkins et al. 2016, Wilkinson 2014).)

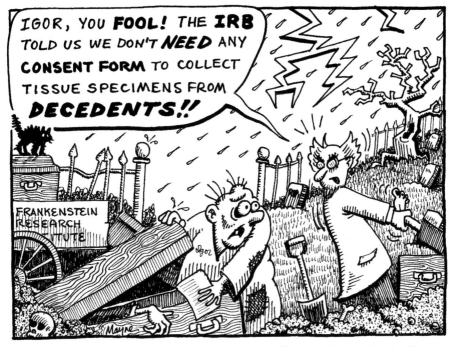

Figure 16.2 Research in those without capacity (© Don Mayne. Used with permission)

An amendment to the Clinical Trials Regulations (2008) specifically permits research to occur in situations such as this – so long as an ethics committee has approved the study. The patient or their surrogates (e.g. family) may be approached later for permission. This is sometimes referred to as 'deferred consent' or 'retrospective consent'. However, this seems to be a misnomer, since it is not possible to consent to something that has already happened (obviously if the patient or proxy declines to consent, that cannot change the past!). Instead, such situations are regarded more accurately as a waiver of the usual consent requirement. At a later stage, permission is sought to use information collected in the initial phase of the research, as well as (potentially) for ongoing involvement in the trial.

In less urgent situations, consent may be obtained from a proxy who represents the presumed wishes of the participant. For drug trials (CTIMPs, covered by the Clinical Trials Regulations), the proxy is called a 'personal legal representative' (if she is a close friend or relative who is willing to act on the adult's behalf) and is able to consent or refuse consent to the trial. If there is no such person, the proxy can be a 'professional legal representative' (e.g. the person's doctor). The proxy cannot be anyone associated with the trial. Participation in the trial is not permitted if the patient has previously (at a time when he or she had capacity) made an advance refusal to take part. For non-drug trials (covered by the Mental Capacity Act (MCA)), proxies can be consulted about the participant's wishes (which should be taken into account), but cannot formally consent. If the participant (lacking capacity) indicates that they do not wish to take part in the research, this should be taken into consideration; for non-therapeutic research, the MCA indicates that the patient should be 'withdrawn without delay' if they indicate a desire not to be in the study.

Even if proxies might consent, there are restrictions on when research would be permitted in adults lacking capacity. These restrictions are designed to protect vulnerable individuals and to prevent exploitation of those who cannot decline to participate. However, excluding vulnerable patients from research may leave them worse off overall, as research into alleviating their medical conditions will not take place, or they will be subject to treatments that have been inadequately tested.

There are some differences between the various regulations (Shepherd 2016). They generally only allow research in patients without capacity if studies would not be possible in patients with capacity. They vary in the level of risk they allow.

The Clinical Trials Regulations only permit *therapeutic* research in patients lacking capacity. There must be a prospect of benefit for the participant, or *no risk*. The trial must relate directly to a life-threatening or debilitating condition suffered by the participant.

The MCA specifies that the research must be connected with an 'impairing condition' affecting the adult. For example, if the capacity of a participant is impaired as a result of dementia, then the research must be aimed at helping our understanding of dementia. If the research is non-therapeutic, the risks must be *negligible* and not interfere significantly with the participant's freedom or privacy, or be unduly invasive or restrictive.

The incoming European Clinical Trials Regulations indicate that the research should either be therapeutic (offering direct benefit to the participant outweighing the risks and burdens) or, if non-therapeutic, pose *minimal risk* to the participant, while offering direct benefit to patients who suffer from the same life-threatening or debilitating condition.

When is research ethical in children?

The law regulating research on children and young people is now a complex mix of common law, statute (the Family Law Act 1967, Mental Capacity Act 2005) and Regulations (the Clinical Trial Regulations 2004).

The same general principles relating to medical decisions in children that were discussed in Chapter 11 can be applied to research in children and young people, though with some additional restrictions. Unless the research is therapeutic, the risks should be minimal.

For young people aged 16 or 17, a similar approach applies as in adults. If they have capacity, it appears that they may consent to participate in research (or, obviously, refuse to). If they lack capacity, someone with parental responsibility may provide proxy consent.

For children and young people under 16, consent requirements depend on whether the research is a drug trial (CTIMP) or a non-drug trial. For CTIMP research, the Clinical Trials Regulations specify that consent is required from a person with parental responsibility, even if the young person is Gillick competent. If the research is not a clinical trial, a Gillick competent young person might be able to consent (there is no directly relevant case law), though it would usually be wise to also obtain consent from a parent. Royal College of Paediatrics and Child Health guidance gives the example of research in sensitive situations (e.g. relating to sexual health or contraception), where parental consent should be 'carefully considered' (Modi et al. 2014).

In Scotland, consent by children to medical treatment has a different legal structure (see Chapter 11). In the setting of medical research, it may be the case that the Age of Legal Capacity (Scotland) Act 1991 allows 'mature' minors under the age of 16 years to consent to participation in research.

For further discussion about the ethics of experimental treatments in children, see Wilkinson and Savulescu (2018).

How much payment for research is permitted?

Guidelines indicate that payments either to researchers or to participants must be declared to the REC.

If doctors receive payment for the research according to the number recruited, ethics committees may be concerned that undue pressure will be brought to bear on patients to take part in the research. There is evidence that participants in research wish to be informed about any financial conflicts of interest (Kirkby et al. 2012).

Is it ethical for participants to be paid for taking part in research? There is concern that large payments may act as 'undue inducements', leading individuals to do something that they would ordinarily object to (Health Research Authority 2014). However, it appears to be paternalistic to disallow payments for riskier studies (for example Phase I trials) (Jones and Liddell 2009). In other areas of life, we allow competent adults to decide for themselves whether they wish to take risks for the sake of financial gain (Savulescu 2001). Given that ethics committees will normally only allow non-therapeutic research to take place if it is 'minimal risk', it is unclear why participants may not receive reasonable compensation for participation. Health Research Authority guidance indicates that, if the risks and burdens involved in research are such that a competent adult might reasonably take part even if unpaid, it would not be *undue inducement* to provide financial or other incentives (Health Research Authority 2014).

Can confidential patient information be used for research?

Most medical research involves collecting information concerning individuals that should be kept confidential. Researchers will be expected to communicate to potential participants how their information will be stored and how it will be used. Then participants may consent (or not) to use of their information.

Sometimes, however, research requires use of patients' details prior to consent, or without consent. For example, research may be based on the collection and analysis of existing information in medical records. Seeking individual consent from each patient for access to health records may not be possible in the case of large studies or studies involving records from a long time ago. Researchers who wish to use confidential patient information without consent in England and Wales need to apply to the Confidentiality Advisory Group of the Health Research Authority. This group will assess whether use is in accordance with section 251 of the National Health Service Act. Use of information is potentially acceptable if it has a medical purpose (including medical research); is in the public interest or in the interest of improving patient care; and is compliant with the Data Protection Act 1998 (see Chapter 9).

Is it ethical to use a placebo?

Placebos are widely used in clinical research to help assess whether a response to a particular therapy is because of the intrinsic properties of that intervention, rather than (for example) because of the influence of patient expectations. Outside research, placebos are often thought to be ethically problematic, as they usually involve deception. In trials, though, participants consent to receiving a placebo, so there is no issue of deception.

The principle ethical question around placebos is related to the issue of equipoise (discussed above). It is generally accepted that the control group in a treatment trial should receive standard treatment (i.e. they should not be disadvantaged by taking part in the trial compared with people who are not in the trial). The issue can be whether there is sufficient evidence about a new treatment that it would be unethical to withhold it from some patients (and to give them a placebo instead). Alternatively, the concern may be that there is a standard therapy that is known to be beneficial, and the new treatment should be compared with standard therapy instead of with placebo. This question has sometimes arisen in relation to research that is planned (or has been performed) in developing countries.

There is a strong argument that research subjects in any part of the world should be protected by an irreducible set of ethical standards (Angell 1988). However, sometimes researchers have proposed research in the third world that would not be permissible in developed countries.

Case 16.4

In 1994, research in the US and France strongly suggested that a regimen of treatment with zidovudine (known as the ACTG 076 regimen) reduced the chance of vertical transmission (i.e. from mother to child) of human immunodeficiency virus (HIV) by as much as 2/3 (from 25% to 8%). The regimen involved oral doses for the mother while pregnant, intravenous doses during labour and further doses to the newborn infant. However, this regimen was too expensive to be generally available in the third world, and there was interest in determining whether a cheaper regimen (a short oral course of zidovudine) would be effective in preventing babies in the third world from being infected with the HIV.

At the time of the research, the ACTG 076 regimen had become the standard of care in the US.

Two possible designs of study to be carried out in third world countries were considered. The first was to compare the cheaper regimen with placebo. The second was to compare the cheaper regimen with the expensive one (ACTG 076). The first design would have aimed to answer the question: Is the cheap treatment better than nothing (placebo)? The second design would have aimed to answer the question: Is the cheap regimen as effective as the expensive regimen?

Researchers decided to embark on placebo-controlled trials of the short course of zidovudine in Thailand. Were these trials ethical (Up for Debate Box 16.2)? This case sparked intense debate following editorials in the *New England Journal of Medicine* in 1997. See for example Lurie and Wolfe (1997).

Up for Debate Box 16.2 Is it unethical to conduct a placebo-controlled trial in a developing country if there is a proven treatment?

For

1. It would have been unethical to conduct the zidovudine trial in the sponsoring country (the US), because this had become standard treatment. Research ethics committees would not allow such a trial to proceed. It is unethical for research in a third world country to have a lower standard than that in the sponsoring country: a double standard is operating.
2. If we allow such double standards, this is a form of exploitation of people in the third world – using them as 'research fodder'.
3. The Declaration of Helsinki states that new interventions should be tested against the 'best proven intervention'. Placebos can only be used where there is a proven intervention if there are 'compelling and scientifically sound methodological reasons' to justify this.
4. There is no scientific reason for preferring this placebo-controlled design to the alternative design, in which controls receive the expensive regimen. The study could be done using the standard treatment as comparison.

Against

1. If it were not for the trial, no-one in the third world trial would be receiving treatment. No-one, therefore, receives worse treatment as a result of the trial taking place than they would if the trial did not take place (in contrast to the situation if the trial were being carried out in the sponsoring country). There is no-one who has been harmed as a result of the trial.
2. Although it would be better to provide controls with the expensive regimen, this would cost the sponsoring country (or a pharmaceutical company, or whomever) extra money. It would be good for wealthy countries to support health care in developing countries; however, we do not think that is the job of pharmaceutical companies (or research agencies). If we do not think that the sponsoring country, or the pharmaceutical company, should be forced to provide the expensive treatment outside any trial, then why should it be forced to provide such treatment inside the trial?
3. The exploitation argument is wrong. Those who receive the (cheap) treatment as part of the trial are better off than they would be if the trial did not take place. It is in the interests of those in the third world for as many such trials to take place as possible. Some of those who take part in the trial are benefited; some are neither better off nor worse off. No-one is being exploited.
4. A placebo-controlled trial may generate a more rapid answer to the question – as the effect of treatment (compared with placebo) is potentially greater. The sample size required would be lower. This would allow research agencies to perform more research and to generate answers sooner (translating into better treatment).
5. A placebo-controlled trial would answer the question that is most relevant to those in developing countries. Suppose that short-course zidovudine were shown to be less effective than (the more expensive) standard-course zidovudine. That does not help those in developing countries. They need to know whether the short course is effective compared to no treatment, and whether it is cost-effective.

(In early 1998, the CDC-sponsored trial of zidovudine in Thailand reported that the placebo-controlled trial had demonstrated a 51% reduction in perinatal HIV transmission (Shaffer et al. 1999). The CDC and Thai government announced that further use of placebos would cease in ongoing studies.)

Is gene therapy research ethical?

Case 16.5

On 27 November 2018, it was reported that a Chinese researcher, Jiankui He of Shenzhen, had gene-edited two healthy embryos, resulting in the birth of baby girls born that month, Lulu and Nana. The babies' father was apparently HIV-positive, while their mother was HIV-negative. The parents had apparently consented to the research study. He edited a gene to make the babies resistant to HIV. One girl has both copies of the modified gene, while the other has only one (making her still susceptible to HIV) (Marchione 2018).
Was this research ethical?

In Chapter 18, we will discuss the ethics of gene editing in more detail. However, the principal ethical issues in the above case are issues that relate to research ethics, not to specific genetics or gene editing questions (Savulescu 2018, Schaefer 2018).

One of the biggest criticisms of He relates to the risks of the research. We discussed above the idea that risks to participants (particularly for those who are unable to consent, such as embryos) need to be minimized and proportionate to benefits. Lulu and Nana were exposed to significant risk of off-target mutations and cancer. (The gene editing technology has a potential risk of causing damage to other areas of the genome.)

There would have been less expected harm if embryos with lethal disorders were used. Any child produced would stand to derive a very significant benefit: having their life saved. The severe form of Tay-Sach's disease is almost invariably lethal by 5 years of age. Another candidate might be Leigh Syndrome. However, there are likely even more severe, lethal, single-gene disorders which would be even better candidates (Savulescu 2018). The benefits to Lulu and Nana, though, are not proportionate to the risk. They derive no direct benefit: HIV can be prevented in numerous ways, including by protected sexual intercourse.

At the time of writing, the full details of the study are not clear, but other questions include the ethical oversight of the study, the consent process and whether there may have been undue inducement to participate (Schaefer 2018).

REVISION QUESTIONS

1. When is research ethical in a patient who lacks capacity to consent?
2. What are CTIMPs? How are these regulated differently from other forms of research in the UK?
3. Can children or young people consent to research in the UK?

4. What does it mean to lack equipoise? Would it be ethical for a doctor to enrol a patient in a study if they lacked equipoise?
5. Should there be a 'risk threshold' for research in adults who have capacity? Why? Why not?

Extension case 16.6

A randomized study had been performed in South Africa which showed that a topical gel (tenofovir) reduced the risk of acquiring HIV in sexually active women by 50%. The researchers then arranged a further study for those who had been in the trial (as part of a post-trial access scheme). They provided the tenofovir and aimed to collect additional data. The safety of this intervention in pregnancy was not known, and participants had to agree to use barrier contraception and have regular urine pregnancy tests during the study.

During the course of the study, researchers discovered that one of the participants had been pregnant for several months. She had wanted continued access to the study drug, as she believed that she was at risk of HIV (she had an abusive partner) and could not obtain it any other way. She had provided substitute urine samples. Research nurses had not detected her pregnancy.

Do researchers have an ethical obligation to provide study drugs that have been proven to be effective to participants at the end of a study (post-trial access)? (If so, can they impose restrictions or time limits on access?)

Is it fair to exclude pregnant women from research?

Is provision of a study medication a form of 'undue inducement'?

This case is based on Mngadi et al. (2017).

REFERENCES

Angell, M. 1988. "Ethical Imperialism?" *The New England Journal of Medicine* 319 (16): 1081-3. doi: 10.1056/nejm198810203191608.

Binik, A. 2014. "On the minimal risk threshold in research with children." *The American Journal of Bioethics* 14 (9): 3-12. doi: 10.1080/15265161.2014.935879.

Chalmers, I. and Lindley, R. I. 2001. "Double standards on informed consent to treatment Edited by: 2000." In *Informed Consent in Medical Research*, edited by L. Doyal and J. S. Tobias. London: BMJ Books: 266-76.

European Medicines Agency. 2017. "Guideline for good clinical practice E6(R2)." EMA, accessed 28/02/2018. http://www.ema.europa.eu/docs/en_GB/document_library/Scientific_guideline/2009/09/WC500002874.pdf.

Eyal, N. 2017. "The benefit/risk ratio challenge in clinical research, and the case of HIV cure: an introduction." *Journal of Medical Ethics* 43 (2): 65-6. doi: 10.1136/medethics-2016-103427.

Glasziou, P. and Chalmers, I. 2015. "How systematic reviews can reduce waste in research." BMJ.com, accessed 26 Feb 2018. http://blogs.bmj.com/bmj/2015/10/29/how-systematic-reviews-can-reduce-waste-in-research/.

Health Research Authority. 2012. "Governance arrangements for research ethics committees." HRA, accessed 28/02/2018. https://www.hra.nhs.uk/planning-and-improving-research/policies-standards-legislation/governance-arrangement-research-ethics-committees/.

Health Research Authority. 2014. "Payments and incentives in research." HRA, accessed 28/02/2018. https://www.hra.nhs.uk/documents/274/hra-guidance-payments-incentives-research.pdf.

Health Research Authority. 2018. "UK Policy Framework for Health and Social Care Research." HRA, accessed 28/02/2018. https://www.hra.nhs.uk/planning-and-improving-research/policies-standards-legislation/uk-policy-framework-health-social-care-research/.

Jones, E. and Liddell, K. 2009. "Should healthy volunteers in clinical trials be paid according to risk? Yes." *BMJ* 339: b4142. doi: 10.1136/bmj.b4142.

Kirkby, H. M., Calvert, M., Draper, H., Keeley, T. and Wilson, S. 2012. "What potential research participants want to know about research: a systematic review." *BMJ Open* 2 (3): e000509. doi: 10.1136/bmjopen-2011-000509.

Lurie, P. and Wolfe, S. M. 1997. "Unethical trials of interventions to reduce perinatal transmission of the human immunodeficiency virus in developing countries." *The New England Journal of Medicine* 337 (12): 853-6.

Marchione, M. 2018. "Chinese researcher claims first gene-edited babies." Associated Press, 26 November 2018. Accessed 30/11/18. https://www.apnews.com/4997bb7aa36c454 49b488e19ac83e86d.

Medical Research Council. 2018. "Policies and guidance for researchers." accessed 23/02/2018. https://www.mrc.ac.uk/research/policies-and-guidance-for-researchers/.

Mngadi, K. T., Singh, J. A., Mansoor, L. E. and Wassenaar, D. R. 2017. "Undue inducement: a case study in CAPRISA 008." *Journal of Medical Ethics* 43 (12): 824-8. doi: 10.1136/medethics-2016-103414.

Modi, N., Vohra, J., Preston, J., Elliott, C., Van't Hoff, W., Coad, J., Gibson, F., Partridge, L., Brierley, J., Larcher, V., Greenough, A. and Paediatrics Working Party of the Royal College of, and Health Child. 2014. "Guidance on clinical research involving infants, children and young people: an update for researchers and research ethics committees." *Archives of Disease in Childhood* 99 (10): 887-91. doi: 10.1136/archdischild-2014-306444.

Perkins, G. D., Quinn, T., Deakin, C. D., Nolan, J. P., Lall, R., Slowther, A. M., Cooke, M., Lamb, S. E., Petrou, S., Achana, F., Finn, J., Jacobs, I. G., Carson, A., Smyth, M., Han, K., Byers, S., Rees, N., Whitfield, R., Moore, F., Fothergill, R., Stallard, N., Long, J., Hennings, S., Horton, J., Kaye, C. and Gates, S. 2016. "Pre-hospital Assessment of the Role of Adrenaline: Measuring the Effectiveness of Drug administration In Cardiac arrest (PARAMEDIC-2): Trial protocol." *Resuscitation* 108: 75-81. doi: 10.1016/j.resuscitation.2016.08.029.

Royal College of Paediatrics and Child Health: Ethics Advisory Committee. 2000. "Guidelines for the ethical conduct of medical research involving children." *Archives of Disease in Childhood* 82: 177-82.

Royal College of Physicians. 2007. *Guidelines on the practice of ethics committees in medical research with human participants.* London: RCP.

Savulescu, J. 2001. "Harm, ethics committees and the gene therapy death." *Journal of Medical Ethics* 27 (3): 148-50.

Savulescu, J. 2018. "The fundamental ethical flaw in Jiankui He's alleged gene editing experiment." Practical ethics blog, accessed 30/11/18. http://blog.practicalethics.ox.ac.uk/2018/11/the-fundamental-ethical-flaw-in-jiankui-hes-alleged-gene-editing-experiment/.

Savulescu, J., Chalmers, I. and Blunt, J. 1996. "Are research ethics committees behaving unethically? Some suggestions for improving performance and accountability." *BMJ* 313 (7069): 1390-3.

Savulescu, J. and Hope, T. 2010. "Ethics of research." In *The Routledge companion to ethics*, edited by J. Skorupski. Abingdon: Routledge: 781-95.

Savulescu, J. and Spriggs, M. 2002. "The hexamethonium asthma study and the death of a normal volunteer in research." *Journal of Medical Ethics* 28 (1): 3-4.

Schaefer, G. O. 2018. "Rogue science strikes again: the case of the first gene-edited babies." *The Conversation*, 27 September 2018. https://theconversation.com/rogue-science-strikes-again-the-case-of-the-first-gene-edited-babies-107684.

Shaffer, N., Chuachoowong, R., Mock, P. A., Bhadrakom, C., Siriwasin, W., Young, N. L., Chotpitayasunondh, T., Chearskul, S., Roongpisuthipong, A., Chinayon, P., Karon, J., Mastro, T. D. and Simonds, R. J. 1999. "Short-course zidovudine for perinatal HIV-1 transmission in Bangkok, Thailand: a randomised controlled trial. Bangkok Collaborative Perinatal HIV Transmission Study Group." *Lancet* 353 (9155): 773-80.

Shepherd, V. 2016. "Research involving adults lacking capacity to consent: the impact of research regulation on 'evidence biased' medicine." *BMC Medical Ethics* 17 (1): 55. doi: 10.1186/s12910-016-0138-9.

Wilkinson, D. 2014. "Please randomise me, but don't tell my family that you did." Practical ethics blog. http://blog.practicalethics.ox.ac

.uk/2014/08/please-randomize-me-but-dont -tell-my-family-that-you-did/.

Wilkinson, D. and Savulescu, J. 2018. *Ethics, conflict and medical treatment for children: from disagreement to dissensus*. Elsevier.

World Medical Association. 2013. "Declaration of Helsinki: ethical principles for medical research involving human subjects", accessed 04/12/2008. https://www.wma.net/policies-post/wma-declaration-of-helsinki-ethical -principles-for-medical-research-involving- human-subjects/.

16

RESEARCH

Part 3

Extensions

Chapter **17**

Neuroethics

Neuroethics is a relatively recent specialty field within ethics that examines the ethical implications of advances in the neurosciences, including cognitive sciences more generally. It includes psychiatric ethics. Neuroethics also involves the neuroscientific (and broader cognitive scientific) study of moral decision-making. Moral decision-making here includes prudential decision-making, which includes decisions about risk and health. In this chapter, we will outline a small selection of interesting recent topics in neuroethics.

ADDICTION AND FREE WILL

Case 17.1

Dr Jones is a GP. He has been researching the most cost-effective treatments for addiction. He discovers that paying addicts to stay off their drug is an effective intervention. He uses NHS funds to incentivize abstinence and institutes regular testing. After successful results, Dr Jones plans to extend this weight loss and obesity.

  Should addicts and the obese be paid to adopt healthier lifestyles?

  This case is based on Heyman (2009).

Case 17.1 overlaps with some issues that we raised in Case 10.5 (whether obese patients and smokers should have to change their lifestyle before being eligible for elective surgery). Partly, the answer depends on utilitarian considerations: is the intervention (paying patients) overall effective, or the most cost-effective? However, the answer also partly depends on whether we think addicts, the obese and others who adopt unhealthy lifestyles are acting freely and have responsibility for their choices.

If we think that addicts are deciding freely when they smoke or consume drugs, it might seem unreasonable to pay them to stop, and fair to demand that they do so prior to access to certain types of treatment. On the other hand, if addicts (or obese patients) lack free will, then maybe they are not responsible for their condition. Perhaps paying them to change their behaviour is ethically acceptable?

What is addiction? And how can neuroscience help us answer these questions? There are two dominant concepts, each with different implications for freedom of the will (Foddy and Savulescu 2010).

The willpower view

Perhaps the oldest view of addiction maintains that some part of an addict wishes to abstain, but that their will is not strong enough to overcome an immediate desire towards temptation. According to this view, addicts lose 'control' over their actions. Most versions of the willpower view characterize addiction as a battle in which an addict's wish for abstinence seeks to gain control over his behaviour.

Adherents of the willpower view might see it as ethically dubious to pay people to exert their own will. Michael Sandel has argued that we should not pay people to adopt healthy lifestyles or to preserve public goods (Sandel 2012).

The disease view

In contrast to the willpower view, the most popular view is that addiction is the direct result of some physiological change in the brain caused by chronic use of the drug. The disease view states that there is some 'normal' process of motivation in the brain, and that this process is somehow changed or perverted by brain damage or adaptation caused by chronic drug use. According to this theory of addiction, the addict is no longer rational; she uses drugs as a result of a fundamentally non-voluntary process, and not responsible.

Alan Leshner argues that an addicted person's actions are the direct result of brain adaptations caused by chronic drug use – that their actions are more like reflexes than normal rational behaviours (Leshner 1997, 1999). One objection to this kind of argument is that planning and thought are part of the drug-seeking process. A heroin user needs to locate and martial the heroin, the needle, the spoon, the flame and a tourniquet. As Perring points out, it is the 'reward systems' of the brain that are mostly affected by drugs, and not the planning and motor systems, so it does not make sense to say that drug adaptation actually controls the drug-seeking process (Perring 2002). Indeed, addicts are responsive to the price of their drug (tobacco taxes have been most effective in reducing consumption) and to positive rewards (Heyman 2009).

For this reason, a softer, more defensible, version of the disease view is also sometimes advanced. Hyman, for example, claims that it is not the chronic brain changes which alter the process of motivation, but the fact that drugs directly stimulate the pleasure pathways, which he says 'hijacks' the normal motivational process (Hyman 2005).

According to the disease view, payment of addicts might seem reasonable, as they are not fully responsible for their behaviour.

The broader context of addiction

Addictive behaviour extends beyond drugs such as heroin and cocaine. The same pattern of pleasure, intoxication, habituation and even addiction can be produced for a normal pleasurable behaviour, such as eating sweet food.

When we eat any palatable food, there is a release of endorphins. These endorphins bind to the same opioid receptors in the brain that heroin binds to. Just like heroin, this process causes an analgesic sensation and a release of dopamine in the reward centres of the brain. Sugar sensitizes both the opioid and dopamine receptors in the brain in the exact same way as heroin. Our brains adapt to sugar in much the same way as they adapt to heroin. One can become addicted to sugar, and it even has its own withdrawal syndrome which is identical to heroin withdrawal (Foddy and Savulescu 2010).

The only fundamental difference between sugar and heroin is that sugar elicits a release of endogenous opiate chemicals, while heroin directly activates the opioid receptors with no intermediary step. But a number of non-drug substances can also directly activate the brain's reward pathways. Beta carotene (found in carrots), milk, over-eating, sex, gambling, shopping and other behaviours elicit changes that are biologically and behaviourally almost identical to addictions (Earp et al. 2017, Foddy and Savulescu 2010).

Partly because of this wider context of addiction, one of us has offered a more minimal account of addiction which is called the 'liberal view' (Foddy and Savulescu 2010).

Grounding the more minimal liberal view is the idea that addiction is the consequence of habit, which is a result of learning and the nature (and limitations) of the reward system. The learning system is very loose: it is not closely tied to behaviours that are good for us in the long term. It just says: 'keep repeating that'. According to this view, we are prone to bad habits because of the limitations of the reward system. Addiction is a consequence of this, and in a sense 'normal'.

These different concepts of addiction overlap and may represent different ways of viewing the same issue. All agree that it is difficult for addicts to change their behaviour unless there are significant rewards or disincentives – social and personal – to change. All question the degree to which we are free. If freedom exists, we are less free than we commonly believe ourselves to be. People need considerable support to become free and to be responsible. It is difficult to be fully autonomous.

Nudge, incentives and disincentives (see also Chapter 20) are based on a view that people's choices are dominated by social forces, personal biases and psychological limitations. If we are not fully free, we may as well be healthy, as long as our capacity to be autonomous is substantially preserved (Savulescu 2018).

NEUROETHICS

DISORDERS OF CONSCIOUSNESS

Detecting consciousness

Case 17.2

A 23-year-old woman, Gillian, was struck by a car while crossing the road and sustained severe brain injury. Five months after the injury she remained unresponsive. Although she had periods of being awake and asleep, Gillian did not show any purposeful movements or responses to stimulation. She met clinical criteria for a persistent vegetative state.

A neuroscientist, interested in assessing consciousness in patients with severe brain disorders, used functional magnetic resonance imaging (fMRI) to assess Gillian. He used a protocol that could identify different forms of brain activity. When normal patients are asked to imagine walking around their house, one area of the brain is active on fMRI; when they are asked to imagine playing tennis, a different area lights up.

The neuroscientist asked Gillian to imagine playing tennis, and then to imagine walking around her house. The patterns of brain activation were the same as in normal volunteers.

How should consciousness be assessed in patients with severe brain injury?

This case is based on Owen et al. (2006) and Highfield (2014).

With the growing sophistication of modern medical interventions, patients are increasingly being kept alive in states of severely diminished consciousness following injuries that would have, in the past, often been fatal. These are called disorders of consciousness. They include coma, vegetative state (VS) and minimally conscious state (MCS). A relevant state that is clinically related, although consciousness is preserved, is locked-in syndrome (LIS) (this can occur with some brain-stem strokes, for example).

The case of Gillian raises the prospect that some patients who appear to be in a VS may actually be in something that is more like LIS. It is not unheard of for family members of patients with severe brain disorders to have a strong feeling that their loved one has much more awareness than they are given credit for. Doctors sometimes attribute such reports to wishful thinking; but the case of Gillian suggests that perhaps the families are right.

When her case was first reported, there was vigorous debate about what this meant for the assessment of patients with disorders of consciousness. How should we assess consciousness? Do the results of brain scans really mean that the patients are conscious? Some argued that the types of responses in Gillian's case might be more like a reflex, a pattern of retained brain response that does not actually mean that she is aware.

In a further study, scientists reported using these tests in 54 patients with either VS or MCS. Five of the patients (~10%) appeared to be able to obey instructions, and activated different areas of the brain on fMRI. One was even able to correctly answer questions using the technique (he was asked to imagine playing tennis for 'yes', and to imagine walking around his house for 'no'). This sort of evidence convinced many that there could be some (perhaps rare) cases of patients who were from the outside unresponsive, but were actually conscious. But what ethical difference would it make if the patients were conscious?

The ethical significance of consciousness

Case 17.3

A 43-year-old woman, Mrs M, was due to go for a skiing holiday when she was found by her partner to be drowsy and confused. She was rushed to hospital and diagnosed with viral encephalitis.

Mrs M was left with a severe disorder of consciousness and diagnosed to be in a persistent vegetative state. Her family believed that Mrs M would not wish to be kept alive in such a condition. They sought permission from the court to withdraw the artificial nutrition and hydration keeping Mrs M alive.

However, during the process of further investigation for the court, Mrs M was discovered to actually have some intermittent response to basic commands. She was diagnosed with a minimally conscious state.

What is the ethical significance of minimal consciousness for life and death decisions?

This is based on the case of W v M [2011].

In Chapter 14 we discussed the legal framework for cases like that of Mrs M. In her case, the judge concluded that, despite clear evidence that she would not have wished to remain alive in her severely disabled state, life-prolonging treatment should continue. Subsequently, other judgements have placed more emphasis on the previous wishes of the patient and allowed withdrawal of artificial nutrition in patients with a MCS (Chapter 14).

But her case raises an important general question: what is the value of consciousness? The case of Tony Bland (see Case 14.3) and the similar US case of Terri Schiavo were intensely controversial at the time, though both individuals were assumed to lack consciousness. If there had been evidence in either of those cases that Tony or Terri had been conscious, that might have led to even more consternation (and may have led to different judicial decisions).

Higher levels of consciousness are clearly of value. Self-consciousness, rational consciousness, moral consciousness and so on are of paramount importance to what matters most in life. They define persons and personhood.

Lower levels of consciousness are also ethically relevant. Of great importance in the case of Mrs M was the assessment that she could experience pleasure and did not seem to be in pain. Just as non-self-conscious animals can have lives that are worth living if the balance of positive mental states (such as pleasure, happiness, contentment, care, affection, etc.) outweigh negative mental states (pain, suffering, abandonment, fear, loss, etc.), so too can humans with disorders of consciousness. While consciousness exists, life can have value if the balance of positive mental states outweighs the negative. This is separate to the autonomous desires of the previously competent person about whether they should continue to exist in that state (advance directives or living wills – see Chapter 7).

However, the presence of consciousness could also mean that it is a harm to a patient to continue to live. There is a general problem with probing the experiences of those with lower level of consciousness: they cannot competently report their quality of life. While patients who are truly in a VS are thought not to be able to feel pain, there is neuroimaging evidence that those who are in a MCS experience pain (Boly et al. 2008).

Neuroimaging might indicate that a patient who appears to be in a VS is actually fully conscious and 'locked-in'. Some people might hold the view that we are morally required to do our best to preserve the life of a patient in this state. Because they are conscious, there is a moral imperative to prolong life. However, others might ask whether such a life is worse than death (Kahane and Savulescu 2009). Evidence from patients with LIS indicates that some express a desire not to go on living (Bruno et al. 2011), and some request euthanasia (Kompanje, de Beaufort, and Bakker 2007). On the other hand, the capacity of humans to adapt to their condition, no matter how adverse, has been amply documented in other contexts. Indeed, the self-scored perception of mental well-being in one survey of patients with LIS was not significantly lower than that of age-matched normal subjects (Laureys et al. 2005), However, surveys of patients able to communicate may not be relevant to a more severely affected population of patients with full LIS and an apparent VS. Many may also have been in such a state for a long time. Their situation might be compared unfavourably with the worst form of solitary confinement in prison.

There are also highly relevant considerations of distributive justice in the life-prolonging medical treatment of disorders of consciousness. Even if life is worth living, the quality is reduced, raising questions of whether such treatment is just on utilitarian, cost-effectiveness or other grounds of justice (Chapter 10).

NEUROREDUCTIONISM AND BIOPSYCHOSOCIAL PSYCHIATRY

Case 17.4

Jane is in her thirties and is in a long-term loving and supportive relationship. She has two young children. Jane confides to her GP that she has experienced a loss of sexual desire since the birth of her second child.

Jane's GP diagnoses her with hypoactive sexual desire disorder (HSDD). He refers her to a research study that he has seen advertised. The study involves functional neuroimaging while watching a series of television programs (either regular television or erotic videos). The researcher reports that women without a diagnosis of HSDD had increased activity in the insular cortices when watching the erotic videos, while those with the diagnosis did not. The researcher claimed that this provided evidence that HSDD is a neurobiological disorder, rather than a social construct.

Should we interpret changes in brain activity as evidence of pathology?

This case is based on Savulescu and Earp (2014).

Neuroimaging can provide powerful insights into brain function and dysfunction. However, sometimes neuroscientific evidence is misinterpreted or overinterpreted.

Case 17.4 illustrates what we could call 'neuroreductionism': the practice of seeking crude neurobiological explanations for complex biopsychosocial phenomena, and the tendency to over-estimate the contribution of neurobiology (Roache and Savulescu 2017). Because women with HSDD are experiencing the world differently, or behaving differently, there must be differences in their brain activity. This provides no evidence that this is pathological. It is the necessary consequence of materialism (or physicalism) regarding the nature of brain and mind: any difference in mental activity must be underpinned by a difference in brain activity.

The contrasting theory – dualism (held by the philosopher Rene Descartes) – holds that the mind and brain are separate, disconnected entities. Dualism is widely discredited, but the community (and doctors) are still sometimes drawn to the idea that brain scan changes are evidence of a brain problem. In stating that this study provides evidence that HSDD is a 'genuine physical problem', the researcher confuses correlation for causation.

Although we have given the example above of HSDD, there are many examples of neuroscience evidence being used to infer pathology – including a range of different sexual behaviours, but also addiction, psychopathy, bereavement and political orientation. The important point is that these differences in brain activity tell us nothing about what actually caused the differences in brain activity, or whether those differences are pathological, or bad.

There are four causes of brain activity or disorders of the mind:

1. biological
2. psychological
3. social
4. natural circumstances.

The biopsychosocial theory of psychiatry seeks to stress the importance of the first three factors in causation and intervention (Davies, Savulescu, and Roache, forthcoming). The brain is the final common pathway to all neurological and psychiatric disorders. However, the causes of pathological brain activity can be any of these four, or combination of them.

AUTHENTICITY AND DEEP BRAIN STIMULATION

Case 17.5

A 62-year-old man, DM, had severe Parkinson's disease that left him bedbound, severely physically disabled, dependent on others and depressed. Medical treatment had not been able to relieve his symptoms. DM consented to deep brain stimulation (DBS), a non-ablative neurosurgical procedure that implants electrodes into the basal ganglia.

When the stimulator was switched on, DM experienced a dramatic reduction in his Parkinson's symptoms. However, he also experienced a significant personality change with mania, ran up huge debts and got into trouble with the police.

Should the deep brain stimulator be switched off?

This case is based on Kraemer (2013).

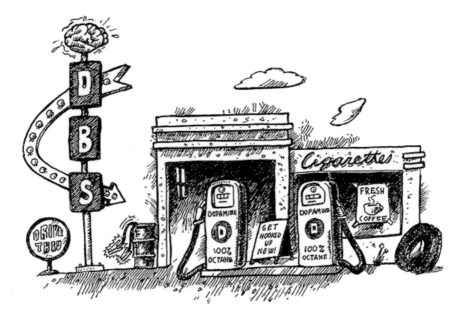

Figure 17.1 Deep brain stimulation (© Marty Bee, reproduced with permission)

Deep brain stimulation (DBS) (Fig. 17.1) has been supported by NICE for more than 15 years. It is being increasingly considered as an experimental therapy for a wide range of neurological and psychiatric conditions, including (amongst others) chronic pain, depression, epilepsy and anorexia nervosa. Preliminary evidence from the experimental use of DBS in these contexts suggests that the procedure may be highly beneficial for treatment-refractory patients. Furthermore, DBS has advantages over existing treatment methods since it is reversible, and levels of stimulation can be tailored to the needs of the individual patient and stopped at the request of the patient.

However, these applications of DBS also raise a number of novel ethical issues that need to be resolved. Case 17.5 raises the issue that direct brain stimulation may change the nature of a person's desires; is this an impediment to autonomy? How is well-being and quality of life to be assessed during stimulation? What if a patient apparently continues to desire DBS, but treatment appears to have altered the patient's motivation or is causing other serious harm? This requires new ethical thinking around the nature of authenticity and autonomy; well-being; and how technology that directly affects the brain can undermine or augment agency (Maslen et al. 2018, Pugh, Maslen, and Savulescu 2017, Pugh et al. 2019).

(In the real case of DM, the patient (when the stimulator was switched off and he was judged to have capacity) decided that he would like the DBS to remain switched on, even if he needed to reside in a psychiatric institution.)

Questions of authenticity have also arisen relating to the use of DBS for the treatment of anorexia nervosa. Just as in the Parkinson's case, there may be significant changes in behaviour after treatment. Is the new behaviour authentic?

To be authentic is to live in accordance with one's 'true self'. The key question for a theory of authenticity is how we should identify those features that are 'true' and those that are peripheral. People tend to identify their positive and moral characteristics as true (Strohminger, Knobe, and Newman 2017).

According to the *essentialist* conception of authenticity, to live authentically is to live in accordance with this deep essence: the path to authenticity is one of *self-discovery* of this (usually positive) essence. Another view is the existentialist conception: to live authentically is to choose the person that one wishes to become, after reflection. There is no fixed essence, just what we rationally choose to be; this is also known as *self-creation.* The truth of essentialism is that we may have certain elements of our character that are more or less fixed, whereas the truth of existentialism is that we may be able to choose which of these elements to bring to the fore, and which to downplay in developing our selves (Erler and Hope 2014, Pugh, Maslen, and Savulescu 2017).

These different accounts have important implications for psychopharmacology and the modification of emotional traits (e.g. in DBS for anorexia). One criticism of antidepressants such as SSRIs (Selective Serotonin Reuptake Inhibitors) is that they undermine authenticity as understood by the essentialist conception (Elliott 2004), though others have responded that patients treated with SSRIs have discovered their 'true self' (Kramer 1997). According to the self-creation or existentialist view, we are free to recreate ourselves according to our values.

According to both the essentialist and existentialist models of authenticity, changes to a person's own character, desires, feelings or behaviour must be intelligible to that person. Interventions that serve to directly induce psychological changes, such as psychoactive drugs or DBS, may in some cases result in feelings of alienation, because they cause the patient to undergo changes that are unintelligible to them in the light of their other values and beliefs. The depressed patient who takes Prozac may feel alienated from their elevated mood if the drug serves only to increase their positive affect without engaging with other elements of the patient's character system that may play a role in their condition (such as apathy and feelings of worthlessness). This stands in contrast to indirect interventions that aim to evince changes in the patient's mood by rationally engaging with them, say, in talking therapy. Changes brought about via such interventions will more likely be intelligible to the patient in so far as they are brought about by changes that the patient herself has decided to make to her modes of thinking (Pugh, Maslen, and Savulescu 2017).

Authenticity has much in common with autonomy. Autonomy has become a central value in modern medical ethics. Today, people value authenticity because it plays a central role in 'giving meaning to their lives'. This understanding of the value of authenticity fits with Mill's famous observation that:

> If a person possesses any tolerable amount of common sense and experience, his own mode of laying out his existence is the best not because it is the best, but because it is his own mode. (Mill 2011)

MORAL BIOENHANCEMENT

One of the central elements of neuroethics is the neuroscience of moral decision-making. This involves trying to understand why people make the normative (including health) decisions they make, and what factors affect those decisions.

This began with the pioneering work of Joshua Greene studying the different neurobiological mechanisms in utilitarian versus deontological (rule-based) decisions relating to trolley problems (Edmonds 2015, Greene 2015), which now capture popular imagination in relation to driverless cars (Awad et al. 2018).

In Oxford, we have studied the effects of moral psychology on vaccination behaviour and during epidemics. For example, we have shown how uncertainty about impact on people has more effect on changing risky behaviour (including spreading infections) than uncertainty about the probability of a bad outcome occurring (Kappes et al. 2018). We have developed a scale for measuring how utilitarian people are (you can try it here: http://www.jimaceverett.com/test/oxford-utilitarianism-scale/). We have also been interested in the biological causes and effects on moral behaviour. Sylvia Terbeck showed that propranolol could reduce unconscious racism (Terbeck et al. 2012), and we outlined the side-effects of drugs that are commonly employed in medicine on moral decision-making (Levy et al. 2014).

Since 2008, the field of moral bioenhancement has become a topic of ethical debate (Douglas 2008, Persson and Savulescu 2008). This involves the use of biological interventions (drugs, transcranial electrical stimulation, brain–computer interfaces, etc.) to improve moral decision-making. Up for Debate Box 17.1 summarizes some of the arguments for and against moral enhancement.

Specifically, examples of moral bioenhancements include the following (see Earp, Douglas, and Savulescu (2018) for an overview):
1. exogenous administration of neurohormones such as oxytocin (in combination with appropriate psychological therapy or social modification) to potentially increase pro-social attitudes like trust, sympathy and generosity
2. alteration of serotonin or testosterone levels to mitigate undue aggression, while at the same time ostensibly enhancing fair-mindedness, willingness to cooperate and aversion to harming others
3. application of newly developed brain modulation techniques, such as non-invasive transcranial electric or magnetic stimulation, or even DBS via implanted electrodes, for example, to reduce impulsive violence by psychopaths.

More ecologically valid results pertain to the administration of methylphenidate or lithium to violent criminals with ADHD or to children with conduct disorders to reduce their aggressive behavioural tendencies, as well as the administration of antilibidinal agents to convicted sex offenders to reduce their sexual desire (see extension case below).

 Up for Debate Box 17.1 Should we pursue moral bioenhancement? (Persson and Savulescu 2012, Specker et al. 2014)

For
1. Human society faces a series of existential threats – threats that could wipe out human life on this planet. This includes terrorist use of dirty bombs or development of biological weapons, as well as the increasingly apparent dangers of pollution, climate change and resource depletion. Whilst education, institutions and good policing are important, we may need to think more radically.

Up for Debate Box 17.1 Should we pursue moral bioenhancement? (Specker et al. 2014) (Persson and Savulescu 2012)—cont'd

17

NEUROETHICS

2. We have been dramatically successful at modifying various moral characteristics of non-human animals. Over ten thousand years or so, we have turned wolves into dogs by selective breeding, and have turned those dogs into breeds with behavioural as well as physical characteristics. There is no reason, in principle, why humans could not be genetically modified using gene editing, or their brains modified in other ways, to make them kinder, happier, more conscientious, altruistic and just (Savulescu 2016). We are already morally modified. This is widely accepted when it comes to negative effects. For example, we all know that alcohol can lead people to behave in aggressive or other destructive ways that they would not have countenanced sober. There is also evidence that we can be morally modified in a more positive direction. For example, SSRIs (a class of drugs widely used to treat depression) like Prozac have been shown to make healthy volunteers more cooperative and less critical.

3. While there may be moral disagreement, there are many areas of agreement, for example, increased altruism and a reduction in unjustified bias.

4. Individual autonomy may already be compromised by our biology (for example, our preference for those like ourselves).

Against

1. Moral bioenhancement is a pipe dream: even if it is acceptable to do this, it is so unlikely to be achievable that it is not worth pursuing. Human psychology and biology are extremely complex. The idea that a simple intervention could improve moral behaviour is unrealistic.

2. We need the negative aspects of our human character. We need people who can fight wars. We need to be able to blot out the suffering of the wider world: to experience it as we would if it applied to our nearest and dearest would be unbearable.

3. Ethical debate in many areas is intractable. It will not be possible to reach consensus on what moral bioenhancement is desirable.

4. Moral bioenhancement might reduce or threaten the freedom of individuals – it might endanger individual autonomy.

5. There is a danger that such interventions would be abused.

REVISION QUESTIONS

1. Is addiction a disease? If addicts do not have free will, do they have the capacity to consent to treatment (e.g. to methadone prescription)? (See Charland (2002).)

2. Functional neuroimaging has shown that heroin addicts have different patterns of brain activation in response to stimuli. What does this imply about the cause of addiction?

3. Recent lab-based work with 'organoids' (neurons grown as 3-D structures in culture) have shown some electrical activity that is similar to patterns seen in extremely premature infants. What is the moral significance of consciousness in organoids? (See Koplin and Savulescu (2018).)

Continued

REVISION QUESTIONS—cont'd

4. A patient with long-standing anorexia consents to deep brain stimulation. This results in a significant improvement in her symptoms. She reports being happy with the results of the treatment. However, subsequently, she has a period when the DBS is switched off, and her symptoms of anorexia return. She no longer wishes for the DBS to be switched on. Which wishes are authentic? Whose wishes should be respected?

Extension case 17.6

Paedophiles throughout the world are sometimes chemically castrated using cyproterone acetate. This is sometimes obligatory, or can be administered in return for shortened prison sentences. Sometimes it is offered without any alteration in custodial sentence. In some jurisdictions (e.g. Czech Republic), surgical castration is employed.

Chemical castration is a form of crude moral bioenhancement. It not only aims to change immoral behaviour, but reduces motivation to do so. It raises many ethical issues.

The most basic principle of medical ethics is that doctors should offer interventions which are plausibly in the best interests of patients. Whether it is in a paedophile's overall interests will turn on the nature and centrality of sexual desire in the good life; the side-effects of medication; the role of social conformity in the good life; the impact of medication on the ability to function in work, wider social life and society; etc.

A second raft of issues surrounds autonomy. Would hormonal castration promote the autonomy of paedophiles? When chemical castration is offered in return for a shorter sentence, some have argued that this is coercive and undermines autonomy (McMillan 2013).

Justice requires weighing the interests of people. Even if hormonal castration harms paedophiles and undermines their autonomy, it might be justified according to principles of justice in virtue of its protective effects for innocent children. This raises issues of the justice of profiling and predicting risk which is commonly used in psychiatry (Douglas et al. 2017).

Should doctors chemically castrate paedophiles?

REFERENCES

Awad, E., Dsouza, S., Kim, R., Schulz, J., Henrich, J., Shariff, A., Bonnefon, J. F. and Rahwan, I. 2018. "The Moral Machine experiment." *Nature* 1: doi: 10.1038/s41586-018-0637-6.

Boly, M., Faymonville, M. E., Schnakers, C., Peigneux, P., Lambermont, B., Phillips, C., Lancellotti, P., Luxen, A., Lamy, M., Moonen, G., Maquet, P. and Laureys, S. 2008.

"Perception of pain in the minimally conscious state with PET activation: an observational study." *The Lancet. Neurology* 7 (11): 1013-20. doi: 10.1016/S1474-4422(08)70219-9.

Bruno, M. A., Bernheim, J. L., Ledoux, D., Pellas, F., Demertzi, A. and Laureys, S. 2011. "A survey on self-assessed well-being in a cohort of chronic locked-in syndrome patients: happy majority, miserable minority." *BMJ Open* 1 (1): doi: 10.1136/bmjopen-2010-000039. e000039.

Charland, L. C. 2002. "Cynthia's dilemma: consenting to heroin prescription." *The American Journal of Bioethics* 2 (2): 37-47. doi: 10.1162/152651602317533686.

Davies, W., Savulescu, J. and Roache, R. forthcoming. *Rethinking the biopsychosocial model*. Oxford: Oxford University Press.

Douglas, T., Pugh, J., Singh, I., Savulescu, J. and Fazel, S. 2017. "Risk assessment tools in criminal justice and forensic psychiatry: The need for better data." *European Psychiatry* 42: 134-7. doi: 10.1016/j.eurpsy.2016.12.009.

Douglas, T. 2008. "Moral enhancement." *Journal of Applied Philosophy* 25: 228-45.

Earp, B. D., Douglas, T. and Savulescu, J. 2018. "Moral neuroenhancement." In *The Routledge handbook of neuroethics*, edited by L. Syd, M. Johnson and K. S. Rommelfanger. New York: Routledge: 166-84.

Earp, B. D., Wudarczyk, O. A., Foddy, B. and Savulescu, J. 2017. "Addicted to love: what is love addiction and when should it be treated?" *Philosophy, Psychiatry, & Psychology: PPP* 24 (1): 77-92.

Edmonds, D. 2015. *Would you kill the fat man?: the trolley problem and what your answer tells us about right and wrong*. Princeton: Princeton University Press.

Elliott, C. 2004. *Better than well: American medicine meets the American dream*. New York: W.W. Norton & Company.

Erler, A. and Hope, T. 2014. "Mental disorder and the concept of authenticity." *Philosophy, Psychiatry, & Psychology* 21 (3): 219-32.

Foddy, B. and Savulescu, J. 2010. "A liberal account of addiction." *Philosophy, Psychiatry, & Psychology* 17 (1): 1-22. doi: 10.1353/ppp.0.0282.

Greene, J. 2015. Moral tribes: emotion, reason and the gap between us and them.

Heyman, G. M. 2009. *Addiction: a disorder of choice*. Cambridge, Mass.: Harvard University Press.

Highfield, R. 2014. "Reading the minds of the "dead"." *BBC Future*, 22 April 2014.

Hyman, S. E. 2005. "Addiction: a disease of learning and memory." *The American Journal of Psychiatry* 162 (8): 1414-22. doi: 10.1176/appi.ajp.162.8.1414.

Kahane, G. and Savulescu, J. 2009. "Brain damage and the moral significance of consciousness." *The Journal of Medicine and Philosophy* 34 (1): 6-26.

Kappes, A., Nussberger, A. M., Faber, N. S., Kahane, G., Savulescu, J. and Crockett, M. J. 2018. "Uncertainty about the impact of social decisions increases prosocial behaviour." *Nature Human Behaviour* 2: 573-80.

Kompanje, E. J., de Beaufort, I. D. and Bakker, J. 2007. "Euthanasia in intensive care: a 56-year-old man with a pontine hemorrhage resulting in a locked-in syndrome." *Critical Care Medicine* 35 (10): 2428-30.

Koplin, J. and Savulescu, J. 2018. "Fresh urgency in mapping out ethics of brain organoid research." The Conversation, accessed 26/11/18. https://theconversation.com/fresh-urgency-in-mapping-out-ethics-of-brain-organoid-research-107186.

Kraemer, F. 2013. "Authenticity or autonomy? When deep brain stimulation causes a dilemma." *Journal of Medical Ethics* 39: 757-60.

Kramer, P. 1997. *Listening to Prozac: a psychiatrist explores antidepressant drugs and the remaking of the self*. New York: Penguin Books.

Laureys, S., Pellas, F., Van Eeckhout, P., Ghorbel, S., Schnakers, C., Perrin, F., Berré, J., Faymonville, M. E., Pantke, K. H., Damas, F., Lamy, M., Moonen, G. and Goldman, S. 2005. "The locked-in syndrome : what is it like to be conscious but paralyzed and voiceless?" *Progress in Brain Research* 150: 495-511. doi: 10.1016/S0079-6123(05)50034-7.

Leshner, A. I. 1997. "Addiction is a brain disease, and it matters." *Science* 278 (5335): 45-7.

Leshner, A. I. 1999. "Science-based views of drug addiction and its treatment." *JAMA: The Journal of the American Medical Association* 282 (14): 1314-6.

Levy, N., Douglas, T., Kahane, G., Terbeck, S., Cowen, P. J., Hewstone, M. and Savulescu, J. 2014. "Are you morally modified?: the moral effects of widely used pharmaceuticals." *Philosophy, Psychiatry, & Psychology* 21: 111-25. doi: 10.1353/ppp.2014.0023.

Maslen, H., Cheeran, B., Pugh, J., Pycroft, L., Boccard, S., Prangnell, S., Green, A. L., FitzGerald, J., Savulescu, J. and Aziz, T. 2018. "Unexpected complications of novel deep brain stimulation treatments: ethical issues and clinical recommendations." *Neuromodulation* 21: 135-43. doi: 10.1111/ner.12613.

McMillan, J. 2014. "The kindest cut? Surgical castration, sex offenders and coercive offers." *Journal of Medical Ethics* doi: 10.1136/medethics-2012-101030.

Mill, J. S. 2011. *On Liberty*. Luton: Andrews UK Limited.

Owen, A. M., Coleman, M. R., Boly, M., Davis, M. H., Laureys, S. and Pickard, J. D. 2006. "Detecting awareness in the vegetative state." *Science* 313 (5792): 1402. doi: 10.1126/science.1130197.

Perring, C. 2002. "Resisting the temptations of addiction rhetoric." *The American Journal of Bioethics* 2 (2): 51-2. doi: 10.1162/152651602317533712.

Persson, I. and Savulescu, J. 2008. "The perils of cognitive enhancement and the urgent imperative to enhance the moral character of humanity." *Journal of Applied Philosophy* 25: 162-77.

Persson, I. and Savulescu, J. 2012. *Unfit for the future : the need for moral enhancement.* Oxford: Oxford University Press.

Pugh, J., Maslen, H. and Savulescu, J. 2017. "Deep brain stimulation, authenticity and value." *Cambridge Quarterly of Healthcare Ethics* 26: 640-57. doi: 10.1017/S0963180117000147.

Pugh, J., Pycroft, L., Maslen, H., Aziz, T. and Savulescu, J. 2019. "Evidence-based neuroethics, deep brain stimulation and personality – deflating, but not bursting, the bubble." *Neuroethics.*

Roache, R. and Savulescu, J. 2018. "Psychological disadvantage and a welfarist approach to psychiatry: an alternative to the DSM paradigm." *Philosophy, Psychiatry, & Psychology* 25: 245-59.

Sandel, M. 2012. *What money can't buy: the moral limits of markets.* Farrar, Strauss, and Giroux.

Savulescu, J. 2016. "Why we should fine-tune the DNA of future generations." *Cosmos Magazine,* 17 August 2016.

Savulescu, J. 2018. "Golden opportunity, reasonable risk and personal responsibility for health." *Journal of Medical Ethics* 44 (1): 59-61. doi: 10.1136/medethics-2017-104428.

Savulescu, J. and Earp, B. D. 2014. "Neuroreductionism about sex and love." *Think (London, England)* 13 (38): 7-12. doi: 10.1017/S1477175614000128.

Specker, J., Focquaert, F., Raus, K., Sterckx, S. and Schermer, M. 2014. "The ethical desirability of moral bioenhancement: a review of reasons." *BMC Medical Ethics* 15 (1): 67. doi: 10.1186/1472-6939-15-67.

Strohminger, N., Knobe, J. and Newman, G. 2017. "The true self: a psychological concept distinct from the self." *Perspectives on Psychological Science* 12 (4): 551-60. doi: 10.1177/1745691616689495.

Terbeck, S., Kahane, G., McTavish, S., Savulescu, J., Cowen, P. J. and Hewstone, M. 2012. "Propranolol reduces implicit negative racial bias." *Psychopharmacology* 222: 419-24. doi: 10.1007/s00213-012-2657-5.

W v. M [2011] EWHC 2443 [Fam].

Chapter 18

Genethics

Advances in genetics and genomics have led to grand claims about the impact on the practice of medicine – as well as leading to widespread ethical concerns. However, few of the ethical issues discussed in the context of medical genetics are unique; many overlap with issues that we have covered in earlier chapters. We will consider here some of the more distinctive ethical issues relevant to modern medical genetics: genetic confidentiality, genetic information (including incidental findings), reproductive choice, gene editing (GE), cloning and mitochondrial transfer.

GENETIC INFORMATION AND CONFIDENTIALITY

Case 18.1

Mrs R has been diagnosed with breast cancer. She has a family history of breast cancer, and genetic testing reveals that she carries the autosomal dominant cancer gene *BRCA1*. Mrs R has a large extended family, including a number of young women who may be at risk of early-onset breast cancer. However, Mrs R does not get on well with her family, and does not wish them to be informed of their genetic risk.

Should Mrs R's doctors breach her confidentiality to alert other family members?

In Chapter 9, we discussed issues of confidentiality and genetic testing. The case of ABC v St George's Healthcare [2017] (Huntington's disease in a family member, Case 9.3) suggests that doctors may, in some cases, have a legal duty to pass genetic information on to family members.

In the absence of any specific legislation or case law concerning genetic confidentiality, the law could take several approaches. Herring (2018, pp. 260-3), for example, suggests the following options:

1. *The traditional confidentiality approach.* According to this approach, only where there is a high risk of significant harm to another would a breach of confidentiality be justifiable. Factors to be taken into account in reaching a decision would therefore include the risk of Mrs R's relatives suffering from the illness, the severity of the illness, the availability of a cure or treatment and so on.

2. *A human rights approach.* Under a rights-based approach, the central question would be the extent to which the exception contained in Article 8(2) of the Human Rights Act would justify breaching confidentiality. Very strong reasons would be required to justify disclosure, given that genetic information might be regarded as even more private than other medical information, because it is related to arguably the most intimate part of a person.

3. *A property approach.* Such an approach reflects a widely held belief that a person's genetic information belongs not just to them, but also to their relatives. This means that Mrs R's relatives could claim (under the Data Protection Act 1998) that information about Mrs R is information about them.

4. *A public health approach.* This would focus on what response would promote public health generally. It might be argued that delaying testing and treatment for the family will impose extra costs on the NHS, and that it would be more cost-effective to tell them now.

Parker and Lucassen (2004) propose an alternative model for genetic information: the 'joint account model'. This is similar to the property approach. According to this model, 'genetic information is shared by more than one person, much like information about a joint bank account' (Parker and Lucassen 2004). Thus, the analogy is that, when a patient asks a doctor not to reveal information to family members, it is like someone asking their bank manager not to reveal information about a joint account to fellow account holders.

The best approach in Mrs R's case would be to gain the patient's consent to inform her relatives of genetic information that may be important to them. If she cannot be persuaded to share information, the General Medical Council (GMC) view that a breach of confidentiality is justified 'where failure to do so may expose the patient or others to risk of death or serious harm', may support alerting her relatives.

Case 18.2

John and Sarah attend the genetics clinic after the diagnosis of an autosomal recessive condition in their newborn baby. The disorder is severe and debilitating, and there is a high chance that the child will die in the first year. The couple have genetic tests to establish risks for future children. These tests show that John is not the biological father of the child.

Case 18.2 cont'd

Should the geneticist disclose the finding of non-paternity to the parents when they come back to the clinic as part of their ongoing counselling? Although they did not seek information about paternity, it is of direct relevance to their understanding of the probability of an affected child in future pregnancies (Lucassen and Parker 2001).

Genetic tests often raise issues of confidentiality that are unusual with other medical tests. The geneticist in Case 18.2 may be tempted to tell a white lie to John and let Sarah know the implications of the test. Lucassen and Parker (2001) argue against this practice, on the grounds both that it does not sufficiently respect the man's interest in knowing the facts, and that it is contrary to the principle that doctors should not lie to patients, except in most unusual circumstances.

GENETIC TESTING AND INFORMATION

Genetic tests are medical tests. One thing that makes them unusual (although not unique) is that some forms of testing (particularly whole genome or whole exome screening) may provide information about health conditions other than the one being investigated, as well as about risk in the distant future.

Case 18.3

Barbara participates in a genetic research study investigating the genetics of multiple sclerosis (her son is affected by this condition). She has whole genome sequencing as part of the study.

Several months after the study, Barbara is contacted by the researchers. Her genomic test has identified something unrelated to her son's condition. She is a carrier of a dominant mutation in the PSEN (presenilin) 1 gene. This is a gene associated with early-onset Alzheimer's disease, and she has almost a 100% chance of developing this condition. There is no treatment or prevention available. Barbara is devastated by the information.

Should this genetic test result have been revealed?

This case is based on Easler and Rivard (2013).

Whole genome analysis can identify the risks of developing major and minor disorders, now, but also in the medium- and long-term. It can provide information about disorders which are preventable, treatable or neither treatable nor preventable. Should such information be provided?

The traditional (paternalistic) approach has been only to reveal information relevant to a disease under investigation, or only one which is treatable or preventable in the future.

Incidental findings are genomic, radiological or other test results which are secondary to the disease under investigation. In 2013, and later in 2015 and 2016, the American College of Medical Genetics and Genomics published recommendations about reporting incidental findings. They identified (as of 2018) mutations in 59 genes that they believed should be reported because of their importance (Kalia et al. 2016). Some of these identify conditions which are neither treatable nor preventable. These include various genetic disorders, inherited cardiovascular conditions (including cardiomyopathies and arrhythmias) and inherited cancers (though the list does not include the PSEN1 gene).

One reason given not to disclose incidental findings is the so-called 'right not to know'. Barbara's case is a good example. She may have preferred not to know that she will develop early-onset dementia. On the basis of interests, privacy and autonomy, people may have a right not to know such information. However, such information may also be important to career planning, retirement, family planning (including prenatal and pre-implantation genetic diagnosis) and for other reasons (Shkedi-Rafid et al. 2014). It can facilitate autonomy. Recently, there have been arguments for a comprehension standard, which proposes that findings should be disclosed according to the patient's ability to comprehend them (Schaefer and Savulescu 2018).

Perhaps what is most important is that, before undertaking a genomic test, there is a discussion with the patient about incidental findings. Ideally, patients should be given choice over what range of findings they wish to be informed of. The situation is more complicated in children (and infants, fetuses and embryos).

Such predictive information has implications for insurance, particularly life insurance. It is important that the implications are made clear prior to undertaking a genomic test. In 2018, a Code on Genetic Testing in Insurance was agreed by the British government and the Association of British Insurers. The code commits insurance companies to:

1. Treat applicants fairly and not require or pressure any applicant to undertake a predictive or diagnostic genetic test
2. Not ask for, or take into account the result of, a predictive genetic test, except when the life insurance is over £500,000 and the applicant has had a predictive genetic test for Huntington's Disease
3. Not ask for, or take into account, the result of any predictive genetic test obtained through scientific research.

Adults lacking capacity

The same principles apply to genetic testing as to other medical testing in adults lacking capacity (see Chapter 7). On rare occasions, it may be desirable to perform genetic testing on incompetent adults solely for the benefit of members of the family. The British Medical Association (BMA) has stated that this may be ethically justified (1998), taking account of the following factors:

1. The potential harm of the test to the individual
2. The degree of harm or benefit to others
3. Any previous expressed wishes of the incompetent individual
4. Whether the information can be obtained by other means, e.g. testing other relatives
5. Whether there are grounds for believing that most competent adults would wish to help others in this way.

The BMA notes that such testing of incompetent people, even if ethically justified, may constitute battery in law (unless it is carried out according to the principles of the Mental Capacity Act 2005). If time permits, it would be desirable to obtain court authorization for such testing. The testing of previously obtained specimens, or of specimens obtained for therapeutic purposes, would not be battery, and may be lawful as long as any relevant provisions in the Human Tissue Act 2004 are followed.

Genetic testing and children

Case 18.4

Peter has a genetic condition (familial adenomatous polyposis, FAP) that is associated with a high risk of colonic polyps and needs close surveillance with regular colonoscopies. Both Peter and his father had bowel surgery in their 20s.

Peter has requested that his 1-year-old son Ethan has testing for this condition. He has indicated that, if the geneticists will not do the test, he will seek testing from other clinics, or online.

Should the test be performed?

This case is based on one in the BSHG report (British Society for Human Genetics 2010).

Should predictive testing be carried out on children, or should such tests be offered only once the person is adult and can decide for herself (Robertson and Savulescu 2001, Savulescu 2001a)? The British Society for Human Genetics (2010), like other professional bodies, has recommended a cautious approach: advising against genetic testing in childhood for adult-onset conditions (unless surveillance, pre-emptive medical treatment or definitive medical treatment is available during childhood). In general, testing should be deferred, to give the child the opportunity to make a decision about testing. However, the guidelines acknowledge that there may be particular children and families where the benefits of earlier testing would outweigh the risks.

In Case 18.4, testing might be delayed until Ethan is 9 or 10 (when colonoscopies would need to begin if he has the gene). However, it seems unlikely that Ethan will be able to meaningfully engage in the decision at that stage (if he refused testing, it is likely that it would be regarded as in his best interests to override him). In practice, almost all at-risk adults elect to have the genetic test for familial adenomatous polyposis (FAP). On that basis, it may be ethical to undertake the testing now for Ethan.

Case 18.4 also raises the challenge for regulators in the current era. Direct-to-consumer testing for a wide range of genes (including for FAP) is readily available on the internet. Although professional guidelines might try to limit tests undertaken by doctors, families may choose to circumvent those limits.

REPRODUCTIVE CHOICE

Genetics allied to modern reproductive technologies can potentially provide would-be parents with enormous reproductive choice. What should be the limits on such choice? We will consider three issues: prenatal selection in general, sex selection in particular and the issue of whether reproductive choice can amount to discrimination against the disabled.

Prenatal genetic testing

Prenatal genetic tests aim to detect genetic abnormalities such as cystic fibrosis in an embryo or fetus, with a view to termination of pregnancy or, in the case of preimplantation diagnosis, to be used to guide selection of an embryo for implantation. Box 18.1 outlines some ethical issues raised by the possibility of prenatal genetic testing.

Case 18.5

Mr and Mrs Whittaker have a young child, Charlie, with a rare autosomal recessive genetic disorder causing bone marrow failure. The only hope of cure for Charlie is for him to have a bone marrow transplant; however, neither parent is a match. Mr and Mrs Whittaker want another child. Although the condition affecting Charlie is not inherited, they wish to have IVF in the hope that the new baby might be able to donate stem cells for Charlie.

Is it ethical for parents to use IVF to select a 'saviour sibling'?
This is based on a real case (Levin 2011).

There have been several legal cases involving the issue of 'saviour siblings'. This situation occurs when a child who exists has a serious condition that could be treated through a bone marrow or umbilical cord stem cell transplant from a close relative with compatible tissue.

In the case of the Whittaker family, the HFEA (Human Fertilisation Embryology Authority) declined permission for the in-vitro fertilization (IVF) clinic to select a saviour sibling. (The family travelled overseas to access treatment, and Charlie later received a bone marrow transplant from his brother's cord stem cells.) The HFEA later changed its policy. In Quintavalle v HFEA [2005], the House of Lords unanimously agreed that a treatment license could be granted (i.e. one designed to produce a child who would be a compatible tissue donor).

Sex selection

What limits, if any, should be placed on reproductive choice? This question is particularly pertinent as more and more genetic tests become available for minor abnormalities and for characteristics that are not disease states at all, such as physical and intellectual abilities or psychological characteristics. One key example is sex selection. Should couples be allowed to select the sex of their child?

The issue of sex selection has taken on greater significance with the advent of non-invasive prenatal testing (NIPT), since couples may identify fetal sex early in pregnancy (and may do so through direct-to-consumer tests). There have been claims that NIPT is being used for sex-selective abortions. This led the Nuffield Council to recommend not reporting sex in NIPT results unless there was a concern about sex chromosome disorders (Nuffield Council on Bioethics 2017).

Box 18.1 Four ethical issues raised by prenatal genetic testing

The ethics of termination of pregnancy

At this point in time, the only intervention available to prevent a child being born with a genetic disorder is termination of the pregnancy. Those who have objections to abortion are likely to be opposed to prenatal testing (see Chapter 13). Preimplantation genetic testing, followed by embryo selection, does not require termination of a pregnancy, although it does usually involve the use of IVF and discarding embryos, which may be of concern for those who believe that early embryos have full moral status.

Which conditions should be tested for?

Termination of pregnancy, or embryo selection, following genetic testing is normally limited to either chromosomal abnormalities, such as Down's syndrome, or single-gene disorders, such as cystic fibrosis or Duchenne muscular dystrophy. How significant should the disability be in order to justify either termination of pregnancy or embryo selection? Is it for the parents to decide, and, if so, should there be any restrictions on the grounds used for their decision? Should parents be allowed to select any embryo on the basis of its sex (see text), and should they be able to choose an embryo whose genetic profile suggests that the child is likely to have what they see as desirable characteristics (e.g. high intelligence), or to avoid what they see as undesirable characteristics (e.g. aggressive behaviour, colour blindness)? Should testing for adult-onset conditions be permitted? (If such testing is permitted, and a pregnancy is continued, that may breach the child/future adult's right not to know – see main text.)

Cost-effectiveness

Should prenatal genetic testing be evaluated for its cost-effectiveness, and, if so, what should the outcome measures be? Some argue that clinical genetics is about providing education and choice, and so it is difficult to evaluate its cost-effectiveness. Others argue that the reduction in the proportion of people born with disability is an important outcome, and the savings from not having to treat disability can be included in the evaluation of its cost-effectiveness (Beaudet 1990).

Public health and coercion

Is public health, or the public interest, a legitimate goal of clinical genetics? Should the state encourage, or even enforce, genetic testing in some circumstances for the purpose of reducing the number of people born with some disease or disability?

Consider testing for the carrier state of thalassaemia in Cyprus, where the Church must authorize marriage. Prior to such authorization, couples must have thalassaemia carrier testing. There is no obligation to have prenatal diagnosis on the basis of the result. However, the vast majority of those tested choose to have prenatal diagnosis, and today virtually no babies with thalassaemia are born in Cyprus.

There is an element of coercion in the carrier testing programme in Cyprus, as people who want to marry must have such testing. However, the programme increases informed decision-making about reproduction, and thus increases autonomy. The carrier testing programme is also in the public interest. Some would argue that coercion may be justified in the public interest if:

- there is a significant health problem
- the intervention will be an effective way of promoting the public interest
- there is no effective, or less coercive, alternative.

However, sex is regularly reported using other prenatal tests, and there is no legal ban on providing such information.

Up for Debate Box 18.1 summarizes some of the arguments for and against prohibiting sex selection.

Discrimination against the disabled

Prenatal diagnosis followed by termination of pregnancy, or embryo selection, has been the object of considerable criticism on the general grounds that it discriminates against the disabled (for further discussion of disability, see Chapter 12). Newell (1994) has claimed that prenatal diagnosis is 'a technology of oppression and control' which 'devalues' the lives of those with disabilities. We will consider three arguments in support of this view (Buchanan et al. 2000).

The expressivist objection

According to this objection, prenatal testing and pregnancy termination express a negative judgement about the life value of people with impairments. For example, this argument has been used by people who argue that screening for Down syndrome involves prejudice and failure to respect diversity and inclusion.

There are two responses to these arguments. The first is that it conflates judgements about people with impairments and judgements about impairments.

Up for Debate Box 18.1 Should sex selection be prohibited?

For
1. Sex should not be a reason to value one person over another.
2. Sex selection may contribute to gender stereotyping and overall gender discrimination.
3. Sex selection may lead to imbalance in the population between males/females.
4. It is morally wrong to terminate a pregnancy purely on the basis of the sex of the fetus.
5. It may represent a misuse of limited medical resources – in the use of IVF/prenatal testing and pregnancy termination.

Against
1. We should respect couples' procreative autonomy. In many jurisdictions, women are permitted to terminate a pregnancy (at least early in pregnancy) for a wide range of reasons not relating to the well-being of the fetus.
2. Sex selection would not necessarily lead to sex imbalance. Some 90% of couples in the West who come forward for sex selection do so in order to balance sex within the family, and in both the US and the UK, just over half of such couples choose a girl (Batzofin 1987, Lui and Rose 1995).
3. Discrimination against women should be tackled through changing the social and legal arrangements that result in such discrimination, rather than through controlling reproduction (Savulescu 2001b).
4. Sex selection is not a misallocation of medical resources if it is funded privately.
5. There is no evidence of harm to the child from sex selection (who, in any case, would not otherwise exist; see Chapter 13).

We can have a negative attitude towards deafness (and seek to prevent it) without having a negative attitude towards people who are deaf. People with impairments can lead full and worthwhile lives, and are clearly entitled to equal concern and respect, but that does not imply that we cannot value impairments negatively.

The second response is to argue that the expressivist objection assumes that embryos or fetuses are persons with a right to life, and that selection through prenatal testing is like eliminating impairments by killing children or adults. This is a controversial assumption (see Chapter 13). Indeed, more than 95% of terminations are for social reasons, and not on the basis of impairment. Imagine that a woman decides to have an abortion because she is unemployed and has insufficient financial resources: this does not express a view that it is better to be dead than poor.

Loss of support argument

According to this argument, a reduction in the number of people with impairments will result in a loss of public support for those with impairment. There is little empirical evidence to support this claim (the opposite might be the case, as a reduction in the number of individuals with a particular disability may mean that there is more funding available per person). Indeed, increased resources were given to those with thalassaemia in Greece following the introduction of carrier testing (Politis 1998). Moreover, the appropriate response to the loss of support argument is to devote more resources to those with the relevant disability and to increase public education (to reduce bias and prejudice against them).

GENE THERAPY AND GENE EDITING

Case 18.6

A 44-year-old man, BM, with an inherited genetic metabolic disorder (Hunter syndrome) currently requires regular injections of an enzyme that he is missing. The enzyme is rapidly degraded, and he requires weekly injections. BM enrols in a trial of a new gene therapy. It involves injection of a viral vector that inserts a copy of the missing gene into his own liver cells. The modified liver cells will then produce the missing enzyme.

Are therapeutic gene modifications ethical (Kaiser 2017)?

Above, we have discussed genetic testing and genetic selection. However, recent scientific advances raise the prospect of editing the genome of existing or future people. The most powerful current GE technology is the CRISPR-Cas9 system. In 2012, a team at UC Berkeley showed that CRISPR-Cas9 could be modified in the lab so that it could target virtually any DNA sequence. This allowed researchers to cut DNA anywhere in the genome. Furthermore, they demonstrated that, after the DNA was cut, DNA repair mechanisms could be recruited to add novel genetic material to the site of the cut. This gave researchers the ability to delete, add or modify DNA sequences.

Gene therapy for existing patients (like in Case 18.6) tends to raise issues that are similar to other therapies – for example issues relating to the use of experimental treatments, the possibility of side-effects and the costs of the therapy. While gene therapies are still in their early stages, there have been some success stories (Mendell et al. 2017).

GE of embryos might be thought to be different, however. In 2015, a lab based in China caused a massive uproar when it was the first to use GE on human embryos. Scientists and public interest groups in the US called for an international ban on any GE research in human embryos. *Nature* published a commentary calling for such research to be strongly discouraged. The US-based National Institutes of Health said that such research 'was a line that should not be crossed'. However, recently, groups like the Nuffield Council of Bioethics have argued that GE could be used if it promotes human well-being and social solidarity (Bioethics 2018). As mentioned in Chapter 16, in November 2018 a Chinese researcher was reported to have used GE to edit a gene, thereby leading to HIV resistance, in a pair of twins (Marchione 2018).

Should we manipulate human DNA?

Case 18.7

A couple who are both carriers for a severe autosomal recessive single-gene disorder have had a previous child affected by the illness. They use IVF to conceive; however, they have limited success. The only viable embryo available for transfer has the genetic disorder.

They ask whether gene editing could be used to undo the mutation in their embryo. Would gene modification in an embryo be ethical?

Six reasons in favour of editing human DNA

1. Therapeutic gene editing – understand and treat disease

    GE of human embryos could be used to gain greater understanding of disease and new treatments. For example, gene-edited embryos could be used to study human development and the origin of disease. They could be used to create embryonic stem cell lines that themselves contain gene-edits that cause or protect against disease, to study the way disease occurs. Or they could be used to create stem cells with edited genes which could be used to treat disease, for example, blood cells that kill and replace leukaemic cells.

    There are valid concerns about applying GE to create live-born babies at present (as requested in Case 18.7 and as allegedly performed in Case 16.5), because of off-target mutations – where the technique introduces genetic damage in other areas of the genome. But such reproductive applications could be banned, and the technology could be used for therapeutic research, to understand disease and develop new treatments. As we understand more about this technology, the constraints on it could be relaxed.

2. Cure single-gene disorders

    Further into the future, once the safety concerns have been addressed, reproductive GE could be used to cure genetic diseases like cystic fibrosis or thalassaemia major. At present, there are no cures for such diseases. They cause much suffering and early death. Objectors say that genetic selection of healthy embryos or fetuses is preferable. But such genetic testing requires either abortion or embryo destruction, which is objectionable to some.

Moreover, genetic selection does not benefit anyone – it is not a cure. It merely brings a different person into existence who is disease-free. Future people will be grateful if their disease is cured, rather than their being replaced by a different (healthier or non-disabled) person. (In Case 18.7, if the embryo were successfully treated, they would have benefited from the therapy.) GE is the ultimate cure for genetic disorders.

3. Address polygenic predisposition to common diseases

Most common human diseases, like heart disease or schizophrenia, have not one gene which is abnormal (such as in Huntington disease or cystic fibrosis), but are the result of many, sometimes hundreds, of genes combining together with environmental effects. Such polygenic diseases are among the world's biggest killers. It is not possible to use genetic selection technologies to eliminate such common genetic dispositions to disease.

As genome editing technologies can target many genes at one time, it may become possible to use them to reduce an individual's polygenic risk at the embryonic stage.

4. Delay aging

The fourth reason is related. Each day, 100,000 people die from age-related causes. Aging kills 30 million people every year. It is the most under-researched cause of death and suffering relative to its significance.

Human aging could be delayed or arrested by GE. This has been achieved in mice. The genetically modified Methuselah mouse lives twice as long as a normal mouse. There are also mice that have been genetically engineered to be resistant to cancer or obesity. GE might offer the prospects of humans living twice as long, or perhaps even for hundreds of years, without loss of memory, frailty or impotence.

5. Correct natural inequality

Most human characteristics, including personality, have a substantial genetic contribution (often up to or exceeding 50%). Some are born gifted and talented, whereas others have short, painful lives or severe disabilities. While we may legitimately worry about the creation of a genetic master race, we should also be concerned about those who draw the short genetic straw. Currently, diet, education, special services and other social interventions are used to correct natural inequality. GE could be used as a part of public health care for egalitarian reasons: to benefit the worst off.

6. Human enhancement

GE could in the future be used to confer resistance to disease. In 2016, the same Chinese groups which first gene-edited a human embryo attempted to engineer HIV resistance using a natural mutation. This mutation, which modifies an immune-cell gene called CCR5, makes humans that carry it resistant to the HIV virus (Kang et al. 2016). (As noted in Chapter 16, in late 2018, there were unconfirmed reports that two infants had been born after GE of the CCR5 gene).

As discussed in the previous chapter, moral bioenhancement might help to address some of the unprecedented challenges facing humanity.

Objections to gene editing

1. Genetic selection is sufficient

    Given the ability to diagnose genetic disorders in the early embryo, some may feel that gene therapy is unnecessary. However, PGD (Preimplantation Genetic Diagnosis) has significant limitations. Its ability to avoid disease is directly related to the number of embryos that can be created through IVF. As in Case 18.7 above, sometimes couples will produce only one or two embryos, in which case PGD will not be effective for avoiding even simple genetic diseases.

    Moreover, genetic selection is of limited value currently in dealing with polygenic conditions. Under a reasonable set of assumptions, a typical couple would be capable of having a child with 15 of the 20 genes that contribute to the polygenic trait (in many cases, having 15 of the 20 genes would be enough to have a significant effect on phenotype). The chance of a couple having such a child would be just over 1% with traditional IVF plus selection (Bourne, Douglas, and Savulescu 2012). However, GE can be used to make multiple changes to a single embryo.

2. Design by another

    As human beings, we each have a unique identity, and a very important part of it, is our biological inheritance, our genetic identity. If we are designed by somebody else, then, in an important way, we are an instrument of that person's will. This is the argument of the German philosopher Jürgen Habermas (Habermas 2003). He said that you have to have non-contingent origins; that is, you have to come into existence through chance, in order to be free, in order to feel that at any point in your life you can go back and remake yourself. If somebody has designed you, then you are not free, and you are not equal to the designer. So, the right to equality is infringed. Another philosopher, the late Hans Jonas, argued that embryos have a right to an open future – that right may be compromised by genetic modification (Jonas 1974).

    One response is that whether parents constrain a child's freedom is not necessarily determined by the genes that they started life with. Modifying a child's genes may actually give a child a more open future (for example, by removing the negative effect of a serious genetic disorder). What would constrain a child's freedom is if his parents 'hyper-parent' the child, for example, by forcing them to develop a particular interest or skill. That is indeed a terrible thing to happen to child, but it is to do with parents' behaviour, not the genes that a child is born with.

3. Genetic essentialism

    At the heart of objections to GE is often a kind of 'genetic essentialism' or genetic determinism: that we are our genes, and by changing our genes, we are changing ourselves in some fundamental sense. This may or may not be the case. If genetic modification were to change fundamental aspects of personality and character, it might change identity. But for lesser degrees of modification, it would not change identity. Giving a child a better memory or better impulse control is not changing that child's identity.

4. Inequality

Lee Silver predicted that cloning might result in two separate human species emerging. Concerns of genetic inequality and discrimination are the heart of public concern about new genetics, as depicted in the film *Gattaca*, which involved genetic selection.

However, if GE were targeted at natural genetic inequality, it would reduce existing inequality. Secondly, whenever new therapies are developed, they might increase inequality because they are only available to the rich. However, the response to that should be to make them available to the poor – not to prevent them from being used (see Chapter 10).

5. Loss of diversity

A final common objection to GE is that it will reduce genetic diversity. This could be bad in two ways. First, it could reduce our resistance to new infectious threats. Secondly, loss of genetic diversity could compromise the social integration and functioning of society. Some mix of genetic traits may be best for society overall. For example, it may be better that there is a distribution of IQ; or a range of responses of empathy; or a mixture of introverts and extroverts. Whether this is true is an empirical issue. Moreover, one would have to balance the social advantages against the personal advantages or disadvantages in terms of well-being.

CLONING (FIG. 18.1)

Case 18.8

A scientist proposes to develop a source of patient-matched stem cells as a treatment for Parkinson's disease. This would involve taking a somatic cell from an affected patient and transferring the nucleus into a donated egg (which had had its nucleus removed) – a process called somatic cell nuclear transfer. This egg is then stimulated to develop into an early embryo that will be genetically virtually identical to the patient (a clone). At a very early stage of development, embryonic stem cells would be removed from the cloned embryo to be used to develop treatment. The embryo would be destroyed.

Would therapeutic cloning be ethical?

A cloned cell has a genome that is a near-identical copy of the genome of its parent or 'progenitor' cell. There are two methods of genome cloning: fission and fusion (Box 18.2) (Savulescu 2005). Cloning can be divided into *therapeutic cloning* and *reproductive cloning*. Therapeutic cloning involves using cloning processes to produce embryonic stem cells, tissues or whole organs for research and transplantation (Case 18.8 is an example of this). Reproductive cloning is the use of cloning to grow a living person who shares the DNA of the progenitor.

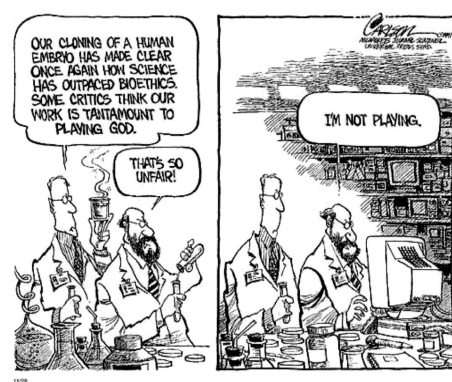

Figure 18.1 Cloning (© Stuart Carlson, reproduced with permission)

Box 18.2 Two methods of cloning

Cloning by fission

Blastocyst division

Twinning is induced in a blastocyst by the application of heat or mechanical stress. The blastocyst splits in two, and the two halves continue to grow into complete embryos. At most, two identical embryos can be created using this method.

Blastomere separation

The coating of an early embryo (blastocyst) is removed, and the cells (blastomeres) are placed in a solution that separates them. Each of these blastomeres is undifferentiated and can grow into an embryo. This technique can produce eight embryos at most, but can be repeated for each new embryo to produce larger number of cloned embryos.

Cloning by fusion

Fusion is achieved through the process of somatic cell nuclear transfer (SCNT). The nucleus is removed from a somatic cell and implanted into the cytoplasm of a denucleated egg. The egg reprogrammes the somatic cell's DNA so that a complete embryo can be grown out of this cell. Using this technique, a theoretically endless number of clones can be created from the same individual. SCNT is the only method currently available that might be used to clone existing or pre-existing people.

Therapeutic cloning

The possibility of therapeutic cloning centres on the concept of stem cells. Stem cells have the ability to develop into different mature cell types. *Totipotent* stem cells are cells with the potential to form a complete animal if placed in a uterus. They are early embryos. *Pluripotent* stem cells are immature stem cells with the potential to develop into any of the mature cell types in the adult (liver, lung, skin, blood, etc.), but cannot by themselves form a complete animal if placed in a uterus.

Ethical issues associated with therapeutic cloning often relate to the use of embryos. For example, some may object to the proposed procedure in Case 18.8 because it would involve destruction of embryos. If the embryo is considered to have a moral status similar to, say, that of a child, then embryo research would normally be wrong. According to this view, IVF, and almost any termination of pregnancy, would also be wrong (see Chapter 13). Those who support such embryo research argue that, if some of the embryos produced during IVF would be otherwise discarded (as normally they would), then what could be wrong with using those embryos for research and then destroying them? This counter-argument is less persuasive if the embryos are created solely for the research and would not otherwise exist. Views about the moral status of the embryo (see Chapter 13) are then more crucial.

Some of the potential uses of therapeutic cloning discussed in the early years of cloning have now been achieved in other ways. For example, 'induced pluripotent stem cells' (where adult somatic cells are reprogrammed to become stem cells) are being tried in patients with Parkinson's disease (Normile 2018). This avoids ethical or legal concerns about cloning in embryos. There are some types of research, however, that cannot be carried out using adult stem cells. Adult stem cells are not immortal and cannot be used to develop cellular models of disease in the way that embryonic stem cells can.

The use of non-human animal eggs to develop cellular models of human disease can overcome some of these objections. These models would require few or no human eggs in order to produce vast amounts of tissue for the study of disease (because this tissue, once produced, is potentially immortal).

The use of non-human eggs, however, raises another possible moral objection: that we should not create human clones using animal eggs or new human–non-human hybrids or chimeras, because they are unnatural and cross some kind of ethical line. In fact, scientists have been inserting human genes into animals to create animal models of human disease for over 20 years. More recently, scientists have introduced human embryonic cells into animals to study development and disease.

A final objection to therapeutic cloning is that, although not wrong in itself, it will lead down a slippery slope (see Chapter 1) to reproductive cloning. One response to this objection is to argue that there is a clear distinction between the two types of cloning; that is, there is a clear barrier that will prevent slipping down the slippery slope. The UK has already banned reproductive cloning, and any scientist in the UK who clones a human person would face criminal charges. But is reproductive cloning necessarily unethical?

Reproductive cloning

Reproductive cloning is the production of a (near-identical) genetic copy of an existing or previously existing person. Live animals have been cloned using both fission methods (in the cattle industry) and somatic cell nuclear transfer (SCNT; see Box 18.2), in cases such as the one that produced Dolly the sheep. In January 2018, the first primates (a pair of macaques) were successfully cloned. So far there have been no confirmed cases of the deliberate cloning of a human embryo that has developed into a live baby.

The Human Reproductive Cloning Act 2001 aims to prevent human reproductive cloning by making it a criminal offence to place a human embryo in the womb of a woman unless the embryo has been created by fertilization. Reproductive cloning is illegal in many other countries (e.g. Australia), and several international declarations prohibit it.

Up for Debate Box 18.2 summarizes some arguments for and against reproductive cloning.

MITOCHONDRIAL TRANSFER

Case 18.9

A woman is diagnosed as a carrier of a rare, potentially serious mitochondrial disorder MERRF (Mitochondrial Epilepsy with Ragged Red Fibres). While she is not, herself, seriously affected by the disorder, she would transmit the disorder to all children she conceives naturally. There is a risk that the children would be severely affected, and prenatal genetic diagnosis would not be able to detect this. Although this could be avoided by using donor eggs, the woman would prefer to have a genetically related child. Her IVF clinic offers her the option of mitochondrial transfer, in which would transfer her own nuclear DNA, but the mitochondria from another woman. (This is sometimes referred to as 'three-parent IVF'.)

Should mitochondrial transfer be permitted?

This case is based on Sample (2018).

Mitochondrial transfer has been suggested as an option in rare situations like Case 18.9, where women are at high risk of transmitting genetically abnormal mitochondria to all of their offspring. In the process, a donor egg has its nucleus removed and replaced by the nucleus from the mother. The hybrid egg is then fertilized and reimplanted in the mother (Poulton and Oakeshott 2012).

Mitochondrial transfer is sometimes misleadingly described as 'three-parent IVF'. While IVF is necessary to transplant the organelles, this is perhaps more accurately described as a form of microscopic transplantation – organelle transplantation (Savulescu 2015). The child who is conceived would have a tiny proportion of (mitochondrial) DNA from another woman. Solid organs like a liver or kidney also contain DNA from a donor. But we would not say that a child who receives a liver or kidney transplant now has 'three parents'. Certainly, in terms of the

Up for Debate Box 18.2 Should reproductive cloning be permitted?

18

GENETHICS

For

1. Liberty – we should be free to reproduce however we choose.
   Response: The harm to a clone and to society in general justifies constraint on this freedom.
2. For medical reasons – clones could be created as a compatible source of protein, cells, tissue or organs. This is already taking place without cloning through the creation of 'saviour siblings' (see above). Cloning would ensure the best possible match.
   Response: Such a use, as with 'saviour siblings', is wrong, because it uses people as an *instrument* for the benefit of others (see 'instrumentalization' below).
3. Freedom of scientific enquiry – the knowledge gained by human cloning will be invaluable in gaining scientific understanding.
   Response: The potential for harm to the clone and society constrains the pursuit of knowledge.
4. To achieve a sense of immortality – while we may die, our clone may live on. This would give us a greater sense of connectedness with the future.
   Response: Clones are different people. Any sense of connectedness with the future would be based on false assumptions about personal identity.
5. Eugenic selection – cloning could be used to reproduce especially gifted individuals, such as Einstein.
   Response: Clones will be different people from the 'original'. Eugenic selection is based on a crude genetic determinism which suggests that people are merely the product of their genes.
6. Treatment of infertility.
   Response: Cloning is necessary for the treatment of infertility only in the case of mitochondrial disease. Such diseases are rare. Moreover, there are other ways for people to have a baby using donor gametes (see also discussion of mitochondrial transfer below).
7. Replacement of a dead relative.
   Response: The relative will not be replaced (even if this were desirable), as the clone will be a different person – a sibling rather the same person.
8. Negative attitudes to cloning represent a new form of discrimination: *clonism.* To label the creation of a clone as an affront to human dignity (see below) is like saying that creating a black person is an affront to human dignity. People deserve equal concern and respect regardless of the origin of their genome.
   Response: This analogy is unconvincing. No one is saying that a person who is a clone should in any way be discriminated against. But from that it does not follow that it was not wrong to have used cloning in the first place. In believing that it is wrong to clone humans, one is not 'expressing' a negative view towards individuals created by cloning (see also 'expressivist argument', above).
9. Most arguments against cloning assume that the clone is the same person as the 'original', but, just as identical twins are not the same person, neither are clones. Much opposition to cloning is also based on a crude genetic determinism that underplays the importance of environment (and, perhaps, freedom of the will) in determining the kind of person we are.
   Response: Many arguments against cloning do not make these assumptions. Cloning will reduce originality, as clones will be more similar to one another than non-clones.

Continued

Up for Debate Box 18.2 Should reproductive cloning be permitted? — cont'd

Against

1. Cloning is an affront to human dignity – this claim has been made by the European Parliament, UNESCO and the World Health Organization. The *Additional Protocol to the Convention for the Protection of Human Rights and Dignity of the Human Being with regard to the Application of Biology and Medicine, on the Prohibition of Cloning Human Beings (1998)* (http://conventions.coe.int/treaty/en/treaties/html/168.htm), for example, states in its preamble that: 'the instrumentalisation of human beings through the deliberate creation of genetically identical human beings is contrary to human dignity and thus constitutes a misuse of biology and medicine', and goes on to say in Article 1: 'Any intervention seeking to create a human being genetically identical to another human being, whether living or dead, is prohibited'.

   Response: What is human dignity, and how is cloning an affront to it? Approximately 1 in 300 live births are identical twins (and therefore clones), and this does not seem to represent any threat to human dignity. Are identical twins an affront to human dignity?

2. Cloning is liable to abuse – dictators and other evil people will clone multiple copies of themselves, or use cloning technology to produce large armies of clones.

   Response: This argument assumes genetic determinism. A different time and different circumstances will ensure that the clone is not a replica. Moreover, it would be an inefficient means for a dictator to impose his will. We have much more to fear from dictators than cloning – such as their distortion of the truth, oppression of minorities, manipulation of the media, introduction of illiberal laws, use of military force, etc.

3. Cloning allows eugenic selection – this criticism has been put forward by the European Parliament.

   Response: Many other current techniques could be used for eugenic purposes, such as preimplantation diagnosis, prenatal testing, abortion and sterilization. Should these also be prohibited? The eugenics practised by the Nazis was an atrocity, both because it was motivated by racism and because it was imposed by the state on individuals without their agreement. The choice by parents to have a child without a serious genetically determined disease is quite different from what the Nazis did.

4. Instrumentalization – cloning uses people as a means.

   Response: People have children for a variety of motives. What is important is how a child is treated and loved, not the reasons her parents had for conceiving her.

5. Clones will live in the shadow of the 'original' person.

   Response: Many people live in the shadow of their parents, or others, without excessive untoward effect. In any case, cloning does not significantly increase risks from high expectations. A clone may well *benefit* from fore-knowledge of his genetic inheritance – his talents, limitations and disease propensities.

6. Cloning would reduce genetic variation.

   Response: Identical twins occur at a rate of 3.5 per 1000. This does not affect genetic diversity. It is likely that only a small proportion of any population would be clones, and so cloning would have little impact on genetic diversity.

Up for Debate Box 18.2 Should reproductive cloning be permitted?—cont'd

7. Right to genetic individuality – the European Parliament claimed, in the context of cloning, that the individual has a right to his or her own genetic identity.
   Response: It is clear that twins are autonomous individuals. Identical twins do not seem deficient in any way, as is manifested by the absence of objection to drugs that increase the rate of twinning, and by the fact that little research into preventing twinning is carried out.
8. Safety – cloning increases the risk of serious genetic malformation, cancer or shortened lifespan.
   Response: This is currently a valid objection, because the science of cloning is in its infancy. Reproductive cloning of primates has been very difficult (only a tiny proportion of attempts have succeeded). Further research on cloning and improved techniques are likely to reduce the risks.

law (The Human Fertilisation and Embryology (Mitochondrial Donation) Regulations 2015), the provider of the mitochondrial DNA will not be recognized as a parent.

In 2015, the UK became the first jurisdiction to make mitochondrial transfer legal. A healthy baby was born in Mexico in 2016 after using the technique. In January 2018, the first patients in UK were offered this procedure (Case 18.9 is based on that situation).

What ethical issues are raised by mitochondrial transfer? As with any new medical procedure, there are risks. However, the evidence so far suggests this procedure is safe. Moreover, it has certain advantages over other forms of transplantation. Mitochondrial transplantation would be curative, whereas conventional transplantation often only works for a finite period of time. While conventional transplantation requires the administration of dangerous drugs to suppress the body's immune system, mitochondrial transplantation would not.

Importantly, by doing this transplant at the very early stage of embryo development, the children of the offspring of this procedure will themselves be free of mitochondrial disease. It would be eradicated forever in this family. Germ-line modifications have the potential to magnify the benefit of an intervention (as the benefit is passed on). However, if there are unforeseen harms, those too will potentially be passed on to offspring.

REVISION QUESTIONS

1. James is interested in genetics, and sends off a cheek swab to an online company offering whole-genome sequencing. To his horror, he discovers that he has the gene for Huntington's disease. Does James have an obligation to share this news with his siblings and other members of his family? Does the genetic testing company have an obligation to find out whether James has informed the rest of his family? James has told his GP

Continued

about the test result. Does the GP have an obligation to pass on the result to others in the family if James will not?

2. James decides to take out life insurance in order to look after his family. Is James obliged to reveal his genetic test results to his insurer?

3. James is concerned that perhaps there was an error in the testing. Should the public health system bear the cost of repeating James' whole-genome sequencing, and of providing him with genetic counselling? (This is not really a revision question, as we did not cover it in the chapter – but it is an interesting one!)

4. What is the expressivist objection to prenatal genetic testing? Do you agree with this objection? What implications should it have for prenatal testing?

5. What is the difference between therapeutic and reproductive gene editing? Is there an ethical difference between these?

6. What forms of cloning are legal? Is the law around cloning justified?

7. Would gene editing of embryos (as in Case 16.5) be legal in the UK? Should it be?

Extension case 18.10

Recent scientific developments suggest that some of the tools used to reprogram stem cells can be used to generate cells for a different purpose. Somatic cells could be induced to form pluripotent stem cells. These could then be introduced into an ovary or testicle, where they would develop into gametes. In mice, cells from a mouse tail have been transformed, using this sort of technique, into eggs that then generated eight healthy offspring (Vogel 2016).

In-vitro–generated gametes might have several important uses. They could be used as treatment for infertile couples (who lack suitable gametes). They could avoid the need for invasive procedures in egg donors. They could make it possible for same-sex couples to have offspring that are genetically related to both parents. Further, they could be used to facilitate gene editing – preventing transmission of genetic mutations (or facilitating genetic enhancement). Gene modification of gametes may be technically (and ethically?) easier than modifying embryos.

Should in-vitro gametogenesis be permitted?

Read Suter (2015), Bourne, Douglas, and Savulescu (2012), Sparrow (2014).

REFERENCES

ABC v St. George's Healthcare NHS Trust and others [2017] EWCA Civ 336.

Batzofin, J. H. 1987. "XY sperm separation for sex selection." *Urologic Clinics of North America* 14: 609-18.

Bourne, H., Douglas, T. and Savulescu, J. 2012. "Procreative beneficence and in vitro gametogenesis." *Monash Bioethics Review* 30 (2): 29-48.

British Medical Association. 1998. *Human genetics: choice and responsibility*. London: BMA.

British Society for Human Genetics. 2010. "Report on the genetic testing of children."

BSHG, accessed 21/11/18. http://www.bsgm. org.uk/media/678741/gtoc_booklet_final_new .pdf.

Buchanan, A. E., Brock, D. W., Daniels, N., Wikler, D. and Sober, E. 2000. *From chance to choice: genetics and justice*. Cambridge: Cambridge University Press.

Easler, J. and Rivard, L. 2013. "Case study in incidental findings." Nature Education, accessed 21/11/18. https://www.nature.com/ scitable/forums/genetics-generation/case -study-in-incidental-findings-103821707.

Habermas, J. 2003. *The future of human nature*. Cambridge: Polity Press.

Herring, J. 2018. *Medical law and ethics*. 7th ed. Oxford: Oxford University Press.

Jonas, H. 1974. "Biological engineering – a preview." In: *Philosophical essays: from ancient creed to technological man*. Cambridge: University of Chicago Press.

Kaiser, J. 2017. "A human has been injected with gene-editing tools to cure his disabling disease. Here's what you need to know." *Science* accessed 21/11/18. http://www .sciencemag.org/news/2017/11/human-has -been-injected-gene-editing-tools-cure-his -disabling-disease-here-s-what-you.

Kalia, S. S., Adelman, K., Bale, S. J., Chung, W. K., Eng, C., Evans, J. P., Herman, G. E., Hufnagel, S. B., Klein, T. E., Korf, B. R., McKelvey, K. D., Ormond, K. E., Richards, C. S., Vlangos, C. N., Watson, M., Martin, C. L. and Miller, D. T. 2016. "Recommendations for reporting of secondary findings in clinical exome and genome sequencing, 2016 update (ACMG SF v2.0): a policy statement of the American College of Medical Genetics and Genomics." *Genetics in Medicine* 19: 249. doi: 10.1038/gim.2016.190. https://www.nature.com/articles/gim2016190. supplementary-information.

Kang, X., He, W., Huang, Y., Yu, Q., Chen, Y., Gao, X., Sun, X. and Fan, Y. 2016. "Introducing precise genetic modifications into human 3PN embryos by CRISPR/Cas-mediated genome editing." *Journal of Assisted Reproduction and Genetics* 33: 581-8. doi: 10.1007/s10815-016-0710-8.

Levin, A. 2011. "I know I was born to save Charlie instead of being born just for me: Incredible story of the saviour sibling who sparked an ethical furore." Daily Mail, 22 May 2011. Accessed 21/11/18. https://www .dailymail.co.uk/health/article-1389499 /I-know-I-born-save-Charlie-instead-born-just-Brotherly-love-saviour-sibling .html.

Lucassen, A. and Parker, M. 2001. "Revealing false paternity: some ethical considerations." *Lancet* 357 (9261): 1033-5. doi: 10.1016/ S0140-6736(00)04240-9.

Lui, P. and Rose, G. A. 1995. "Social aspects of over 800 couples coming forward for gender selection of their children." *Human Reproduction* 10: 968-71.

Marchione, M. 2018. "Chinese researcher claims first gene-edited babies." *Associated Press* Accessed 30/11/18. https://www.apnews.com /4997bb7aa36c45449b488e19ac83e86d. 26 November 2018.

Mendell, J. R., Al-Zaidy, S., Shell, R., Arnold, W. D., Rodino-Klapac, L. R., Prior, T. W., Lowes, L., Alfano, L., Berry, K., Church, K., Kissel, J. T., Nagendran, S., L'Italien, J., Sproule, D. M., Wells, C., Cardenas, J. A., Heitzer, M. D., Kaspar, A., Corcoran, S., Braun, L., Likhite, S., Miranda, C., Meyer, K., Foust, K. D., Burghes, A. H. M. and Kaspar, B. K. 2017. "Single-dose gene-replacement therapy for spinal muscular atrophy." *The New England Journal of Medicine* 377 (18): 1713-22. doi: 10.1056/NEJMoa1706198.

Newell, C. 1994. "A critique of the construction of prenatal diagnosis and disa." In *Ethical issues in prenatal diagnosis and the termination of pregnancy*, edited by J. McKie. Clayton Victoria, Australia: Centre for Human Bioethics, Monash University: 89-96.

Normile, D. 2018. "First-of-its-kind clinical trial will use reprogrammed adult stem cells to treat Parkinson's." *Science* accessed 21/11/ 18. http://www.sciencemag.org/news/2018 /07/first-its-kind-clinical-trial-will-use -reprogrammed-adult-stem-cells-treat -parkinson-s.

Nuffield Council on Bioethics. 2017. "Noninvasive prenatal testing: ethical issues." NCB, accessed 21/11/18. http://nuffieldbioethics. org/wp-content/uploads/NIPT-ethical-issues-full-report.pdf.

Nuffield Council on Bioethics. 2018. *Genome editing and human reproduction: social and ethical issues*. London: Nuffield Council on Bioethics.

Parker, M. and Lucassen, A. M. 2004. "Genetic information: a joint account?" *BMJ* 329: 165-7.

Politis, C. 1998. "The psychosocial impact of chronic illness." *Annals New York Academy of Sciences* 850: 349-54.

Quintavalle v Human Fertilisation And Embryology Authority [2005] UKHL 28.

Poulton, J. and Oakeshott, P. 2012. "Nuclear transfer to prevent maternal transmission of mitochondrial DNA disease." *BMJ* 345: e6651.

Robertson, S. and Savulescu, J. 2001. "Is there a case in favour of predictive genetic testing in young children?" *Bioethics* 15 (1): 26-49.

Sample, I. 2018. "UK doctors select first women to have 'three-person babies'." The Guardian, 1 February 2018. Accessed 21/11/18. https://www.theguardian.com/science/2018/feb/01/permission-given-to-create-britains-first-three-person-babies.

Savulescu, J. 2001a. "Predictive genetic testing in children." *The Medical Journal of Australia* 175 (7): 379-81.

Savulescu, J. 2001b. "In defense of selection for nondisease genes." *American Journal of Bioethics* 1: 16-9.

Savulescu, J. 2005. "The ethics of cloning." *Medicine* 33 (2): 18-20. https://doi.org/10.1383/medc.33.2.18.58382.

Savulescu, J. 2015. "Mitochondrial disease kills 150 children a year. A micro-transplant can cure it." *The Guardian*.

Schaefer, G. O. and Savulescu, J. 2018. "The right to know: a revised standard for reporting incidental findings." *Hastings Center Report* 48: 22-32. doi: 10.1002/hast.836.

Shkedi-Rafid, S., Dheensa, S., Crawford, G., Fenwick, A. and Lucassen, A. 2014. "Defining and managing incidental findings in genetic and genomic practice." *Journal of Medical Genetics* 51: 715-23.

Sparrow, R. 2014. "In vitro eugenics." *Journal of Medical Ethics* 40: 725-31.

Suter, S. M. 2015. "In vitro gametogenesis: just another way to have a baby?" *Law and the Biosciences* 3 (1): 87-119. doi: 10.1093/jlb/lsv057.

Vogel, G. 2016. "Mouse egg cells made entirely in the lab give rise to healthy offspring." *Science* accessed 21/11/18. http://www.sciencemag.org/news/2016/10/mouse-egg-cells-made-entirely-lab-give-rise-healthy-offspring.

FURTHER READING

Agar, N. 2003. *Liberal eugenics*. Blackwell: Oxford

British Medical Association. 1998. *Human genetics: choice and responsibility*. Oxford: Oxford University Press. *The British Medical Association's position on ethics and genetics.*

Buchanan, A., Brock, D. W., Daniels, N. and Wikler, D. 2000. *From chance to choice: genetics and justice*. Cambridge: Cambridge University Press. *One of the best books on ethics and the new genetics which covers the literature thoroughly. Highly recommended.*

Harris, J. 1998. *Clones, genes and immortality*. Oxford: Oxford University Press. *An updated version of Harris's influential 'Wonderwoman and superman' (Oxford University Press, Oxford, 1992).*

Mehlman, M. J. and Botkin, R. 1998. *Access to the genome: the challenge to equality*. Washington, DC: Georgetown University Press.

Chapter **19**

Information ethics

In the first part of the 21st century, the enormous growth in digitization of information and in the internet has had a huge influence on medical practice – much as it has on the rest of society.

Some of the ethical questions arising from these changes overlap with the issues relating to medical information and confidentiality that we covered in Chapter 9. Here, we will focus on the distinctive ethical or legal questions for health professionals arising from digital information, big data, the internet and social media.

ACCESS TO INFORMATION

Case 19.1

Stefan is a Swedish post-graduate student who is in the UK for three years. He also has long-standing type I diabetes. Soon after arriving in the UK, Stefan has a hospital admission following gastroenteritis, and has a number of tests. After his discharge from hospital, Stefan asks his GP for access to his full test results from the hospital stay, as well as to the results from all of the tests that the GP arranges. The GP appears put out by the request. She tells him that the results are normal, and she will let him know of any significant results.

Does Stefan have a right to his medical information?

In the UK, a series of Acts give patients the legal right to see their medical notes, medical reports, computerized personal data and personal files held by social services. Patients might want this information because they are unhappy with the care they have received (that might be the doctor's suspicion in Stefan's case). However, they may wish for the information in order to inform decisions about their health. (For example, online access to medical records has been associated with improved glycaemic control in some patients with diabetes (Mold et al. 2018).) It may facilitate communication if the patient is seeing different health professionals (e.g. if they are moving). Or they may simply feel that the information relating to their health belongs to them. In the future, they may be able to use it in decision-making algorithms for diagnostic or therapeutic purposes.

The Access to Medical Reports Act 1988 gives patients the restricted right of access to any medical report relating to them that has been supplied by a doctor (medical practitioner) for employment or insurance purposes.

Another Act (with a similar name), the Access to Health Records Act 1990, has largely been replaced by the Data Protection Act 1998, except in relation to the records of deceased persons. The executor or administrator of a deceased person's estate may apply under this act for access to health records.

The Data Protection Act 1998 sets out eight principles that apply to both computer records and records held in manual form (e.g. patients' medical notes). These principles are designed to ensure that personal data held by health professionals are accurate and relevant, held only for specific defined purposes for which the user has been registered, not kept for longer than is necessary and not disclosed to any unauthorized persons (Box 19.1).

In Stefan's case, he therefore has a right to his medical records, and might apply to his GP informally or formally (in writing). If he applies formally, he should expect to receive a copy of his records within 6 weeks, though he is likely to have to pay a fee for this. If his request is refused, Stefan could approach the Information Commissioner's office.

GP surgeries in many parts of the UK offer patients online access to parts of their record, including letters and results. Stefan could apply to his surgery for access to that, though it would not provide his hospital test results, unless they were in his discharge summary.

But should it be so difficult for Stefan to access his records? One reason that he asked might be his experience in Sweden. Since 2017, there has been universal access of Swedish patients to their electronic medical records, in a manner akin to online banking (Armstrong 2017). Health professionals were initially wary of this, as they were concerned that it would increase patient anxiety or consultation time (due to patients asking additional questions). Those concerns have generally not been borne out in trials of open patient access to medical records (Walker, Meltsner, and Delbanco 2015). In the UK, there are plans to make something similar possible within the next 5 years, though there are concerns about the security of information and possible data breaches.

Recording patients

The widespread availability of recording devices (on mobile phones) has made cases like Case 19.2 (below) much more common. Doctors are obliged to obtain patient consent before any form of recording that includes them (with the exception of investigations like an ultrasound, where consent is implied by consent for the

> **Box 19.1** The Data Protection Act 1998
>
> A key term is 'data subjects'. These are the people to whom the data apply, e.g. patients or participants in research. The Act gives statutory right for data subjects to have access to personal information held on them, subject to certain exceptions (see below).
>
> The Act enables data subjects:
> 1. to be informed as to whether personal data are processed
> 2. to be given a description of the data held, the purposes for which they are processed and the persons to whom the data may be disclosed
> 3. to be given a copy of the information constituting the data
> 4. to be given information on the source of the information.
>
> NB: The Act defines the 'processing' of data as 'obtaining, recording, or carrying out any operation including retrieval or consultation, or use of information, and disclosure'.
>
> The data subject also has the right of rectification, i.e. the right to have inaccuracies in the data corrected. Data subjects may seek compensation for any harm suffered as a result of the inaccuracy.
>
> For a patient to gain access to his personal health record, a request must be made in writing. A response must be given by the appropriate person or institution within 40 days of the request, or the applicant must be informed that there are grounds for withholding the information. Information can be withheld in certain circumstances, for example:
> - when access 'would be likely to cause serious harm to the physical or mental health or condition of the data subject or any other person'
> - where the request for access is made by another person on behalf of the data subject, such as a parent or child, and if the data subject had provided the information in the expectation that it would not be disclosed
> - where '[g]iving access would reveal the identity of another person, unless that person has given consent to the disclosure or it is reasonable to comply with the access request without that consent. This does not apply if the third party is a health professional who has been involved in the care of the patient unless serious harm to that health professional's physical or mental health or condition is likely to be caused by giving access'.

> **Case 19.2**
>
> A patient, Mr B, records a pre-operative consultation with his surgeon on his mobile phone, as he wishes to be able to listen to the conversation afterwards. However, partway through the conversation the surgeon becomes aware of the recording and becomes upset. He tells Mr B that he had no right to record the conversation without his permission. He would never contemplate recording Mr B without Mr B's consent. He asks Mr B to switch off the recording.
>
> Is the surgeon right?

procedure). Covert recordings of patients would, in almost all circumstances, be regarded as unethical (and probably unlawful). However, the reverse does not apply. Patients are regarded as having a right to record conversations with their doctors. While (as in the first case) doctors may interpret the attempt to record as a lack of trust, recordings may be sought for more practical reasons – including the possibility of revisiting information later. The Data Protection Act (s36) states that '[p]ersonal data processed by an individual only for the purposes of that individual's personal, family or household affairs are exempt from data protection principles'. It may be that patients *should* seek the doctor's consent before recording their conversation, but they are entitled to record even without consent.

One pragmatic response for the surgeon in Case 19.2 would have been to welcome the recording, but to ask for a copy of it at the end of the consultation so that it can enter the medical record (Zack 2014).

ETHICS AND BIG DATA

Case 19.3

Mr A has been diagnosed with acute leukaemia. As part of the work-up for his treatment, a blood sample was sent to analyze the genetic profile of his cancer. He was asked at the time if he would be happy for any leftover specimen to be stored in a biobank that could be used for research. He was promised that no identifying information would be recorded in the biobank. Mr A agreed to his specimen being used.

However, some time later Mr A started to wonder what he had agreed to. Could his specimen be used for commercial research that might generate a patent, or by a company that he didn't agree with (like a tobacco company)?

Digitization of information, as well as the collation of medical information from large numbers of patients, has enormous potential value for medical research. Analysis of trends and patterns in health-related 'big data' could generate vital insights into health and disease. Repositories – 'biobanks' – sometimes include biological material. Or they may be simply large information repositories that contain medical data.

To prevent harm to patients from research databases, there are two ethical approaches often taken. The first is to obtain consent from patients prior to retaining specimens or information. The second is to ensure anonymization of patient information.

Consent

We discussed consent for medical research in Chapter 16, and consent to sharing of data in Chapter 9. However, as Mr A's case shows, one of the challenges around research databases is that information or specimens may be kept for a long period. Some potentially beneficial uses might not be initially anticipated. Should patients consent specifically for each and every piece of research involving their data, or is a generic consent enough? Alternatively, perhaps consent should be dynamic – so that patients and researchers can have ongoing interaction, and patients can alter their consent choices over time (Kaye et al. 2014).

Obtaining consent can be time consuming and complex. Because of the potential benefits from collecting data, researchers, policy makers and ethicists have sometimes been keen to reduce the requirement for consent to entry in research in situations where specimens or data will be stored anyway and will be anonymized. For example, since May 2018, the NHS has applied an opt-out system for use of confidential patient information in research or planning (Armstrong 2018). The ethical basis for such a system is similar to the justification cited in opt-out organ donation policies (see Chapter 15). There is a large benefit to the community from involving most or many people. Status quo bias (a general preference for the current state of affairs) means that opt-out rates will often be low (Samuelson and Zeckhauser 1988). And those who do care about the use of their data can always vote with their feet.

The use of data by outside organizations or companies can raise ethical concern. In early 2018, Public Health England was criticized for releasing data on 180,000 patients with lung cancer to a US consulting firm linked to tobacco companies (Hughes 2018). A London hospital that transferred data from more than 1 million patients to a subsidiary of the tech company Google was found not to have complied with the Data Protection Act (2017b). Decisions to share information are not necessarily subject to research ethics committee review.

Anonymization

Case 19.4

A young man, MM, is suspected of the murder of a politician, but police are unable to link him directly to the crime. They obtain a blood specimen that had been collected from MM when he was a newborn, and which had been stored in a national database. The blood specimen matches DNA from the crime scene. When presented with this evidence, MM confesses to the murder.

Is forensic use of biobank specimens lawful?

This case is based on the case of Mijailo Mijailovic and the murder of Swedish politician Anna Lindh (Dranseika, Piasecki, and Waligora 2016).

Biobanks usually stipulate that they will only share information with bona fide researchers, and will not release information to insurers or to the police. However, they might be compelled to do so by a court. There are no cases to date of this occurring in the UK. A case like that of MM would be unlikely to occur in the current era, as most jurisdictions will permit police to obtain samples from suspects for DNA. However, if police did not have specific suspects, they might seek access to DNA databases to help identify one. One reason to not allow this sort of forensic use of biobanks is that this would be likely to discourage people from donating their specimens.

Some databases (for example, newborn screening databases) maintain patient-identifying details so that they can contact the patient if a significant diagnosis is discovered. As noted, to avoid possible harms, other databases may be completely anonymized. However, this can cause the opposite ethical concern – if tests on a specimen yielded a potentially important diagnosis, that information could not be fed back.

There is also concern about the fallibility of anonymization. Even if the patient's name is not recorded, it may be possible to put together different pieces of information to identify someone ('jigsaw identification'). Studies have suggested that surnames might be able to be identified in some cases by matching someone's DNA specimen to patterns in publicly accessible genealogy databases (Gymrek et al. 2013).

Given the possibility that even anonymized data might lead to identification, the security of data repositories is crucial. Lack of trust in data security (as well as lack of understanding about how information would be used) led to many patients opting out of a previous NHS data repository (care.data) (Temperton 2016).

The General Data Protection Regulation (GDPR), an EU regulation which came into effect in May 2018, governs anyone who holds personal information about another. This means that hospitals and doctors' surgeries will need the explicit consent of the individual to process their data.

DIGITAL DOCTORS AND ARTIFICIAL INTELLIGENCE

There have been very substantial advances in the application of machine learning and artificial intelligence (AI) to medical tasks, including particularly diagnostics. For example, deep-learning algorithms appear to perform as well as humans in the diagnosis of illness or prediction of cardiovascular risk from retinal examination. A neural network trained on a database of more than 129,000 clinical photographs was able to correctly identify skin cancers as well as dermatologists. In other areas, the machines seem to already be better than human doctors, correctly identifying malignant tumours in 89% of breast cancer images (compared with 73% by a human pathologist) (Loh 2018).

If computers are better than human doctors, that appears to be ethically a good thing. Could there be any ethical concerns?

One question relates to errors or adverse events that arise from the use of AI to diagnose or manage health conditions. Who would the patient sue for negligence if the computer makes a mistake? It is possible that those who wrote the medical program might be found liable, though presumably it would have to be established that they had a duty of care to the patient. If a human health professional acted on the recommendation of a computer (and other responsible doctors would not have relied on the computer), they might be found negligent. The opposite problem might arise if evidence continues to accumulate that computers are outperforming doctors – human health professionals might be found negligent if they failed to take advantage of an AI to assist with diagnosis/management.

As patients can access more of their data and utilize AI, a third party will enter the doctor–patient relationship. The norms which should govern such a relationship are yet to be determined. However, the basic principles of promoting patient well-being and autonomy should continue in the digital relationship.

The other main ethical concern frequently raised in response to the possibility of digital doctors is that patients would miss out on the important therapeutic benefit of human contact. However, at least in the medium-term, it appears that computers are likely to be confined to specific tasks (where they have been shown to be valuable). They will supplement human doctors, rather than replace them.

Dr H is a paediatrician who works with adolescent patients. She establishes a strong bond with many of her patients. One of her former patients (who is now a young adult, and no longer attends Dr H's clinic) contacts her via Facebook with a 'friend' request.
  What should Dr H do?

One of the challenges for professionals in the current era is the blurring of personal and professional boundaries. Professionals may contribute to this; they may have social media accounts (on Facebook, Twitter or elsewhere) where they share information relevant both to their personal lives and their professional lives. Although they might never discuss politics or their taste in music with a patient in person, a doctor may express their views about current topics in the media. A doctor might have a picture of his family on his office desk. However, on Facebook, he might share photos, stories and videos of his children.

Relationships with patients may also become blurred. Patients may follow a doctor's profile on certain social media platforms (e.g. Twitter, Instagram), or they may seek to become an electronic 'friend' (Fig. 19.1).

Would it be ethically a problem for Dr H to friend her former patient? Doctors can and do become friends with patients in the physical world, so it would be inconsistent to prohibit this online. However, where a doctor has an ongoing professional relationship they would usually be advised to separate their roles as far as possible. (If not possible, it may be that the patient's medical care should be provided by someone else.) If the doctor is going to share information on Facebook that they would not want current or former patients to see (for example, pictures of them inebriated), they would be wise to decline friendship requests – though it would not be unethical to accept. One option would be to have separate social media accounts for doctors' professional role and non-professional roles.

DIGITAL PATIENTS

Andy and Jacinta have taken their daughter to a paediatrician for advice for a medical condition. The paediatrician prescribes treatment for the girl. After writing it out, she warns the parents not to look up the medication on the internet, as they will only scare themselves and find inaccurate information. The parents promise that they will do as the doctor suggests.
  On leaving the surgery, Andy and Jacinta instantly Google the medication.
  This case is based on Shrimsley (2014).

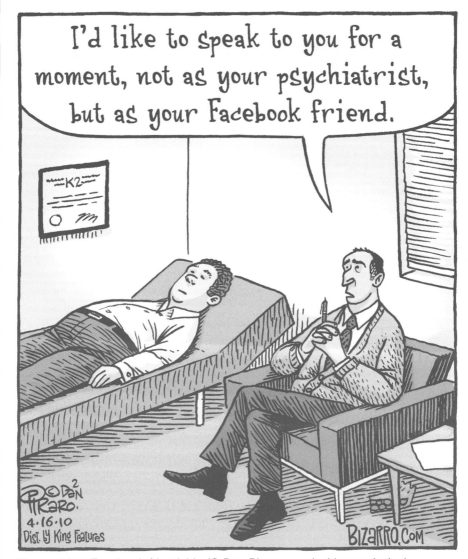

Figure 19.1 Facebook friendship (© Dan Piraro, used with permission)

It is not likely that patients will be replaced by computers. However, computers are already having a significant role in medical consultations. Patients frequently use the internet to attempt to self-diagnose medical symptoms (Fig. 19.2), and often resort to the internet to check information provided by doctors (even, or perhaps especially, when doctors tell them not to). This will become more pronounced as patients access diagnostic algorithms.

There are obvious ethical obligations for those who provide medical information or offer tools for self-diagnosis online. There is an obligation to provide information that is accurate and not misleading, to declare conflicts of interest and to explain the source of information offered. However, the nature of the internet is that a good proportion of those offering health information online will not be medical

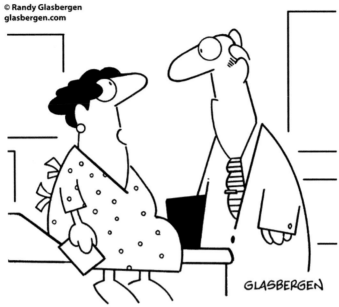

© Randy Glasbergen
glasbergen.com

GLASBERGEN

"I already diagnosed myself on the Internet.
I either have three left kidneys, recurring
puberty or Dutch Elm disease."

Figure 19.2 Internet diagnosis (© Randy Glasbergen, used with permission)

practitioners, and may not acknowledge or recognize these ethical obligations. Patients like Andy and Jacinta may have little or no legal recourse if information that they find online is in fact inaccurate, misleading or even harmful.

How should doctors respond to patients' use of the internet for medical information? Simply telling patients not to go online is unlikely to be helpful. It may be more useful to direct patients to reliable, relevant sources of medical information. Doctors should potentially invite patients to discuss information that they have found online, particularly if that does not match the information provided by their doctor. However, particularly in resource-limited settings, doctors may have little time to discuss information found online. Discussion may therefore not occur, or may displace other important activities.

Case 19.7

Dr G is a keen user of computers, and an advocate of e-health. After a consultation with a young professional Ms J, who has a long-standing history of depression, she asks him a follow-up question by email. Dr G replies by email to Ms J's question, and attaches a copy of his letter from the consultation.

However, Ms J had emailed from a work email address, and her employer has access to her emails. When her employment contract is not renewed, Ms J suspects that her boss had access to her medical history. She seeks legal action against Dr G for failing to protect her confidential medical information.

In the current era, interactions with patients may occur electronically, as well as in person. Doctors may receive communications from patients by email, text message or other online messaging service. There are potential benefits for both patients and doctors in convenience and in access to medical advice (Atherton et al. 2013). UK government policy encourages this ('patients should be able to communicate electronically with their health and care team') (Gunning and Richards 2014). However, there might be several potential harms or risks from electronic medical communication. One of those is highlighted by Ms J's case. Information communicated may not be secure. Even if doctors use secure email servers to send emails, emails may go astray with inadvertent release of confidential information (for example, if the address is mistyped, or if, as in Case 19.7, others have access to the recipient's email account). Communication may not be recorded in the medical record, potentially hindering other health professionals who care for the patient – or leaving the doctor without adequate records if there is a later legal question. There could be a significant workload for doctors in responding to emails. There are also questions about responsibility (how often should doctors check emails, how quickly should they respond?) and accountability (is an electronic communication equivalent to a physical encounter?). Box 19.2 includes some recommendations for mitigating the risks of email communication. Ms J might be best advised to bring a claim against her employer for unfair dismissal, rather than seeking to sue Dr G. Even if a breach of confidence could be shown, it may well be that no remedy could be obtained.

Social media and patients

Patients who are unhappy with the medical care they have received may lodge an official complaint with the doctor or hospital, complain to the General Medical Council or seek legal advice. However, in the current era they may also (or instead)

Box 19.2 Ethics and electronic communication with patients

Consider any electronic communication as equivalent to an in-person encounter. (If you would not say it in person, do not communicate it electronically. If you would require more information before providing advice in person, seek more information before advising electronically.)

Ensure that key communication is recorded in the patient's medical record. (If this communication were by telephone, would you record it in the notes? If so, record a copy of the email/message in the patient notes.)

Use work accounts (not personal accounts) for communicating. Seek patients' consent before communicating with them by email. If they initiate communication, ensure that they are aware of limits of the medium (e.g. confidentiality) and seek their permission before continuing.

Avoid discussion of sensitive topics by email (e.g. disability, psychiatric illness, sexual issues). Use a secure (at both ends) communication tool for such purposes.

Confine exchanges to concise messages. For complex information, or in the face of multiple emails, arrange a face-to-face or telephone conversation.

Dr A is alerted by a friend that a family has been posting heavily on social media, complaining about the medical treatment their child is receiving. They name Dr A in the posts and are highly critical of his care of their child. Dr A feels that the discussion about him is unfair, inaccurate and potentially damaging for his professional reputation.
   What should Dr A do?

vent their dissatisfaction online – in reviews of the doctor on online websites or in social media.

What should a doctor do in such a situation? Should they exercise their right to reply to the criticism? Could they or should they sue for defamation?

Doctors have a disadvantage in replying – in that they may not be able to do so without breaching the patient's confidentiality. In the case of an official review website, it may be useful for clinics or hospitals (but probably not individuals) to post replies that acknowledge patients' concerns, indicate a concrete desire to address the problem and point out how or where the patient can make an official complaint.

When it comes to posts on social media, it is probably unwise for doctors to reply, since that may inflame the conflict and generate more negative attention (Anon 2017a). Dr A could invite the parents offline to come and discuss their concerns. He could ask the relevant website to remove the post if it violates the terms of use. Finally, he could seek legal advice if he believes the information posted is defamatory. However, the risk of legal action is that it may be extremely costly, take a long time, generate more attention for the patient's assertions and increase, rather than decrease, reputational damage.

In some circumstances, doctors can apply for personal data stored on search engines or other sites to be removed. This is found in Article 17 GDPR ('the right to be forgotten'). In addressing such requests, providers must balance individual privacy against the potential public interest in having access to that information. If requests are granted, the websites will not be removed, but will not appear on search results in the EU. (They may still appear in other parts of the world.)

REVISION QUESTIONS

1. A mother dies following a catastrophic complication of childbirth. Afterwards, the family ask the hospital for her complete medical record. The doctors are reluctant to provide this, as they are concerned that it includes information (for example, about previous termination of pregnancy and sexual assault) that the patient would have wanted to keep private. Can they deny the family's request?
2. Police use a publicly accessible genealogy database to identify a suspect in a murder investigation (Creet 2018). Is that ethical? How is it different to using a biobank?

Continued

REVISION QUESTIONS—cont'd

3. A doctor uses a secure electronic messaging service to communicate with a student, including the result of a pregnancy test; however, the student accesses her messages on a computer in a public area, and other people in the room are able to read the message. Has the doctor acted wrongly?
4. A patient seeks medical information online about her medical symptoms (pelvic pain) and is reassured by the information she finds. She delays seeking medical attention, and later has a complicated admission due to an ectopic pregnancy. Can she sue the website?

Extension case 19.9

A patient relates to her GP an extremely traumatic episode from her past. Some years later, her GP refers her to a medical specialist (for an unrelated problem). The patient is shocked to find reference to the past trauma in the referral letter. She asks the GP practice to erase all reference to the past trauma from her medical record. When they decline to do this, she asks the practice to destroy all of her medical records. They also refuse to do this.

Should patients be able to request that part or all of their medical history be destroyed? This is based on the case of ST (Randeep and Dinsdale 2013).

REFERENCES

Anon 2017a. "Dealing with online criticism." Medical Defence Union, accessed 15/11/18. https://www.themdu.com/guidance-and-advice/guides/dealing-with-online-criticism.

Anon 2017b. "Royal Free – Google DeepMind trial failed to comply with data protection law." Information Commissioner's Office, accessed 15/11/18. https://ico.org.uk/about-the-ico/news-and-events/news-and-blogs/2017/07/royal-free-google-deepmind-trial-failed-to-comply-with-data-protection-law/.

Armstrong, S. 2017. "Patient access to health records: striving for the Swedish ideal." BMJ 357.

Armstrong, S. 2018. "Data deadlines loom large for the NHS." BMJ 360: k1215.

Atherton, H., Pappas, Y., Heneghan, C. and Murray, E. 2013. "Experiences of using email for general practice consultations: a qualitative study." The British Journal of General Practice: The Journal of the Royal College of General Practitioners 63 (616): e760-7. doi: 10.3399/bjgp13X674440.

Creet, J. 2018. "How cops used a public genealogy database in the Golden State Killer cas." The Conversation. https://theconversation.com/how-cops-used-a-public-genealogy-database-in-the-golden-state-killer-case-95842.

Dranseika, V., Piasecki, J. and Waligora, M. 2016. "Forensic uses of research biobanks: should donors be informed?" Medicine, Health Care, and Philosophy 19 (1): 141-6. doi: 10.1007/s11019-015-9667-0.

Gunning, E. and Richards, E. 2014. "Should patients be able to email their general practitioner?" BMJ 349: g5338.

Gymrek, M., McGuire, A. L., Golan, D., Halperin, E. and Erlich, Y. 2013. "Identifying personal genomes by surname inference." Science 339: 321-4.

Hughes, O. 2018. "PHE under fire for supplying cancer patient data to tobacco-linked firm." digitalhealth, accessed 15/11/18. https://www.digitalhealth.net/2018/01/public-health-england-cancer-patient-data/.

Kaye, J., Whitley, E. A., Lund, D., Morrison, M., Teare, H. and Melham, K. 2014. "Dynamic consent: a patient interface for twenty-first century research networks." European Journal of Human Genetics 23: 141. doi: 10.1038/ejhg.2014.71.

Loh, E. 2018. "Medicine and the rise of the robots: a qualitative review of recent advances of artificial intelligence in health." *BMJ Leader* 2: 59-63.

Mold, F., Raleigh, M., Alharbi, N. S. and de Lusignan, S. 2018. "The impact of patient online access to computerized medical records and services on type 2 diabetes: systematic review." *Journal of Medical Internet Research* 20 (7): e235. doi: 10.2196/jmir.7858.

Randeep, R. and Dinsdale, P. 2013. "Patient lost £18,000 legal battle over GP medical records." The Guardian, accessed 15/11/18. https://www.theguardian.com/politics/2013/aug/01/patient-legal-battle-medical-records.

Samuelson, W. and Zeckhauser, R. 1988. "Status quo bias in decision making." *Journal of Risk and Uncertainty* 1: 7-59.

Shrimsley, R. 2014. "The computer will see you now." Financial Times, accessed 15/11/18. https://www.ft.com/content/17060096-07be-11e4-8e62-00144feab7de.

Temperton, J. 2016. "NHS care.data scheme closed after years of controversy." wired.co.uk, accessed 15/11/18. https://www.wired.co.uk/article/care-data-nhs-england-closed.

Walker, J., Meltsner, M. and Delbanco, T. 2015. "US experience with doctors and patients sharing clinical notes." *BMJ* 350: g7785.

Zack, P. 2014. "Patients recording consultations." Medical Defence Union. https://www.themdu.com/guidance-and-advice/journals/good-practice-june-2014/patients-recording-consultations.

INFORMATION ETHICS

Chapter **20**

Public health ethics

Case 20.1

Low folate levels during early pregnancy are associated with increased risk of a particular birth defect: spina bifida.

Pregnant women are advised to take supplemental folate during pregnancy, but some women do not realize they are pregnant until too late. Others forget or do not know to take the supplements. The UK has one of the highest rates of spina bifida in Europe – affecting 1000 pregnancies per year.

An intervention has been proposed to supplement flour in the UK with folate (Limb 2018). Similar programs in other countries have been associated with halving of the rates of spina bifida. However, some bakers are concerned about the impact on their industry. Other people have concerns about possible risks from fortification.

Should the UK fortify flour with folate?

WHAT IS PUBLIC HEALTH ETHICS?

Public health ethics is concerned with ethical aspects of individual, collective or institutional behaviours that affect the health of the 'public', rather than the health of any single specified individual. However, the boundaries between public health and individual health are not clear-cut. Since the public is nothing more than the aggregation of individuals, public health is a function of the health of individuals. For example, abortion can be considered a matter of the individual health of women. However, a law that regulates abortion can be seen as a matter of public health, because it has the potential to affect the health of a large number of women within a population, and therefore public health.

Public health ethics is closely related to infectious disease ethics. As contagious diseases potentially affect large numbers of people, the issues are similar. Sexually transmitted diseases, pandemics and highly contagious diseases (such as smallpox) are classic examples.

As the abortion example suggests, rather than drawing a sharp line between public health and individual health issues, it makes more sense to distinguish between the public and the individual aspect of certain health issues. Consider this example. If my child is not vaccinated and gets measles, there is both an individual and a public health aspect involved, since it is my child who gets measles, but my child can potentially infect other people. Furthermore, as the number of unvaccinated individuals gets larger, the risk of others being infected increases, because the population might not achieve 'herd immunity' against a certain infectious disease.

Public health ethics often captures the conflict or relationship between the individual and society. What is characteristic of public health ethics is that it imposes some kind of cost on individuals for the sake of public good, or for the health of populations (Box 20.1). But how much is reasonable?

Individual versus population

In the example of fortifying flour, there are costs that a borne by some for the sake of the well-being of others. Individual autonomy is compromised (a little), as individuals do not get to choose whether or not to take vitamin supplements. There can also be harms imposed on others: one possible risk of folate supplementation is that it can interact with another vitamin deficiency (B12) in the elderly. There is debate about how high this risk might be (Mills, Molloy, and Reynolds 2018), but it is an example of how a public health intervention might cause harm to some in the population, while it benefits others.

Box 20.1 Public health ethics: imposition of a burden on an individual for the sake of others or that individual's future self

Burdens
  Restriction of liberty
  Short-term reduction in well-being
  Invasion of privacy or confidentiality

Ethical issues
  Imposition of risk or burden for the sake of others
  Coercion
  Exploitation
  Justice
  Stigma
  Trust
  Solidarity

As another example, the best way to protect the elderly from influenza is to vaccinate children. This is better than selective vaccination of the elderly or vaccination of health care workers. This may seem to be using children as a means, and thereby violating Kant's dictum to never use people merely as a means (see Chapter 2). But since it also overall protects children (it reduces the risk of mortality of children from flu), it is not treating the child *merely* as a means.

Case 20.2

Henry and Michelle are considering whether or not to immunize their second child. Their older child was diagnosed with autism, and they are terrified of having another child affected by this condition.

Henry and Michelle are scientists and have read extensively the literature on MMR and autism. They are aware that the scientific evidence linking the vaccine to autism is poor. However, they rationalize that their particular concern about autism means that they are justified in withholding the vaccine. They would not be able to live with themselves if they elected to immunize their second child and he developed autism.

The cost to the individual is clearest in the case of vaccination with high levels of herd immunity. In Chapter 5 we considered the case of Rania and James (Case 5.3), who judged that the risk of measles for their daughter was lower than the risk of side-effects from the vaccine.

If Rania and James are correct in their assessment, the vaccine would potentially involve exposing their daughter to the risks of vaccination for the sake of herd immunity. It would then be in their daughter's best interests not to be immunized.

One response to such cases is to point out that individuals are often mistaken in their assessment of the relative risks. For example, the risk of hospitalization from the measles vaccine has been estimated at 0.003%, and the risk of death is 0%. In comparison, the risk of hospitalization from measles is approximately 20%, and the risk of death is 1/350–1/1200. (Thinking only of the risk of hospitalization, there would need to be a <0.02% chance of contracting measles for non-immunization to be safer (Jamrozik, Handfield, and Selgelid 2016).)

However, reflecting on the case of Henry and Michelle, it is clear that evaluating best interests, and whether or not to pursue an intervention, involves values, as well as statistical risks. A doctor might conclude that it would be in the baby's interests to be immunized; however, Henry and Michelle's particular concerns means that they do not share that view.

The problem is that, sometimes, infringing on individual privacy, liberty, values or autonomy, or even sacrificing individual health for the sake of public health, is the only alternative available.

Policy questions

Most ethical issues in public health ethics arise at the level of policy-making, and therefore public health ethics can be conceived of as predominantly an ethics for public health policy. Typical public health ethics issues include: the legitimacy of state coercion (for example, is mandatory vaccination justified? When is it permissible to quarantine or isolate individuals, and on what conditions?); the importance of individual privacy compared to the importance of public health goals (for example, should we require patients whose genomes are sequenced for diagnostic purposes to make their genetic information available for inclusion in genetic databases that can then be used to improve diagnostics for other people?); and state paternalism (for example, is it justified for a state to disincentivize unhealthy behaviours like smoking and drinking?).

At the policy level, there are three different values that we typically want to take into account: the 'expected utility' of a certain policy; individual liberty or autonomy; and some conception of justice (for example, ensuring that everyone contributes their fair share to some public good and that they receive their fair share of benefits of public health). Public health ethics policy-making is fundamentally about how to balance these three values when they come to conflict with one another.

There are two characteristics of public health ethics which differentiate it from many other areas of medical ethics.

First, as public health is affected by a great variety of factors, which include lifestyle choices, not all public health interventions are a matter of *health care*. Mandatory vaccination is a public health policy based on health care interventions, but whether there is resistance depends on public education and trust. A tax on sugar or alcohol or tobacco, or water fluoridation to prevent tooth decay, are public health measures that do not involve standard health care interventions.

Second, these examples suggest that the 'public' aspect of public health, and therefore of 'public' health ethics, can refer either to the actor who brings about certain outcomes or to those who experience the consequences of the actor's behaviour. More specifically, we normally talk of 'public health' to refer either to collective behaviour that has some impact on people's health (for example, the realization of herd immunity is a public health issue in the sense that it requires the aggregate actions of a large number of individuals) and/or to the health impact of a certain behaviour on population at large, rather than on a single individual (for example, herd immunity is a public health issue in the sense that it provides a health benefit to the population at large).

COERCION AND EXPLOITATION

Case 20.3

A woman, Mrs MM, who worked as a cook, was suspected to be an asymptomatic carrier of typhoid fever after public health inspectors identified that there had been typhoid outbreaks in many of the places that she had worked previously. At the time, there were no antibiotics for typhoid. She was quarantined for a period of time, but later released on condition that she did not work as a cook.

After Mrs MM returned to work as a cook (she denied that she was unwell, and felt that she was blamed unnecessarily), there were further typhoid outbreaks. She was subsequently confined to quarantine for a period of more than 20 years.

Is it ethical to quarantine someone to prevent spread of an infectious disease?

This is based on the case of Typhoid Mary (Brooks 1996).

Traditionally, the central ethical issue raised in public health ethics has been coercion. Coercion is an ethical issue precisely because, often, protecting public health and implementing fair policies require infringing upon some individual liberty, and because we rightly value individual liberty. The question, then, is to what extent we should constrain or even temporarily infringe certain individual liberties in order to prevent harm to others. Should individuals be coerced to vaccinate their children, and in what way should they be coerced? Considering that a tax on alcohol and tobacco disincentivizes people from drinking and smoking, how heavy should this tax be? The clearest example of infringement of individual liberty in order to protect public health consists in quarantine and isolation of individuals who, respectively, have been exposed to or have been infected by a certain disease. While the case of Typhoid Mary (Case 20.3) might appear extreme, in a recent case a man was imprisoned for life for deliberately spreading HIV to a number of men through unsafe sex. (The duration of his sentence was partly punitive; however, it also reflected the risk that he appeared to pose to others if released (Rawlinson 2018).)

Coercion is a concept that has been widely debated within moral philosophy. Different philosophical views have different implications for whether certain public health interventions are considered coercive, and whether their being coercive makes them prima facie impermissible. For example, Australia recently implemented the so-called 'no jab, no pay' vaccination policy, whereby parents of unvaccinated children are no longer eligible for certain state child benefits; in other words, state benefits have become a premium for vaccinating parents. Are such offers coercive?

Coercion exists when one person gets another person to do what they want by issuing a threat to make that person worse off. The paradigm case is when a robber says: 'Your money or your life'. Of course, in this case, you want both your money and your life. That option – the status quo – is removed by the robber by force. Typically, coercion results in an individual being worse off (harmed) or having their liberty restricted. Coercion exists when there is a restriction of options by a powerful individual or authority – it never exists when the status quo is still an option.

On this account, offers, such as incentives, cannot be coercive (provided the full status quo is an option). A related concept is exploitation. Exploitation leads to an agent choosing an offer (with the status quo being available), but only because of background injustice or misfortune. The paradigm case is someone selling a kidney or participating in risky research because of debt (see Extension Case 20.5). The way to prevent exploitation is to either ensure background injustice or misfortune are corrected, or pay people sufficiently that the benefits reasonably outweigh the burdens (such as a fair price or wage).

NEW CONCEPTS AND PRINCIPLES: SHAPING THE FUTURE OF PUBLIC HEALTH ETHICS

In this section, we present some concepts that have more recently been introduced in the public health debate in order to address the new challenges of public health of the 21st century.

Duty of easy rescue

As a basic requirement of morality, a duty of easy rescue asserts that, when someone can do something that entails a small cost to herself and a large benefit to others (or averts a large harm to others), then she ought to do it. Examples of easy rescue are donating one's organs after death, donating blood or participating in low-risk research. According to some ethicists, the duty of easy rescue could sometimes be enforceable by the state (Savulescu 2007). At the very least, the fact that a certain duty is a duty of easy rescue provides a reason for state interventions that somehow coerce individuals to contribute to a public health cause.

How 'easy' does rescue need to be for this to be justified? According to one view (a 'comparative' notion of easy rescue), that depends on the size of the benefit that can be brought about or the harm that can be prevented, so that the bigger the benefit or the harm, the larger the sacrifice demanded (Giubilini et al. 2017). In contrast, on an 'absolute' notion of easy rescue, there is an upper limit beyond which an individual sacrifice is no longer a duty, no matter what is at stake. According to this version, individuals should only have to incur small costs (e.g. risks of death commensurate with everyday life) for the sake of some public health benefit. For example, X-ray screening of all passengers at airports for terrorism exposes people to a dose of ionizing radiation equivalent to one short-haul flight. Over millions of passengers, it is possible this will cause low numbers of cancers, but not more than would be regularly attributable to air travel.

The duty of easy rescue plays a prominent role in public health ethics today: one of the ethical questions most frequently raised is about what kind of sacrifices it is acceptable to ask people to make in order to protect public health. For example, is quarantine in case of exposure to certain infectious diseases an 'easy rescue'? Or what kind of diseases would render quarantine a duty of easy rescue? It might depend on how long a period of quarantine is proposed (a 20-year confinement, as in the case of Typhoid Mary, hardly seems easy!).

Collective action problems

Some public health issues raise distinctive collective action problems, particularly the so-called 'free-riding problem' and the 'tragedy of the commons'. As mentioned in Chapter 5, a collective action problem emerges in situations where every individual can rationalize that it would be better for them not to contribute, but, when all or many individuals act in this way, everyone is worse off. These are clear cases in which the individual interest conflicts with the collective interest.

The free-riding problem and the tragedy of the commons occur when the good in question is either a 'public good' or a 'common pool resource'. The two clear examples of such goods in public health are herd immunity and antimicrobial effectiveness. The former is a public good that gives rise to the free-riding problem: if I am not vaccinated, I can still benefit from herd immunity as long as enough other people around me are vaccinated, so I have at least a reason to free-ride; but if too many people are not vaccinated, the good itself is compromised. Antimicrobial effectiveness is a common pool resource that gives rise to a tragedy of the commons. By using antibiotics, I contribute to the erosion of antimicrobial effectiveness, given that the use of antimicrobials determines an evolutionary advantage for resistant microbes, which can then more easily proliferate.

What we need is for people to be vaccinated and keep their antimicrobial consumption to a minimum, even when doing so is not in their interest. How can we guarantee that people behave in this way? Collective action problems need to be solved through some form of state intervention. These interventions are designed to motivate people to contribute to the public good. Such action could be disincentives, incentives or nudges.

Case 20.4

In early 2018, Norway increased its rate of taxation on chocolate products by 83%. All sweets, chocolate and sweet biscuits are taxed at a rate of £3.34/kg, while sweetened drinks are taxed at 43p/litre. This is twice the rate of the tax introduced on soft drinks in the UK in April 2018 (Bloch-Budzier 2018).
   Are taxes on unhealthy foods ethical?

Disincentives

Some have proposed the introduction of a tax or a financial penalty for individuals who could easily contribute to a worthwhile public health objective but fail to do so. In other words, the idea here is punish those who fail to fulfil a duty of easy rescue. One example might be to tax or financially sanction those who fail to vaccinate their children. Such penalties could fulfil either or both the two functions: discouraging the anti-social behaviour, e.g. free-riding on herd immunity; and internalizing the costs individuals produce. For instance, we could think of taxing non-vaccinators or those who contribute to antibiotic resistance, e.g. those who consume products from animals raised using antibiotics. In the first case, the tax would discourage free-riding on herd immunity. In the latter case, it would discourage contributing to the erosion of antimicrobial effectiveness by engaging in behaviour, such as eating meat from factory farms; importantly, in this latter case, revenue from the tax could be used to fund research and development of new antibiotics (Giubilini et al. 2017). Disincentives can also be applied to public health interventions that do not necessarily represent collective action problem, for example, lifestyle diseases like obesity (Box 20.2). Up for Debate Box 20.1 summarizes some of the arguments for and against sugar taxes.

Incentives

Alternatives to disincentives are incentives that encourage behaviours that promote public health at some individual cost. For example, families might receive a cash payment for completing a course of immunization.

The use of incentives, for example in the form of conditional cash transfers (CCTs), is often taken to be problematic when the behaviour in question is seen as a basic moral duty. According to some, paying people for doing what they have a clear moral obligation to do anyway is a way of commodifying morality, and would erode people's motivation to act ethically. Michael Sandel has famously

Box 20.2 Disincentives for lifestyle diseases

Smoking, drinking and sugar consumption

Certain lifestyle choices can have a significant impact on individual and public health. Tobacco consumption and over-consumption of alcohol and sugar all involve some health costs for consumers: tobacco can cause various forms of cancer; alcohol can cause cancer and serious liver damage; and sugar can cause obesity and diabetes. Thus, when many people engage in such unhealthy behaviours, the level of public health drops, and the public health expenditure goes up, which means that individual and easily avoidable lifestyle choices pose a significant cost to society. Should people be disincentivized from engaging in such unhealthy behaviours? And should they be required to internalize the costs they are imposing on society? Most people would say yes to both questions: alcohol, tobacco and, less frequently, sugar are taxed precisely in order to disincentivize unhealthy behaviour and to force people to internalize the costs (which minimizes the costs on the public health system).

However, if we think these kinds of disincentives are ethically justified, or even ethically demanded, then we would need to ask the further question: as many lifestyle choices constitute health hazards and potentially impose a cost on society, which ones should be treated like alcohol, tobacco and sugar? Things like skiing or riding a motorbike on weekends involve health risks that would potentially burden the public health system. Unlike other activities that also involve health hazards, such as doing hazardous jobs or driving to work every day, those hobbies can easily be avoided at no significant cost to individuals. So one might ask what the justification is for treating these different types of activities differently, and for stigmatizing some but not others.

argued we should not pay people to contribute to public good (Sandel 2012). However, sometimes public health interventions, especially in emergency situations, require individuals to make sacrifices that, at least according to the comparative conception of 'duty of easy rescue', go beyond the 'call of duty'. For instance, addressing the problem of antibiotic resistance might soon require doctors to withhold antibiotics from or delay administering antibiotics to certain patients who might need them; and preventing epidemics of serious infectious disease sometimes require quarantining or isolating individuals. Those in quarantine who are not infected may have a higher risk of contracting the disease than if not quarantined. Those isolated and those quarantined have their liberty restricted. These seem to be cases in which individuals are requested to do things that maybe over-demanding for the sake of public health. Perhaps we should pay people for doing these things, considering that we can all potentially benefit from their sacrifice?

Concerns about CCTs include the problem of commodification, inducement and ultimately, once again, exploitation. Some would see incentives as a way of exploiting people, who have no reasonable alternative but to accept the money, by pushing them into making a great sacrifice. According to some philosophical theories, this can constitute coercion (Feinberg 1986, Frankfurt 1973, Held 1972).

Up for Debate Box 20.1 Should there be a sugar tax?

For

Promotes public health by reducing obesity, diabetes, liver disease, etc.

Choice to consume is the product of capitalist and powerful multinational forces that undermine liberty and autonomy

Leads to internalizing of the cost of behaviour (people have to take on board some of the financial costs of the choices they make)

Raises revenue, including for the public health care system

Taxes on smoking have been effective in reducing smoking rates, so a sugar tax might be expected to reduce sugar consumption

This would be likely to cause companies to reduce sugar content

Sugar is addictive, therefore people's choices to consume sugar are not fully autonomous

Processed sugar has no significant nutritional benefits

Children are targeted and addicted before they can make their own choice

Against

Liberty – people should be free to decide what they consume when they are not directly affecting others

Makes food more expensive and increases the cost of living

Regressive taxation has a disproportionate effect on the poor and increases inequality (those who are already disadvantaged are likely to be most affected by a sugar tax)

Substitution of artificial sweeteners is problematic – for example, they might stimulate appetite and increase weight gain (and similar strategies will be used to market products if sugar is reduced)

Causes of sugar over-consumption are multifactorial and social – this does not treat the underlying causes

Sugar taxes stigmatize the poor and obese

Sugar taxes are an example of hard paternalism (i.e. 'doctor knows best'), which is never justified

Nudging health

Nudges are sometimes taken to be a good compromise between pursuing some public health goal and preserving individual freedom. A nudge is a way of presenting the choices that are open to an individual, or the 'choice architecture', in such a way as to make it more likely that an individual would choose a certain option over the other (Thaler and Sunstein 2008). The classic example is the 'cafeteria' one: it has been shown that the way food is displayed and arranged in a school cafeteria influences what kind of food children will pick, without having to change the menus; this means that we can simply nudge individuals to eat healthy food without having to coerce them by removing unhealthy items from menus. Nudges could exploit certain decision biases such as the default effect, e.g. people's tendency to stick with the default option without assessing the pros and cons of opting out, even when they could easily opt out of the default. Apart from the cafeteria case, other examples of possible uses of nudges for public health purposes include default vaccination at school (children are vaccinated unless parents opt out) or an opt-out system for organ donation (see Chapter 15).

Principle of least restrictive alternative

To raise immunization rates, countries might use different strategies (Table 20.1). Disincentives, incentives and nudging constrain individual autonomy to different degrees. Incentives and disincentives might leave certain vulnerable individuals with 'no reasonable choice', and nudging might exploit certain unconscious psychological mechanisms. Another alternative is, of course, outright compulsion (which might not be too different from imposing heavy high penalty). Which of these interventions should be preferred depends to a great extent on the magnitude of the public health issue and which one is more effective at realizing the relevant public health goal. However, when more than one type of intervention would be effective, it is commonly accepted that we should implement the policy, among those that are effective, that is least restrictive of individual liberty (Gostin 2008,

Table 20.1 Public Health strategies to increase immunization rates (Scutti 2018).

Strategy	Example	Country/region
Disincentive	School exclusion – non-immunized children are not permitted to attend school	Oregon
		France
		Italy
Incentive	Parents receive payment for completing immunization/participating in child health programs	'No jab, no pay' – Australian program that provides child welfare payments only to families providing proof of immunization
		(some see this as a 'disincentive' rather than an incentive)
		Conditional cash transfer in rural India for mothers to engage with child health services
Nudging	Default/opt-out program – for example, providing school immunization to all children unless parents opt out, or automatically scheduling immunization appointments	Default flu vaccine appointments for health care workers in a Dutch medical centre
Compulsion	Mandatory vaccination program	Slovenia has a mandatory vaccination program (no non-medical exemptions are permitted), and families are fined for non-compliance (this might be regarded as a 'disincentive' rather than true compulsion)
		Belgian compulsory polio vaccine program

p. 142, Saghai 2013). While this principle seems uncontroversial, it nonetheless raises certain practical and ethical problems. For example, how should we measure restrictiveness (is restrictiveness a matter of liberty from external constraints? Or of autonomy? Or of infringement upon some other right?).

Compensation

Compensating individuals for losses and costs incurred as a consequence of public health measures is a matter of fairness and social justice: existing inequalities and unfair inequalities could be exacerbated by certain public health measures. For example, arguably, people who are quarantined or isolated to prevent or contain outbreaks of serious infectious diseases should be compensated for any loss of income that results for the forced inactivity period. Compensation would fulfil two functions: first, it would avoid over-burdening those for whom forced inactivity represents a significant cost, which is a matter of social justice; second, it would contribute to making submission to public health measures a form of easy rescue, thus strengthening the ethical justification for a coercive policy.

INFECTIOUS DISEASES

Vaccination

Vaccination has become a central concern in public health ethics recently, mainly because of significant drops in vaccination rates and suggestions or implementation of more coercive policies (Table 20.1).

This might be surprising, as vaccination would seem to be one of those cases in which individual interest and collective interest overlap: by getting vaccinated, I acquire immunity from infectious diseases and I contribute to the realization of herd immunity. Still, many people refuse or anyway fail to vaccinate their children for a number of reasons and factors (see Case 10.2 above). In 2017 in Europe, about 40 people died of measles, and the number of cases increased by 400% from the previous year.

The current law does not compel parents to vaccinate their children, but there have been several cases where parents (or parents and children) disagree about whether the children should be vaccinated. These disputes are resolved based on an assessment of what order would be in the welfare of the child. Invariably the courts have determined that the vaccination will promote the child's welfare.

How should policy makers react? Vaccination seems to be a clear case of 'easy rescue', as the burden of vaccination on individuals is minimal, and indeed vaccination comes with significant benefits. For this reason, vaccination also seems one of those cases where incentives are not justified, and where there is a strong case for disincentives such as fines for non-vaccination (as happens in Italy) or prohibition to enrol unvaccinated children in schools (as happens, for example, in the US).

When such coercive policies are implemented, an issue that is likely to arise is that of 'conscientious objection' or non-medical exemptions: some people claim to have philosophical or religious opposition to vaccines, and sometimes, especially in the US, states allow exemptions in the name of 'freedom of conscience'. Striking a balance between collective interest and individual freedom is problematic, not only because too many conscientious objectors would compromise herd immunity, but also because, as herd immunity is a public good, the non-vaccinated would be free-riding on herd immunity, which raises issues of fairness.

Pandemics

Pandemics are epidemics of infectious diseases that spread so widely that they affect large part of the world. Pandemics are some of the most dreaded events in public health. Influenza pandemics are relatively common, striking about three times every century. The most severe in modern times has been the 1918–19 pandemic flu, which killed 40 million people worldwide in less than one year. The most recent example is the SARS pandemic of 2003, which expanded rapidly from Asia to America and Europe, causing more than 8,000 people to get sick worldwide and 774 to die; the total cost of the SARS pandemics for the world economy has been estimated to be at least US$40 billion (Lee and McKibbin 2004).

As the SARS example shows, pandemics represent a challenge for public health ethics because, as the people potentially affected by an infectious disease during a pandemic are many and the health and economic costs of a pandemic are very high, there seems to be a very strong case for infringing individual rights and for compromising individual interests in order to protect the collective good. Restrictions on movement (e.g. isolation or quarantine) may be especially important in the current era, given globalization and the rapid interconnectedness of people all over the world (e.g. by air travel).

Often, pandemic prevention or containment raises issues about social justice: preventing the H5N1 flu strain from becoming pandemic required killing many birds and household poultry, which for many families represented the sole source of income. In other words, poor people were the ones who paid the higher economic costs of the public health measures taken to prevent the pandemic, which raises the question we mentioned above about duties of compensation (Faden and Shebaya 2016).

Antimicrobial resistance

Antimicrobial resistance (AMR) is a looming public health emergency that only very recently – and indeed too late – has started to be taken seriously by policy makers (O'Neill 2016). The fundamental problem is that, while it is true that in many parts of the world people still do not have access to effective antibiotics and other antimicrobials, in other parts of the world people consume too many of them. As explained above, exposure to antimicrobials causes bacteria or parasites to develop resistance and therefore make antimicrobials ineffective. Importantly, it is not only the abuse of antimicrobials (e.g. consumption of antibiotics in case of viral infections), but also their justified use to treat infections that drive resistance. In order to contain AMR and allow research and development of new antimicrobials to keep up with the rate of AMR, we need to collectively, and drastically, reduce the amount of antimicrobials we consume. So, collective responsibility is clearly at stake here, as are its implications for attribution of individual responsibility – for example, should each of us reduce antibiotic consumption, perhaps even to the point of leaving apparently minor and self-limiting infections untreated, in order to preserve the common good of antibiotic effectiveness for those who are in greater need of effective antibiotics? While the traditional ethical issues in public health we have seen above basically required striking a balance between individual autonomy and public interest, AMR raises the even more difficult ethical issue of balancing individual health and risk against public health and risk. At some point, we might have to expose individuals to greater than minimal risk in order to preserve the common good of antibiotic effectiveness, say by delaying administration of last-line antibiotics. This rather extreme solution would require addressing many of the ethical issues that have emerged in this chapter: what are the limits of individual obligations in a context of collective responsibility? Should individuals be compensated for delaying the treatment of certain infections? Which infections can be left untreated in order to remain within the boundaries of a duty of easy rescue? Should consumption of antibiotics in the case of minor and self-limiting infections be disincentivized? Importantly, AMR raises issues about antimicrobial stewardship, not only for policy makers, but for individual medical doctors, who will soon be required to make responsible decisions about whether to prioritize their individual patients' interests (by prescribing them antibiotics) or the collective interests (by refraining from prescribing antibiotics to some of their patients). Will that be politically acceptable? In a recent survey of the general public, 50.3% of participants thought that doctors should generally prioritize individual patients over society. When asked in the context of AMR, 39.2% prioritized individuals, whereas 45.5% prioritized society. People's attitudes were more oriented to society and sensitive to collective responsibility when informed about the social costs of antibiotic use and when considered from a third-person rather than first-person perspective (Dao et al. 2019).

ACKNOWLEDGEMENT

Special thanks to Alberto Guibilini for valuable assistance with background research and preparation of this chapter.

REVISION QUESTIONS

1. What is the 'duty of easy rescue'? How does it apply to interventions in public health?
2. Is it ethical to quarantine patients during a pandemic? How much inconvenience would be acceptable to impose on patients?
3. What strategies might be employed to increase rates of immunization? How should societies evaluate and choose between these?
4. It is unethical to pay people to behave morally. Do you agree? Giving examples, explain why/why not.
5. What are collective action problems in public health? How could they be addressed?

Extension case 20.5

Challenge studies involve deliberately infecting human beings with a microbe (in a controlled environment) in order to study its pathogenesis or to test the efficacy of a vaccine or an antimicrobial medication. Challenge studies offer significant benefits. For example, in the investigation of candidate vaccines, physiological or biochemical signs of infection can be detected before symptoms develop.

Researchers have proposed a study that would deliberately infect volunteers with the Zika virus, a recently emerged arbovirus associated with congenital microcephaly in fetuses.

Is it ethical to deliberately infect volunteers with Zika virus for the sake of greater benefit?

How much risk is acceptable?

How much could participants be paid for involvement in such a study?

Read Miller and Drapkin Lyerly (2018), Anomaly and Savulescu (2019, forthcoming), and Bambery et al. (2016).

REFERENCES

Anomaly, J. and Savulescu, J. 2019 (forthcoming). "Compensation for cures: why we should pay a premium for participation in 'challenge studies'." *Bioethics*.

Bambery, B., Selgelid, M., Weijer, C., Savulescu, J. and Pollard, A. J. 2016. "Ethical criteria for human challenge studies in infectious diseases." *Public Health Ethics* 9: 92-103. doi: 10.1093/phe/phv026.

Bloch-Budzier, S. 2018. "Crossing the border for a sugar fix." BBC News, 12 March 2018. Accessed 20/11/18. https://www.bbc.co.uk/news/health-43245138.

Brooks, J. 1996. "The sad and tragic life of Typhoid Mary." *CMAJ* 154 (6): 915-6.

Dao, B., Douglas, T., Giubilini, A., Savulescu, J., Selgelid, M. and Faber, N. S. 2019. "Impartiality and infectious disease: prioritising individuals versus the collective in antibiotic prescription." *AJOB Empirical Bioethics*. 10(1): 63-9. doi: 10.1080/23294515.2019.1576799.

Faden, R. R. and Shebaya, S. 2016. "Public health ethics." In *The Stanford encyclopedia of philosophy (winter 2016 edition)*, edited by E. Zalta.

Feinberg, J. 1986. *The moral limits of the criminal law: harm to self*. New York: Oxford University Press.

Frankfurt, H. 1973. "Coercion and moral responsibility." In *Essays on freedom of action*, edited by T. Honderich. London: Routledge and Kegan Paul.

Giubilini, A., Birkl, P., Douglas, T., Savulescu, J. and Maslen, H. 2017. "Taxing meat: taking responsibility for one's contribution to antibiotic resistance." *Journal of Agricultural and Environmental Ethics* 30: 179-98. doi: 10.1007/s10806-017-9660-0.

Gostin, L. O. 2008. *Public health law: power, duty, restraint*. Revised and expanded second ed. London: University of California Press.

Held, V. 1972. "Coercion and coercive offers." In *Nomos XIV: coercion*, edited by J. R. Pennock and J. W. Chapman. Chicago: Aldine-Atherton: 49-62.

Jamrozik, E., Handfield, T. and Selgelid, M. J. 2016. "Victims, vectors and villains: are those who opt out of vaccination morally responsible for the deaths of others?" *Journal of Medical Ethics* 42: 762-8.

Lee, J. W. and McKibbin, W. 2004. "Estimating the global economic costs of SARS." In *Learning from SARS: preparing for the next disease outbreak: workshop summary*, edited by S. Knobler. Washington, DC: National Academic Press.

Limb, M. 2018. "Flour to be fortified with folic acid within weeks, say reports." *BMJ* 363: k4348.

Miller, F. G. and Drapkin Lyerly, A. 2018. "Navigating ethics review of human infection trials with Zika." Hastings Center, accessed 20/11/18. https://www.thehastingscenter.org/navigating-ethics-review-human-infection-trials-zika/.

Mills, J. L., Molloy, A. M. and Reynolds, E. H. 2018. "Do the benefits of folic acid fortification outweigh the risk of masking vitamin B_{12} deficiency?" *BMJ* 360: k724.

O'Neill, J. 2016. Tackling drug-resistant infections globally: final report and recommendations. AMR-review.

Rawlinson, K. 2018. "Man jailed for life after deliberately infecting men with HIV." *The Guardian*. https://www.theguardian.com/uk-news/2018/apr/18/hairdresser-daryll-rowe-given-life-sentence-for-deliberately-infecting-men-with-hiv.

Saghai, Y. 2013. "Salvaging the concept of nudge." *Journal of Medical Ethics* 39 (8): 487-93.

Sandel, M. 2012. *What money can't buy: the moral limits of markets*. Farrar, Strauss, and Giroux.

Savulescu, J. 2007. "Future people, involuntary medical treatment in pregnancy and the duty of easy rescue." *Utilitas* 19 (1): 1-20.

Scutti, S. 2018. "How countries around the world try to encourage vaccination." CNN.com, 2 Jan 2018. Accessed 20/11/18. https://edition.cnn.com/2017/06/06/health/vaccine-uptake-incentives/index.html.

Thaler, R. H. and Sunstein, C. R. 2008. *Nudge: improving decisions about health, wealth, and happiness*. New Haven, Conn.; London: Yale University Press.

Index

Page numbers followed by *"f"* indicate figures, *"t"* indicate tables, and *"b"* indicate boxes.